*The Weariness, the Fever, and the Fret*
*The Campaign against Tuberculosis in Canada,*
*1900–1950*

An ancient disease which predates humankind, tuberculosis was one of the earliest chronic life-threatening diseases faced by Canadians. By 1900 "The White Plague" was the number one cause of death for Canadians between fifteen and forty-five years of age. Racked by incessant coughing, barely able to catch their breath, tuberculosis sufferers seemed to literally waste away. In *The Weariness, the Fever, and the Fret* Katherine McCuaig takes an in-depth look at the campaign against TB, from its beginnings as part of the turn-of-the-century urban social reform movement to the 1950s and the discovery of antibiotics that could cure it. Although the bacillus that causes it had been discovered in 1882, at the turn of the century TB was, as Sir William Osler observed, "a social disease with a medical aspect." With "fresh air, good food, good houses, and hope" as the only available treatment, fighting the disease meant not only eliminating the germ but attacking the underlying social problems that predisposed an individual to disease – alcoholism and poor living and working conditions.

By the end of World War I the bacteriological approach had become dominant, with federally expanded sanatoria, increasing provincial involvement and responsibility, and more sophisticated technology to diagnose and treat the disease. The campaign against TB not only influenced the way in which health services were established and the division of responsibility among various levels of government and volunteers but profoundly affected attitudes toward the political and economic development of Canadian health care and the ultimate demand for medicare.

KATHERINE MCCUAIG is a fellow of the Royal College of Surgeons of Canada. A physician with a Masters Degree in Canadian history, she has published in both medical and historical journals.

MCGILL-QUEEN'S ASSOCIATED MEDICAL SERVICES
(HANNAH INSTITUTE)
Studies in the History of Medicine, Health, and Society
Series Editors: S.O. Freedman and J.T.H. Connor

Volumes in this series have financial support from Associated
Medical Services, Inc., through the Hannah Institute for the
History of Medicine program.

# The Weariness, the Fever, and the Fret

## The Campaign against Tuberculosis in Canada, 1900–1950

KATHERINE McCUAIG

McGill-Queen's University Press
Montreal & Kingston · London · Ithaca

*36 2. 196 995*
*M 4 7 w*

Legal deposit third quarter 1999
Bibliothèque nationale du Québec

Printed in Canada on acid-free paper

This book has been published with the help of a grant from the Humanities and Social Sciences Federation of Canada, using funds provided by the Social Sciences and Humanities Research Council of Canada.

McGill-Queen's University Press acknowledges the financial support of the Government of Canada through the Book Publishing Industry Development Program (BPIDP) for its activities. We also acknowledge the support of the Canada Council for the Arts for our publishing program.

Canadä

**Canadian Cataloguing in Publication Data**

McCuaig, Katherine, 1959–
    The weariness, the fever and the fret: the campaign against tuberculosis in Canada, 1900–1950
    (McGill-Queen's/Hannah Institute studies in the history of medicine, health and society; 8)
    Includes bibliographical references and index.
    ISBN 0-7735-1833-9 (bound)
    ISBN 0-7735-1875-4 (pbk.)
    1. Tuberculosis – Canada – History. 2. Tuberculosis – Canada – Prevention. I. Title. II. Series.
    RC314.M33 1999    362.1'96995'00971    C99-900746-7

*AP*

Typeset in New Baskerville 10/12 by Caractéra inc., Quebec City.

*To my mother, June Marie McCuaig*

*And in memory of my father, James Auley McCuaig*

*This book is dedicated with love and gratitude*

# Contents

# Tables and Figures

# Preface

This book originated many years ago as a master's thesis in Canadian history at McGill University. Although it owes much to those individuals who encouraged and supported me in tackling such a subject, many debts have also been incurred throughout the years as it has undergone extensive revisions in format, content, and philosophy.

McGill University funded the early, seminal research as part of my graduate studies with a McConnell fellowship. I owe a tremendous debt to my supervisor, Dr Carman Miller, who offered unfailing support and valuable criticism. The original draft was typed on a history department typewriter loaned to me by the administrative head, Mrs Rubie Napier – and to this day, I'm not sure if some rules were not bent to lend it. The National Archives of Canada (then the Public Archives of Canada) provided me with dozens of rolls of microfilm of the records of the Canadian Tuberculosis Association, while the McGill medical library – where I spent many months – was a fruitful source of local reports and national journals.

While I was undertaking extensive revisions in recent years, Dr Stuart Houston offered detailed and valuable criticism, as did peer reviewers for the Social Science Research Council, who suggested a thematic, rather than a chronological, approach: as a result, I was able to appreciate the development and role of volunteer associations and then make the link, in a more meaningful way, between the campaign and other socioeconomic and political changes occurring simultaneously in North America, drawing parallels between developments in the anti-TB campaign and those in business and society. Because their input was anonymous, I cannot thank them personally, but I am very grateful.

Donna Gerometta, the medical librarian at Mesa Lutheran Hospital in Mesa, Arizona, was unfailingly helpful in doing countless literature searches and providing dozens of articles on TB from both a medical and historical perspective: the assessment of the role of surgery, in particular, would not have been possible without her and the hospital library's support. Winnie Wong at Alberta Word Processing Services in Edmonton did an excellent job typing my first handwritten revisions into a readable form on a computer disk. Connie Novak, at Personalized Word Processing in Tempe, Arizona, uncomplainingly took a manuscript with multiple – frequently unreadable – revisions, additions, note changes, and tables and cheerfully and competently turned it into a readable book, offering valuable advice along the way.

The staff at McGill-Queen's University Press are owed a special thanks for their professional and personal support – especially in guiding me through the land mines of peer review in the social sciences and tolerating my dilatory behaviour in completing promised revisions. Peter Blaney, my original editor, and Philip Cercone, who subsequently assumed responsibility for the manuscript and its author, are owed a special debt of gratitude for their professionalism, advice, good humour, and forbearance. I also deeply appreciate Ron Curtis' painstaking work in editing and revising the final draft. I was fortunate to have his aid and advice, which improved the manuscript immensely.

I would like to express heartfelt thanks to Dexter and Karlene Mapel of The Book Island, an antiquarian bookstore and search service in Phoenix, Arizona. It was they who searched all over North America for every out-of-print text I needed, tracked down and ordered monographs from specialized publishers, discovered a California dealer of old medical texts who provided me with multiple rare sources (some of which are found, if at all, only in rare-book rooms), and listened with endless patience and provided psychological support when the stress of my medical practice made it appear foolish to continue a project that seemed not only to be costing me a great deal of money but was also eating away at my very limited free time. If not for their support, I might have abandoned the project on several occasions.

Equally importantly, friends and family have encouraged me to complete this manuscript – particularly Anne Stevens, who not only provided the champagne in a Crescent Street bar, celebrating the completion of the thesis but also suggested I consider revising it as a book. Stephanie Conoley also had to listen to many theories on the subject and was unfailingly patient and encouraging. I am also very grateful to my parents, June and Jim, and my sisters and brothers – Paul, Diane, Jack, and Jill – for their support and encouragement.

Which leads me to a final, personal note. This study was influenced by my work in both history and medicine. As William Carlos Williams once commented on his dual career in medicine and writing, "the one nourishes the other." In turn, my life was profoundly altered by my research for this book. I had intended to proceed to a PHD and a career as a history professor; instead I completed my master's degree, left university, found a job, picked up science courses at night, and applied to medicine. It seemed no more absurd to think I could do that than that a handful of doctors would believe they could finally conquer a disease. This book might have been quite different if I were not a doctor with a background in historical studies; but I would probably not be a surgeon today if it were not for this book.

# Introduction

Fade far away, dissolve, and quite Forget
What thou among the leaves hast never known,
The weariness, the fever, and the fret
Here, where men sit and hear each other groan;
Where palsy shakes a few, sad, last grey hairs,
Where youth grows pale, and spectre – thin, and dies;
Where but to think is to be full of sorrow
And leaden-eyed despairs;
Where Beauty cannot keep her lustrous eyes,
Or new Love pine at them beyond to-morrow.

John Keats, "Ode to a Nightingale"

"That drop of blood is my death warrant, I must die."

John Keats, 1820
(A year before his death from tuberculosis)

Like other North Americans born at the tail end of the baby boom, I am a member of the "antibiotic generation" – the first generation in Canadian history not to grow up in the shadow of life-threatening, infectious disease. By the mid-fifties a vaccination had been discovered for polio, and tuberculosis was curable. For a brief moment, it must have seemed like a new millennium.

In less than a decade, AIDS has destroyed this optimism. Perhaps our outrage at the ravages of AIDS stems partially from our innocence and ignorance, our lack of historical perspective. Tuberculosis had reached epidemic proportions in Canada less than a hundred years ago; but memories are short, and few of us can even begin to comprehend the misery and suffering it entailed. Most victims were young adults, to whom the diagnosis meant a fearful, painful, protracted death – ostracized in a sanatorium for years, slowly forgotten by friends, unable to support either themselves or their families.

That is the human tragedy of TB, largely forgotten today. It can be gleaned from chance conversations with Canadians who still remember, but this collective memory is fast disappearing. One elderly woman told me proudly of her experiences in Alberta. "My husband went off to the war and I went into the san. I was in bed for two years, and then they collapsed my lung – but I got out." It was the most important achievement of her life. "I never swam in the lake at Ste Agathe," another informed me. "You know, the san was up there, and the TB might have gotten in the water." Another native of Montreal remembers high school classmates in the forties who had to leave school for two years to take the cure.

Oral history is fascinating, but to be of real value in determining community attitudes, it must be done on a large scale. There is the added problem of reliability. Asking anyone to recall events is tricky enough; asking them how they felt about a disease, and how their attitudes changed over a forty-year period is something else altogether. Can any of us honestly state not only what we remember about cancer twenty years ago but how we regarded it? And how our attitudes changed? Disease is so much a part of our everyday lives that we rarely stop to consider our views about it.

Newspapers and popular periodicals are valuable; but they generally printed information that specialists provided – in the case of tuberculosis, the Canadian Tuberculosis Association or a local league. They are a guide to the public's access to information and the knowledge the specialists wished it would acquire, but not to what the public necessarily *believed*. The community's attitude toward disease can sometimes be guessed at using indirect means; for example, the increasing demand and the resultant shortage of sanatorium beds from the 1920s on perhaps reflects a general belief that the disease could be treated and sometimes cured. And the fear of consumptives that the antituberculosis workers railed against in the early years of the twentieth century suggests that Canadians were beginning to believe that tuberculosis was infectious rather than hereditary. But such conclusions are limited at best. Much of this book is therefore a study of the changing attitudes of those reformers and specialists who directed antituberculosis work in Canada.

I have omitted Newfoundland and the problem of tuberculosis among the native peoples from this study. Newfoundland did not obtain provincial status until 1949 – the end of the period covered by this book. The problem of disease among native peoples, a very serious one, would be better studied as part of the whole issue of health services in general among the native peoples, who were a federal responsibility.

The challenge in a historical study of a disease is that it encompasses both advances in scientific knowledge and social, economic, and political changes peculiar to a specific time and place. Inevitably, each factor influences the others – and resulting attitudes about the disease itself. The origins of the national campaign against tuberculosis in Canada, for example, owed its development both to Koch's discovery of the bacillus in 1882, proving the infectious nature of the disease, as well as to the turn-of-the-century climate of social reform, when, as William Osler observed, TB was "a social disease with a medical aspect."

Advances in technology, notably radiology, but also surgical procedures such as pneumothorax and thoracoplasty, permitted the interwar campaign to focus increasingly on a *bacteriological* approach to the disease. But it would be a mistake to see this purely in terms of scientific knowledge, for the themes of organization and standardization were in the ascendancy in North American political and economic life in general. In many respects, the development of the campaign itself, with a national voluntary association and a leadership of public health experts trying to organize the local service clubs responsible for the Christmas Seal sale, paralleled concurrent developments in business and government, now run by a growing number of expert administrators, managers, and bureaucrats.

The campaign against TB in Canada, therefore, cannot be seen in simple cause and effect terms or even in terms of a classic left-right paradigm. Many of the attitudes touted by those leading the campaign – their focus on science and "scientific management," the promotion of the "expert manager" and the goals of organization, standardization, and efficiency – were espoused both by socialists desiring a new social order and by capitalists such as John D. Rockefeller, whose foundations did so much to promote it. Their *goals* may have differed, but the philosophical *means* were the same.

To best demonstrate the important role changes in Canadian social, political, and economic life played in the campaign, this book is arranged thematically. Beginning with the social reform era, in which the campaign against the disease was yet one more cause in a myriad assortment of reform issues, the anti-TB movement is traced through World War 1, and the role of the federal government and military. Desmond Morton and Glenn Wright's *Winning the Second Battle* was particularly valuable in setting the disease in its context here. The interwar fight against the disease is studied from several perspectives: the specialization and importance of volunteer organizations, from the parochial service clubs to the growing "professional" voluntary associations (the Red Cross, the Canadian Tuberculosis Association), is examined, as are the large-scale philanthropies, most notably the Rockefeller Foundation. The role of the state is addressed, beginning with reluctant municipal then provincial, and finally federal involvement, with the post–World War 2 grants, as it became progressively clearer that the problem of TB was too expensive and extensive to be managed locally. John Thompson and Allen Seager's *Canada 1922–1939: Decades of Discord* was a fruitful source of information regarding interwar changes in Canadian society in general. Angus McLaren's *Our Own Master Race: Eugenics in Canada 1885–1945* and Jay Cassel's *The Secret Plague: Veneral Disease in Canada 1838–1939* greatly aided in studying the campaign's links with other concurrent philosophies and reforms. Childhood TB, with its slightly different forms, is treated in a separate chapter. Again, by helping provide a broader context, Neil Sutherland's work, most notably *Children in English Canadian Society: Framing the Twentieth Century Consensus*, made this possible. C. Stuart Houston's biography of George Ferguson, *R.G. Ferguson: Crusader against Tuberculosis* was invaluable, particularly in assessing the campaign in Saskatchewan; while his work, together with that of Georgina D. Feldberg on the bacillus Calmette-Guérin (BCG) vaccine, *Disease and Class: Tuberculosis and the Shaping of Modern North American Society*, aided immeasurably in addressing the role the vaccine played in the campaign against TB. Heather MacDougall's *Activists and Advocates* and Janice P. Dickin-McGinnis' work on the influenza epidemic and the creation of the federal department of health, together with J.H.T. Connor's work on the London Health Association and Sheila M. Penney's dissertation on tuberculosis in twentieth-century Nova Scotia were also very helpful.

In the concluding chapters, I have attempted to place the Canadian campaign against TB in a somewhat broader context and to assess, as much as possible, the merits and liabilities of the treatment of and attitudes to the disease. Much of this material is controversial: to what extent were sanatoria beneficial – and to whom? How important in the epidemiology of the disease was the bacterial focus – or, as Thomas McKeown argues, was good nutrition the key influence? René Dubos' *White Plague*, McKeown's *Role of Medicine* and Leonard Wilson's rebuttals; Barbara Bates' study of TB in Pennsylvania, *Bargaining For Life: A Social History of Tuberculosis 1876–1938;* Linda Bryder's *Below the Magic Mountain: A Social History of Tuberculosis in Twentieth Century Britain;* and Sheila Rothman's *Living in the Shadow of Death: Tuberculosis and the Social Experience of Illness in American History* were particularly helpful.

In addition to discussing the development of the anti-TB movement from a wider medical perspective, I have attempted to place the campaign in a broader social and political context. Several recent North American studies have helped immeasurably with this. Paul James Croce, in his *Science and Religion in the Era of William James*, discusses the importance of Darwinism not only as a challenge to traditional religion but, in its reliance on plausibility and probability as "proof," as an agent in the transformation of science; Ramsay Cook, in *The Regenerators*, charts the attempts of traditional religion to accommodate the new theories with social reform ideology, while John M. Jordan, in *Machine-Age Ideology: Social Engineering and American Liberalism, 1911–1939*, delineates the results of the application of *engineering principles* to social policy. Jeffrey A. Charles' study, *Service Clubs in American Society*, focuses on a long-neglected area that was most useful in discussing the role service clubs played in the anti-TB campaign; Kenneth Ludmeier's *Learning to Heal* and Paul Starr's *Transformation of American Medicine* aided in discussing the tensions between academic medicine, public health, and community physicians – tensions that Heather MacDougall, in her study of the Toronto health department, *Activists and Advocates*, and Michael Bliss, in *A Canadian Millionaire: The Life and Business Times of Sir Joseph Flavelle, Bart, 1858–1939*, both documented, and tensions that were clearly evident throughout the anti-TB campaign. For explaining such tensions, recent works by Christopher Lasch (*The Revolt of the Elites and the Betrayal of Democracy*) and Robert H. Wiebe (*Self Rule: A Cultural History of American Democracy*) proved particularly useful. Both described the development of a national, educated class of managers, intellectuals, and administrators in the United States, and its consequences; their interpretations proved illuminating in discussing the tensions between the public health advocates and specialists and the general practitioners in dealing with tuberculosis. It appears the campaign merely reflected philosophical attitudes and biases generally current in North American society.

"Every society is an arena of social conflicts," wrote British historian E.H. Carr, "and those individuals who range themselves against existing authority are no less products and reflexions of the society than those who uphold it."[1] This is equally true of scientists and lay persons, experts and generalists. It is in this context that the campaign against TB in Canada must be understood.

The intent of this work is to provide an account of the anti-tuberculosis campaign in Canada during the first half of this century and the complex interaction of social, economic, and political forces that determined its development – and, in turn, its own influence on those same forces in Canadian society. But it is only one book on a huge topic. It cannot possibly be all things to all readers – nor should it be. It is as rational to expect one single study of World War 2 to be the definitive statement about the wartime era. As in every other aspect of Canadian history, I hope and expect that future historians will tackle this subject again and again, in their own way, influenced by their own backgrounds, their own interests and their own times.

The emaciated figure strikes one with terror; the fore-
head covered with drops of sweat; the cheeks painted with
a livid crimson, the eyes sunk; the little fat that raised
them in their orbits entirely wasted; the pulse quick and
tremulous; the nails long, bending over the ends of the
fingers; the palms of the hands dry and painfully hot to
the touch; the breath offensive, quick and laborious, and
the cough so incessant as scarce to allow the wretched sufferer time to tell his complaints.

Thomas Beddoes, *Essay on the Causes, Early Signs of, and*
*Prevention of Pulmonary Consumption*, 1799

What had happened to Ruby? She was even handsomer
than ever; but her blue eyes were too bright and lustrous, and the color of her cheeks was hectically brilliant;
besides she was very thin; the hands that held her hymn-
book were almost transparent in their delicacy.

"Is Ruby Gillis ill?" Anne asked of Mrs Lynde, as they
went home from church.

"Ruby Gillis is dying of galloping consumption," said
Mrs Lynde bluntly.

L.M. Montgomery, *Anne of the Island*, 1915

# 1 The Social Reform Era, 1900–1914: A Social Disease with a Medical Aspect

The Spencervale doctor ... sent a message to Marilla Cuthbert by another person. It was: "Keep that red-headed girl of yours in the open air all summer and don't let her read books until she gets more spring into her step." This message frightened Marilla wholesomely. She read Anne's death warrant by consumption in it unless it was scrupulously obeyed.

L.M. Montgomery, *Anne of Green Gables* (1908)

"This is not merely a campaign against tuberculosis," the president of the Canadian Association for the Prevention of Tuberculosis, J.G. Adami, proclaimed enthusiastically in 1910, "but is the inevitable centre of a great movement making for social betterment ... Everything ... that makes for impoverished health makes for susceptibility to tuberculosis. Everything that makes for better social conditions develops naturally as an object and outcome of our campaign."[1] Such optimism was recent, a result of dramatic advances in scientific and medical knowledge infused with turn-of-the-century intellectual and social reform fervour.

An ancient disease that predates man, Hippocrates (460–377 BC) termed tuberculosis "phthisis," meaning to melt and waste away. "The white plague," "consumption," "scrofula," and "the king's evil" were efforts to describe different forms of the same dreaded malady. Considered largely incurable and probably inherited, TB reached epidemic proportions during the industrialization and urbanization of late-eighteenth- and nineteenth-century Europe. During William Nisbet's lifetime (1759–1822) an estimated one-half of the children born in London died before the age of two, and of that half, one-third died of scrofula. John Bunyan termed it "the Captain of all these men of death." The 1880 death rate for Montreal and Toronto has been estimated to have been approximately 200 deaths per 100,000 population – a figure that likely remained stable until the turn of the century.[2]

A French physician, Théophile Laennec, revolutionized diagnosis with invention of the stethoscope in 1816; but it was Louis Pasteur who ushered in the bacteriological era when he postulated and proved the germ theory. A third French physician, Jean Villemin (1827–92), demonstrated the infectious nature of tuberculosis (*On the Cause and Nature of Tuberculosis and Its Inoculation from Man to Rabbit*, 1865), but it was Robert Koch (1843–1910), a one-time, unknown Prussian country physician, who isolated the tuberculosis bacillus and, on 24 March 1882, proved conclusively to the Berlin Physiological Society that it was responsible for the disease.

Despite initial excitement, it would take over half a century for a cure to be found. Not until 1944, with the announcement of the discovery of streptomycin, would effective chemotherapy be introduced and the already declining death rate plummet. Prior to that, all drugs, including even gold and tuberculin injections, were unsuccessful. Treatment consisted of conservative medical measures – rest, good nutrition, and fresh air – and, increasingly popular in the interwar period, surgical "collapse therapy," ranging from artificial pneumothorax (collapse of a portion of the lung) to disfiguring and often dangerous chest-wall and lung resections. Although adopted widely, the value of such aggressive measures remained in dispute. Some studies suggested that the survival rate continued to hover at a dismal 50 percent at five years.[3]

Despite Koch's discovery, attitudes changed slowly. Many still believed, like Edward L. Trudeau's professor in medical school, that TB was a "non-contagious, generally incurable and inherited disease, due to inherited constitutional peculiarities, perverted tumors and various types of inflammation." Following the example of Hermann Brehmer, who had established a German sanatorium in 1859 that emphasized a cure based on fresh mountain air, a liberal diet, and exercise, Trudeau, a consumptive New York physician, unexpectedly found his health improving in the Adirondack Mountains of upstate New York. In 1885 he opened the Adirondack Cottage Sanitorium at Saranac Lake, which would become the best-known sanitorium in North America and the inspiration for many in the subsequent campaign against the disease. By the turn of the century it began to seem that TB, like smallpox and diphtheria, was indeed contagious – and thus theoretically preventable and curable.[4]

## The Nature of the Disease

As Koch had demonstrated, tuberculosis is a bacterial infection caused in humans by both the *Mycobacterium tuberculosis* and the closely related bovine form (*M. bovis*). Characterized pathologically by a granuloma (a distinct inflammatory and fibrous tissue reaction) in infected tissues, it most frequently involves the lungs (pulmonary TB) but can infect the kidneys, brain, gastrointestinal tract, adrenal glands, lymph nodes (scrofula), bones and joints, and even the eye. A systemic form is termed "miliary."

Bacilli are transmitted from person to person via small inhaled droplets expelled during coughing, sneezing, or speaking, and the likelihood of infectivity corresponds to the number and virulence of organisms in the expectorated sputum, the extent of pulmonary disease, and the frequency of the cough. As mycobacteria are susceptible to ultraviolet irradiation, outdoor transmission is minimized during daylight, while good ventilation reduces environmental infection in general. Historically, transmission of *M. bovis* was associated with the consumption of contaminated cow's milk.

Several factors influence susceptibility, the form the disease takes, and its progressive development: acuteness of infection, the stage at which treatment is begun, natural resistance and heredity (both individual and racial), age (at one time it killed most victims between fifteen and forty-five years), environment, and concurrent disease. Diabetics, for example, especially before the discovery of insulin, were particularly prone.

In the common pulmonary form of the disease, the tubercle bacilli may lodge in the lungs, multiply, and produce a primary tuberculosis pneumonia. Contained to a variable degree by the immune system, the infection spreads initially to regional lymph nodes and then to the rest of the body. With the release of hydrolytic enzymes by sensitized immune cells (lymphocytes and alveolar macrophages), caseation necrosis – local destruction of lung tissue – is seen in the tuberculous lesion, which can go on to heal with fibrosis and calcification. The tubercle bacilli, however, are not destroyed and the disease may be reactivated decades later when the patient's immune status changes.[5]

The initial infection may be asymptomatic, with clinical disease developing weeks to years later in individuals whose immune systems do not successfully contain the focus of infection. In fact, the insidious nature of TB often makes it difficult to diagnose. Initial symptoms are vague – weight loss, fatigue – and are often overlooked or ascribed to another cause. As the disease progresses, the sufferer develops an incessant, wracking cough, spitting up blood-streaked sputum associated with fever and drenching night sweats. Weak and emaciated, the tuberculous individual literally, as Hippocrates had observed, "wastes away."[6]

*Tuberculosis at the Turn of the Century: Social Reform*

Turn-of-the-century advances in knowledge relating to tuberculosis reflected advances both in public health and in science in general.

For most of the nineteenth century public health was equated with control of epidemics: smallpox, cholera, typhoid. British reformers such as Edwin Chadwick had promoted sanitation to clean up water supplies and improve the environment, premised on the belief that the noxious vapors, or "miasmas," from decaying organic matter, animal and human waste, caused disease. This, in turn, encouraged the development of vital statistics and sanitary engineering.

The knowledge that sanitation could prevent disease, coupled with revolutionary bacteriological discoveries, gave reason and impetus to the public health movement in the 1880s and 1890s. The Public Health Act in Britain (1875) served as a model for the Ontario Provincial Board of Health (1884). Other provinces soon followed: Quebec in 1886, New Brunswick in 1887, Nova Scotia, Manitoba, and British Columbia in 1893, and the rest in the first decade of the new century.[7]

Equally significant changes were taking place in Canadian society. Industrialization, urbanization, and immigration were all straining the existing social fabric, promoting the growth of an urban social reform movement that would, in the years before World War 1, alter the way Canadians conceived of both tuberculosis and public health in general. Canada's population grew by 64 percent from 1901 to 1921, while in the Prairies alone urban residents increased from 19.3 percent of the total population in 1901 to 28.8 percent by 1911, with the number of incorporated cities increasing from three in 1901 to seventeen in 1916.[8] With such rapid expansion came almost inevitable problems: urban slums with poor or nonexistent ventilation and sanitation, overcrowding, labour unrest, and distrust of the thousands of immigrants with their "foreign" attitudes and customs. If the twentieth century belonged to Canada, as Sir Wilfrid Laurier had insisted in 1904, many Canadians worried about the manner in which the prophecy was being fulfilled.[9]

Of equal importance, as Ramsay Cook has so convincingly demonstrated in *The Regenerators*, was a profound religious crisis provoked by Darwinian science and the historical criticism of the Bible. Moreover, social and economic injustices of a newly industrializing Canada demanded a reassessment of conventional theological assumptions. Together, these challenges caused religious Canadians to attempt to salvage or "regenerate" Christianity by replacing the traditional religious focus on the individual's salvation through his or her relationship with God with a new "social salvation" that emphasized relationships with other human beings.

Ironically, such an attempt to revitalize religion and adapt it to a "social gospel" – the Christian imperative that infused the social reform with its moral fervour – ultimately led to a substitution of sociology for theology. A new social science and new professional leadership replaced the old Victorian church-based morality. As the twentieth century progressed, appeals would be to the "laws of science" rather than the "laws of God," and those laws would be interpreted by secular, not clerical, experts.

It is this philosophical change that may, as much as concrete developments in bacteriology, account for the burgeoning interest in tuberculosis and public health. Both the anti-tuberculosis and more general public health movements were "scientific," with an ostensible basis in bacteriology, buttressed by physical science with the developments in sanitary engineering. As such, they provided a means by which the new "liberal Christians," as Cook terms them could, with their social gospel, incorporate *science* into their religiously inspired "social gospel." In this way science did not *challenge* religious beliefs, but instead supported the new theology and promoted the urban reform emphasis in the anti-TB campaign before World War 1. Unlike other reform causes, however, the anti-TB campaign was, in the end, secular and scientific – and it would be these qualities that would ensure its expansion and inevitable alteration in the secular 1920s.[10]

Taken together, such socioeconomic and philosophical changes promoted the growth of a turn-of-the-century urban social reform movement. Idealistic and imbued with a moral imperative to create the Kingdom of God on Earth, those involved concentrated on restructuring municipal governments, planning the physical environment, public ownership and the regulation of utilities, and social welfare – improved housing, shorter working hours, temperance, and the abolition of prostitution – all of which were loosely bound together with the ultimate goal of creating a utopian society. As J.S. Woodsworth observed, city life was "like a spider's web – pull one thread and you pull every thread."[11] Public health in general and the prevention of tuberculosis in particular were ideally suited to Woodsworth's view of social reform. With nearly every Canadian infected by adulthood, it seemed obvious, as one Toronto physician observed, that the germ was merely a cause, but not the only cause of tuberculosis.[12] Although no one was immune, the problem seemed worse in the slums; therefore, reformers reasoned, it was the causes that predisposed an individual to breaking down with TB that were the real determining factors. "The death rate from tuberculosis in any family, community or state," Peter Bryce informed the National Council of Women in 1908, "is the most exact measure we have of the social status of the individual family, community or state."[13]

As a result, reformers ambitiously attacked tuberculosis on two fronts: bacteriologically – to reduce or eliminate exposure to the germ itself – and socioeconomically, to increase resistance to the disease by improving social conditions, living standards, and general health. Their focus extended from the personal and individual – indiscriminate spitting, the common drinking cup, dry sweeping – through to more general concerns such as flies, impure milk, poor housing, long working hours, low wages, overcrowding, poor nutrition, and alcoholism. As Sir William Osler observed, TB was preeminently "a social disease with a medical aspect." To cure TB, one had to cure society.[14]

### The Early Years:
### Organizing Antituberculosis Associations

Beginning in 1896 with the National Sanatarium Association in Ontario, lay and medical reformers began to unite to form voluntary antituberculosis associations. Aided by various women's groups – the Imperial Order of Daughters of the Empire (IODE), women's institutes, and local councils of women – by church groups, civic improvement leagues, relief associations, and women's suffrage and temperance societies, these local antituberculosis leagues were organized on a local, patchwork basis.[15] In 1899 the Canadian Medical Association (CMA) appointed a committee that recommended the formation of a national anticonsumptive society.[16] In 1901 the Canadian Association for the Prevention of Consumption and Other Forms of Tuberculosis held its first meeting. The fledgling, impecunious association embarked on two tasks: public education and the establishment of local tuberculosis leagues or associations to provide sanatoria. In this effort, the IODE was particularly helpful, for after the Boer War the organization had remained intact with one of its principle objectives being to fight tuberculosis.

Hamilton, Ontario, provides a typical example of how a variety of social reform groups worked together to found a league or erect accommodation. The City Improvement Society's initial efforts in 1903 to collect funds for a sanatorium were frustrated by public fear of consumptives (phthisiophobia). Unable to find a site acceptable to the community, the society turned the funds already collected over to the National Sanatarium Association to erect a Hamilton pavilion at Gravenhurst. In the end, the Mountain Sanatorium in Hamilton was donated by two prominent businessmen with the support of the local councils of women and the IODE. While the men established the Hamilton Health Association, the ladies' auxiliary, headed by the IODE regent provided relief work (a large part of early antituberculosis efforts).[17]

Like the IODE, other local and national organizations added tuberculosis to their growing lists of concerns. The National Council of

Women formed a committee of public health in 1908. The associated boards of trade of Western Canada passed a resolution supporting the establishment of a sanatorium.[18] The Women's Institutes of Ontario affiliated themselves to the Canadian association in 1907, while the Women's Christian Temperance Union (WCTU) aided the Alberta association by sending Frank Oliver, the minister of the interior, a copy of a petition asking for a grant of money from the dominion government to help the Alberta government support impoverished tuberculous sufferers who arrived in that province. A committee for the prevention of tuberculosis was organized under the Calgary board of trade. The Montreal board of trade and the local council of women agitated for antispitting legislation, along with the cleaning of streetcars to help eliminate the disease.[19]

The women volunteers had a multipurpose agenda, like the campaign itself: demanding the erection of accommodation (usually sanatoria), furnishing new institutions with linen and supplies, working for adequate health legislation, and providing relief work. This was especially true of the IODE – by 1911 they were aiding the tuberculosis campaign in ten Canadian cities. Beginning with the Mountain Sanatorium (Hamilton) after the Boer War, they steadily increased their responsibility – chapters in Vancouver, Kingston, Napanee, London, Ottawa, St Catharines, Windsor, and Winnipeg all furnished sanatoria, supplied tents, and sold Christmas stamps issued by the National Sanitarium Association to aid the free sanatorium at Gravenhurst. The Toronto chapter established and managed a preventorium for infected children. As Mrs Albert E. Gooderham, the IODE regent explained, it was justified by patriotism and the social gospel: "We also feel that it is a *truly* Patriotic work; in our Preventorium we will not only help make the little bodies strong, but minister to the mind and soul as well, as we hope to create the atmosphere of a truly Christian home, endeavoring to live up to one of the most cherished ideals of the British Empire – 'for God, my country and my King.'"[20]

In French-speaking Quebec, women worked through nursing sisterhoods to fight the disease; the Sisters of Providence, for example, supplied the quarters for the French-run dispensary, the Bruchesi Institute, and provided the visiting nurses.[21] This religious involvement was common in health care generally in francophone Quebec, which consequently differed from health care in the English community in Montreal and from anti-TB work in the rest of the country. While anti-TB work in the latter case was almost exclusively organized and funded by lay volunteers, and then later by a combination of lay volunteers and various levels of government, the French community in Quebec, and in particular in Montreal, left tuberculosis work to the religious orders and a very small group of professionals, usually doctors. Philosophically, anti-TB reformers considered tuberculosis itself more than a disease – it was a manifestation of a deeper, underlying social malaise, indicating the rot in urban society; and the prewar fight against the disease was thus, according to one pioneer, J.H. Holbrook, "primarily a humanitarian movement of lay people."[22]

### The Campaign against Bacteriological Causes

Elimination of the germ – the first prong of the campaign – required not only public health legislation but changes in long-standing individual social behaviour. A sufferer should be isolated, sleeping alone, preferably in a separate room, using separate dishes. Kissing was particularly ill-advised. "If you must," sternly instructed M.M. Seymour, the provincial health officer, in a circular published by the Saskatchewan Department of Agriculture, "first wipe your lips with carbolized rosewater and dry them."[23]

At the turn of the century, Canadians spat "a great deal and everywhere": on sidewalks, in post offices, theatres, saloons, schools, and churches – even around stoves and heaters in their homes.[24] As dried, infected sputum caused infection when inhaled, anti-TB reformers promoted stringently enforced municipal antispitting bylaws, easily disinfected compartments in railway cars and steamships, and the availability of cuspidors. As a result of the publicity the Canadian Pacific Railway started an antispitting campaign on its lines in 1910.[25]

Like spitting, the public drinking cup in schools, hotels, railway stations, and other public buildings was considered an obvious purveyor of disease. "A public toothpick," one writer acidly remarked, "would be more unpopular, but not a whit more undesirable,"[26] and various substitutes for the public drinking cup, including disposable paper cups and "bubbling fountains," were promoted.

Milk, too, could transmit tuberculosis. Not only could a diseased cow infect the beverage but the common method of selling it to the urban poor, as "dip tank milk," almost ensured contamination after it was shipped to the city. Milk was stored in large, common tanks, often uncovered, and customers would purchase their required amount by "dipping in" their personal container. As a result the milk became infected not only from customers or their containers but from the ever-present flies swarming about. Pasteurization was no guarantee of purity unless the milk was sold in sealed, preferably nonrefillable, bottles.[27]

It was dust that most aroused reformers' wrath, for they considered dust, blown in the air and mixed up with dried sputa, to be one of the chief means of transmitting the disease. Several methods were

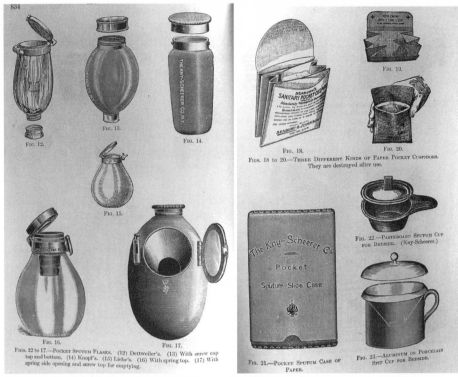

*Left,* pocket sputum flasks; *right,* sputum flasks. Reproduced from Klebs, *Tuberculosis,* 834.

suggested for attacking "the dust menace." Moist sawdust or a wet cloth on a long-handled scrub brush should be substituted for dry-sweeping. Streets should be sprinkled regularly, especially in warm weather. Shoes should be carefully wiped before entering a home. Women's fashionable long trains were a particular irritant – anti-TB crusaders painted a grim picture of a mother innocently infecting a crawling infant by bringing sputum-laden dust into the house on her dress.[28] Flies were also considered dangerous disease vectors transmitting tuberculosis bacilli from sputa to exposed food or milk. Because horses were the main means of transportation, flies were a significant problem. Public health workers demanded that food, whether in the home or in a shop window, be covered.[29]

## The Campaign against Social Causes

While antituberculosis workers attacked the disease from a bacteriological point of view, eliminating exposure to the germ, they fought the disease with almost greater ferocity on another front: the predisposing, underlying social causes, such as poor housing, inadequate light and ventilation, overcrowding and low wages, alcoholism, and even sexual intercourse.[30] In this they joined ranks with other urban reformers striving to improve social conditions. Many, in fact, were members of a variety of reform groups and simultaneously supported several causes. Statistics seemed to justify this approach. Eighty percent of the tuberculosis deaths in Ottawa in 1909 were among earners of a daily wage, while in Montreal the league commented that the average accommodation of its patients was eleven people living in ten rooms, and in some cases, eighteen in four rooms, and fifteen in three.[31]

Since the prohibition movement was one of the key elements of turn-of-the-century social reform thought, it was not surprising that anti-TB workers attacked alcoholism as a key factor not only predisposing alcoholics themselves to the disease but, worse yet, affecting their children by endowing them with a sickly constitution. More generally, as the Quebec Royal Commission of 1910 pointed out, alcoholism bred poverty, which in turn led to overcrowding, a poor diet, and, inevitably, tuberculosis.[32] In 1913 the Bruchesi Institute in Montreal reported that a full 50 percent of its tuberculosis cases had a history of alcoholism (20 percent were alcoholics, 30 percent had a family history).[33] A drunkard was considered unsanitary and irregular in his diet, while an excessive amount of liquor degenerated the stomach, liver, and lungs, forming a good soil for the tuberculosis germs. "L'alcoolisme," one expert succinctly summed up, "fait le lit de la tuberculose."[34]

Not only did alcohol cause children to be "poorly manufactured" but those compelled to work at a young age were at high risk of becoming drunkards themselves. "Alcohol predisposes to tuberculosis in the child as well as in the adult," one American expert, S. Aldolphus Knopf, insisted, "and the prevention of child labor will in many instances prevent both alcoholism and tuberculosis."[35] As the Quebec Royal Commission bluntly stated, "to combat alcoholism is to combat tuberculosis."[36] It was eminently logical for reformers, such as Emily Murphy, a pioneer in the anti-TB movement, to work simultaneously for prohibition, women's suffrage, and a myriad of other reform causes. An anti-TB crusader could work militantly to eliminate "treating" (providing free drinks) in a bar, on the theory that this would ultimately help reduce the disease.

More pragmatically, linking TB and alcohol abuse served a symbiotic purpose: it enabled the anti-TB workers to tap into the organization and rhetoric of the prohibition movement, thus broadening their own base and promoting their own agenda; and in turn this enabled the prohibition movement to justify its campaign on scientific and medical grounds in addition to the moral and social ones.

It must be pointed out, however, that as scientists unravel the puzzles of immunology, the association between alcohol and tuberculosis appears to be based on more than social reform prejudice. Chronic alcohol abuse suppresses the development and expression of cell-mediated immunity, specifically T-cells and pulmonary macrophages, which are essential in controlling tuberculous infection.[37] Epidemiological studies from the United States, Canada, Britain, Denmark, Yugoslavia, and Australia seem to confirm this conclusion, reporting a greater incidence of pulmonary TB in alcoholics than in nonalcoholics. One Australian series demonstrated that, although TB patients smoked and drank heavily, it was alcohol, not tobacco, that was independently linked to the disease.[38] To complicate the issue further, recent studies of immunological markers (antigens) on the cell membranes of pulmonary TB patients have demonstrated a genetic predisposition to breaking down with the disease.[39] In sum, as one American microbiologist stated in a paper commentorating the centennial of Koch's discovery, the current view has evolved into a variant of social reform thought: that microbes are an *essential*, but not necessarily *sufficient*, cause of the disease.[40]

### TB *and* VD

If the anti-TB campaign could broaden its base by association with the prohibition movement, it is not surprising that tuberculosis would be linked to another "social problem" with moral overtones – venereal disease. Again, fear or concern for the epidemic of one disease in Canadian society could increase and legitimize support for a campaign against the other. Middle class morality is evident in the relationship reformers saw between tuberculosis, sex, and venereal disease. As with tuberculosis, recent advances in scientific knowledge had stimulated the campaign against VD: the dark-field microscope to identify *treponema pallidum*, the causative corkscrew organism for syphilis (1905), the Wassermann Test (1906), and finally Salvarsan (1910) to treat syphilis. Now the various venereal diseases – gonorrhea, syphilis, and chancroid – could be identified, diagnosed, and to a limited degree treated. Like TB, venereal disease was linked to other social reform concerns and middle class fears: immigrants, slum living, and "white slavery" or prostitution. However, more than TB, it was still considered a private shame, with resistance to public education. Advocates believed that if newspapers publicized venereal disease as they did tuberculosis, the situation would improve. Linking TB to venereal disease, then, would not only add respectability to a "shameful" problem but promote public discussion of the latter – a bonus to reformers.[41]

As the author of a popular medical reference book for the home warned, "Masturbation, excessive venery" and "fast life in fashionable society" were all predisposing causes of consumption – as was syphilis. In fact, some almost viewed tuberculosis as a punishment for immoral behaviour. One writer linked up alcohol, VD, and TB in the following way: "alcohol excites the passions, and ... the abuse of the same brings about all kinds of exposures. Syphilis brings about, to a certain extent, at least moral degeneration which may be a forerunner of the use of alcohol. The weakening effects of tuberculosis drive one to the stimulating effects to be secured from the use of alcohol. These three diseases, then, are so closely interwoven, in every sphere of influence ... tuberculosis, though generally innocently acquired, follows upon the heels of those two diseases as naturally as does day follow night."[42] The moral was plain. Although everyone might be infected, those who lived a "degenerative" life were especially prone to develop tuberculosis. The patient who hoped to conquer tuberculosis, D.M. King, the brother of the future prime minister, righteously pointed out, needed "a *desire* to be pure."[43]

### Immigration and Eugenics

Immigrants were another social reform concern of the anti-TB movement, demonstrating, together with venereal disease, the intimate linking of the disease with the more general eugenics movement. Again, as with prohibition, this link provided a broader base for the anti-TB movement, which in turn added a scientific, public health rationale to the eugenicists' cause.

Eugenics had been defined in 1883 by Francis Galton (1822–1911), one of its pioneering proponents, as a "study of the agencies under social control that may improve or impair the racial qualities of future generations either physically or mentally."[44] Worried Canadian intellectuals, threatened by the expansion of both big business and the working class, with the associated uncontrolled immigration and urbanization, fostered a movement to protect the "quality" of the race and the "fitness" of the population of Canada. As Dr J.G. Adami, McGill pathology professor, delegate to the International Congress of Eugenics in 1912 and 1921, and president in 1910 of the Canadian Association for the Prevention of Tuberculosis, reasoned, if it was difficult to restrict the breeding of the unfit, at least the reproduction of the fit could be encouraged.[45]

Although aware that tuberculosis was not inherited, many reformers believed people could be predisposed to the disease as a result of inherited traits – both racial and individual. Backed by the biological theory that races "levelled down" (a "defective" parent and a normal one would have "defective children"), anti-TB workers sternly insisted, for genetic reasons, that tuberculous people should never marry. They would merely produce "poor, feeble, miserable members into the world who would have no strength or vitality" and be easy prey to the disease. In fact, reformers asserted, tuberculosis might even be an indirect cause of feeble-mindedness or insanity.[46]

The struggle for existence had national and racial implications. Disease, a few pointed out, although a crude method, still aided natural selection in improving the race. As Sir James Barr, president of the Royal Institute of Public Health, warned members of the Canadian Medical Association at their annual meeting in 1911, "those countries which have to a large extent suspended a selective death-rate, but are not wise enough to establish a selective birth-rate are certain to decay."[47] As proof, he pointed out that since the tuberculosis death rate had fallen, the rate of insanity had risen. Ergo, "Since the insane show such a marked tendency to tuberculosis, it is not improbable that the diminishing death-rate from tuberculosis has played a considerable part in the increase of insanity."[48]

No one was callous enough to advocate a continuation of a natural selection based on disease; besides, most recognized it to be inefficient, especially if the disease was tuberculosis, which seriously damaged survivors. Instead, reformers favoured birth control. Knopf pointed out that the tuberculous individual who came from a large family was often one of the later born children and had inherited a "physiological poverty."[49] "Surely," Mrs Adam Shortt demanded indignantly in 1912, "it is of more importance to have some regulation of grade in our human stock than in our horses and cattle. We spend a thousand dollars to train the intellect of one child, and yet make no laws to prevent his being born without one."[50]

So what was the solution? First, "protective evolution" – have the race develop a resistance to tuberculosis through exposure to the disease. More immediately, reformers wanted a restriction on the marriages of "defectives," particularly the feeble-minded, and they opposed marriage for the tuberculous, especially women (childbearing worsened disease). Birth control was also suggested, to prevent large families with their consequent overcrowding and malnutrition from breeding poor constitutions. And a good environment not only improved the lot of the individual but helped improve "the stock" as well. Linking eugenics to urban social reform concerns gave it national and racial significance, and an added urgency. "When we consider that the food of the child determines the future of the citizen and the physical strength of the potential fathers and mothers," one Ottawa medical health officer reasoned, "we see that in guarding the milk supply we are not confronted solely with the question of infantile sickness and death with possible outbreaks of infectious diseases through the milk, but of the far larger problem, the great social problem, that of the future of the race."[51]

If the future of the race relied on breeding "good stock," it depended equally on not importing "bad stock" – diseased, sickly immigrants – to weaken the population even further. To reformers, this was a chronic, vexing problem, not easily solved – or, more often, inadequately addressed by the governments and steamship companies eagerly promoting and profiting from the new residents. The high mountains and cold, bracing, pure air of Canada had a reputation, especially among the British, of favouring the cure of tuberculosis, which may have encouraged tuberculosis sufferers to immigrate. Hingston, in his *Climate of Canada*, commented on Indian officers who "found that a short residence in Canada restored them to comparative comfort."[52] More often than not, reformers suspected, tuberculous immigrants ended up as public charges who were either sent home at the expense of the municipality or voluntary association or supported until they died.[53] Anti-TB workers found this particularly unfair, and they singled out British immigrants as the worst offenders. According to figures gathered by the Toronto Board of Trade from the National Sanitarium Association, of 243 patients at the Muskoka Free Hospital in 1907, one-third were of foreign birth. At the same time, of the 134 cared for at the Toronto Free Hospital, only 50 percent were born in Canada, while 35 percent were from Great Britain and Ireland, 9 percent from other British possessions, and the remainder from elsewhere.[54] The physician-in-chief clearly expressed the resentment of many reformers when he bluntly stated that "This but emphasizes the necessity for a very rigid scrutiny of all English immigrants before they are allowed to land. They bring with them not only abject poverty, but also well developed diseases. In many cases the history showed that they had been advised to come to this country on account of the bracing climate being so beneficial to persons suffering from pulmonary tuberculosis ... The evidence would seem to show that this country is simply the dumping ground for those afflicted with tuberculosis and other diseases."[55]

Stricter inspection was obviously called for. The Woodstock city council responded to one demand when it passed a resolution to have immigrants inspected properly prior to departure in London – Quebec inspection was futile. Others suggested making the steamship company, instead of the municipality, pay all expenses involved in deporting undesirable immigrants. This shift of responsibility would force the ship's surgeon to inspect more closely. To ensure his objectivity, it was advised that this doctor should be a government appointee, while immigrants should be forced to wait twenty-four hours on each side to be examined properly – a demand that indicated more than anything else how superficial the inspection was.[56]

These measures would do nothing, however, as F. Montizambert, director general of public health for the federal government, pointed out, to stop diseased immigrants from the United States. Shifting responsibility south, the Quebec Royal Commission on Tuberculosis blamed the immigration of Quebec residents who, after working in American factories, returned home in advanced stages of tuberculosis and infected their families. This immigration, "probably more than that of foreigners," contributed to the spread of the disease, the commissioners maintained.[57]

Despite the rhetoric, uncovering tuberculosis in the thousands of immigrants flowing into the country was an impossible task, even for the most zealous and dedicated inspector, for all examinations were clinical. x-ray facilities were technologically too primitive, and with the almost universal rate of infection, tuberculin useless.

Whether the immigrant problem was as critical as publicized was a contentious issue. Peter Bryce, the chief medical officer of the Immigration Branch of the Department of the Interior, pointed out that roughly 100 immigrants out of 350,000 in 1906–7 developed tuberculosis and became public charges – hardly an overwhelming number. This statistic, of course, begged the question as to how many were diseased. Even so, municipalities and voluntary associations resented spending their meager funds on "foreigners" who came to their country only to die. Alberta was especially annoyed, for hearing of its favourable climate, consumptives arrived from all over the country to be cured, usually without funds. The Calgary board of trade and the WCTU both felt that the federal government owed them assistance – it was not an "Alberta problem."[58]

The nativist sentiments underlying the rhetoric were more obvious when irritated anti-TB reformers turned their attention to the shortcomings of the federal immigration policy. It seemed foolish to spend money importing countless strangers while native Canadians were callously neglected. A.J. Richer pointed out in 1903 that probably 48,000 Canadians were invalided each year from tuberculosis – and the federal government had brought in 49,149 immigrants at a cost of $444,730 in 1901 and 67,379 at a cost of $495,842 in 1902. Immigrants were simply replacing the victims of the disease.[59] As the president of the national association, J. George Adami, demanded, with more than a hint of xenophobia: "Is it not better for us in Canada

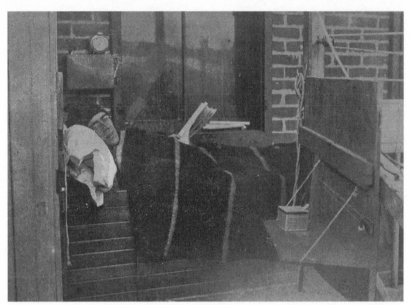

Patient on a roof. Reproduced from Royal Edward Institute, *Annual Report* (1911), 51

to increase our population by saving our own and making them strong and healthy rather than by spending our national money in bringing in Doukhobors, Galacians, Poles and the depressed peoples of Southern and Eastern Europe?" The federal government, he concluded, would "manifest a true statesmanship" if instead it funded the anti-TB campaign and improved sanitation.[60] "In short," according to Angus McLaren, "eugenics arguments provided apparently new objective scientific justifications for old, deep-seated racial and class assumptions," and their success ultimately lay not in impeding the entry of immigrants into Canada but "in popularizing biological arguments to perpetuate the argument – so beloved by the anxious – that the nation's problems were largely the product of the outsider."[61]

### Taking the Cure: Fresh Air, Country Life

It was not surprising that if the causes of TB were seen to be a complex mix of bacteriological, social, and economic conditions, the solutions would reflect this view – particularly if treatment, as William Osler observed, was unspecific at best: "fresh air, good food, good houses and hope."[62] This observation, too, reflected turn-of-the-century urban reform bias. "Foul air" or "air sewage" was found most often in the unsanitary, overcrowded slum dwellings, factories, and narrow city

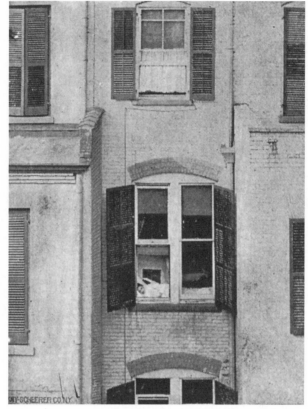

Window tent as seen from the outside. Reproduced from
Knopf, *Report to the United States Government on Tuberculosis*, 40

streets. The stench from the fly-ridden stables, cesspools, and privies could be overwhelming. In 1912 the Toronto health department identified 18,000 privies – and it was not until the following year that the city council passed a bylaw enabling the government to install indoor plumbing, with the cost billed to the individual.[63]

Such noxious air was believed to have a direct physiological effect predisposing people to TB: by causing them to breathe less deeply and ultimately reducing the respiratory capacity of their lungs, it resulted in the typical *habitus phthisicus*, that is to say, a narrow chest, stooping shoulders, and a pale and emaciated appearance. Fresh air was the solution. Slum dwellers were instructed to sleep outside, on the roof if no other space was available. If all did so, predicted Knopf, "tuberculosis would soon be eradicated among the masses."[64]

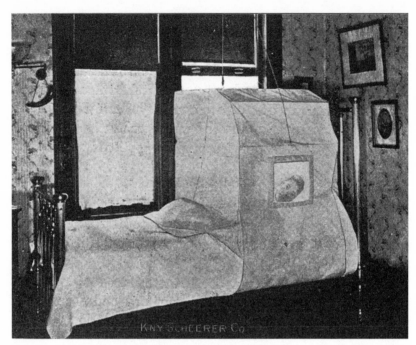

Knopf indoor window tent when in use. Reproduced from Knopf, *Report to the United States Government on Tuberculosis*, 40

Not only slums suffered from poor ventilation – ignorance about the elementary laws of hygiene was rife among the upper and middle classes as well. Montreal churches were condemned as "sanitary death traps,"[65] and the wealthy were faulted for keeping the airiest and sunniest room in their homes as the "best parlour," while their children slept in dark and ill-ventilated bedrooms. Extolling the merits of fresh air and of sunlight as a natural germicide, reformers condemned the prevalent irrational and harmful fear of "night air," exhorting the public to leave their windows open at all times and in all climates.

This emphasis on fresh air, probably the most prominent part of the prewar "cure" for TB, was influenced by both the treatment carried out in the pioneer sanatoria, particularly Saranac Lake, and a more general idealized view of the country itself as a healthy Garden of Eden, unaffected by urban rot. The special committee of the National Council of Women (NCW) on "matters concerning the public health," for example, opined in 1906 that "The health of the rural population is good. The climate of Canada is almost everywhere healthy, and in the older portions of the Dominion at least the people are of a vigorous and rugged stock. Farming, ranching, lumbering, fishing, all

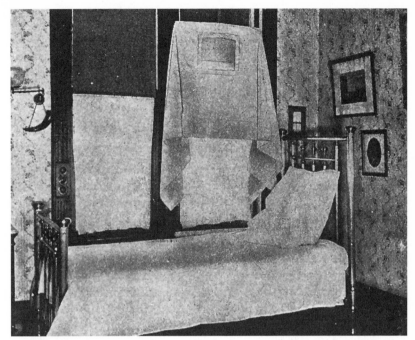

Knopf window tent when not in use. Reproduced from Knopf, *Report to the United States Government on Tuberculosis*, 40

typical Canadian industries, are conducive to health and strength. Except among the poorer city population, good air, comfortable houses, and plenty of nutritious food are within the reach of all who are willing to work."[66]

This idealization of rural life crossed all political lines, from urban reformers involved in the "garden city" movement to imperialists such as G.M. Grant, Andrew Macphail, and Stephen Leacock, the last of whom was a staunch antiprohibitionist.[67] Like them, anti-TB reformers saw, as Peter Bryce pointed out to the NCW in 1898, society evolving from a "natural state" in the country to an unsanitary, urban state, with its attendant evils of overcrowding, improper sewage, poor ventilation, and inadequate lighting inevitably causing disease.[68] As one pioneer anti-TB worker summed up later, "little provision was made for *medical* treatment, for this was very much a back to nature movement."[69]

Such an obsessive belief in fresh air encouraged the construction of sanatoria in the countryside to get maximum benefit from the pure air, while open-air sleeping balconies were added to many larger homes during the period. Reformers advocated agricultural and horticultural colonies and farming as one of the healthiest occupations,

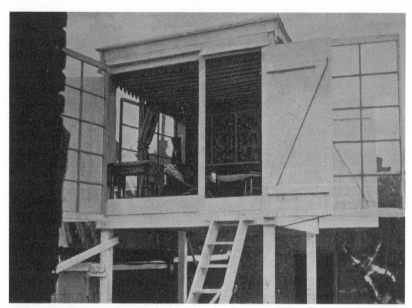

The cure of tuberculosis in Montreal. Shack built by some friends for a patient, and where he is now taking the cure. Elevation 12 feet. Windows arranged so as to be adjusted to wind conditions. Patient has done splendidly in his private sanatorium. Reproduced from Royal Edward Institute, *Annual Report* (1911), 37

and they even went so far as to maintain that it was easier to fight alcoholism in the country because there was a "better class of people" there.[70]

"Taking the cure," then, was only for the hardiest of souls. "I kept comfortable on the coldest days" related one sufferer, "wearing a hockey cap, woollen lined leather mittens, felt boots, and, over my ordinary clothing, a fur coat and two heavy woollen blankets. If the weather was extra cold I had a hot soapstone placed at my feet. At night, sleeping in a bedroom as cold as outdoors, I wore a woollen cap, woollen socks and used the soapstone."[71] For added warmth, the patient slept in a "klondike bed," a complicated affair of layered blankets and pillows.[72]

An abundance of food, especially eggs and milk, was also essential. Both nutrition and fresh air were emphasized to such an extent that the Hamilton relief officer considered medical supervision unnecessary when the sanatorium was first erected in 1906. Local leagues, as part of their curative efforts, dispensed eggs, milk, bovril, fruit, and meat to needy sufferers. Weight gain was the standard method of evaluating progress of a cure, and most early sanatorium reports stressed the number of patients gaining weight and the number of

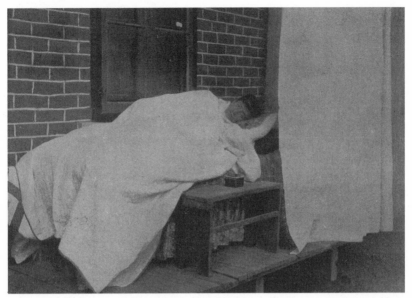

Patient on a verandah. Reproduced from Royal Edward Institute, *Annual Report* (1911), 45

pounds added. "The tubercular patient," insisted one Manitoba group, "should be overfed rather than underfed." Patients were encouraged to eat three hearty meals a day, two or three substantial snacks, with at least a quart of rich milk and as many raw eggs as they could stomach.[73]

Although it would later be the bedrock of treatment, complete rest was not a core element of the cure during the prewar period. In fact, sanatoria advertised a variety of amusements and sports for their patients – a planned sanatorium at Mount Tremblant, Quebec, for example, boasted "fishing, fowling, bathing, canoeing ... snowshoe tramps, toboggan slides, and the agreeable excitement and movement of skating."[74] Practical economics bolstered this philosophy. A change in philosophy would mean that authorities would have to accept the necessity of a lengthy treatment period to cure tuberculosis. This, in turn, would require more permanent buildings – shack-like structures and tents were sufficient for a few months (the average stay in an early sanatorium), but no longer. The authorities would also have to deal with the problem of patients unable to support themselves or their families throughout their cure. And both problems required more money.

Aside from patent medicines, "tuberculin treatment" was the only specific targeted to the disease itself in the prewar period. Robert Koch caused much excitement when he announced in 1890 that he had discovered a cure – a mixture of proteins and antigens derived from a broth in which he had cultured tuberculosis bacilli. An infected guinea pig, when inoculated with the substance, had healed at the injection site. Koch postulated that repeated injections would similarly enable a human subject to slough off infected tissues and recover from the disease. Testing began. Tuberculous patients were injected with measured amounts of tuberculin in an attempt to stimulate natural resistance. Since such a treatment was cheap and possible to administer through a dispensary and since it permitted patients to work while undergoing it, tuberculin quickly became popular.[75] Nevertheless, it shortly proved to be a disappointing failure. Ironically, as a diagnostic tool it would later prove invaluable, for it would enable the identification of infected but not clinically diseased humans – and animals.

The attempt to build up the body's natural resistance with a bacteriological approach not only spawned the use of tuberculin as a curative technique but led to the development of "graduated labour" and its associated "auto-innoculation." First promoted in England in 1911, graduated labour had a limited popularity in Canada, although even at its height many specialists, seeing the value of rest, were dubious about physical exertion.[76] Maintaining that exercise built up antibodies in a patient's system (auto-innoculation), advocates devised a detailed system of graduated work, from walking and watering plants to heavier manual labour, such as pulling down trees and trenching ground. Graduated labour was also lauded as a means of both reducing the duration of the cure and preventing a relapse when the patient returned to work. Results were unimpressive, however, and by 1920 the superintendent of the Manitoba Sanatorium would remark that "we have rest squads where ten years ago we had work gangs."[77]

Before a patient could take the cure, the disease had to be diagnosed. Because x-rays were limited and primitive, a diagnosis of tuberculosis hinged on vague clinical symptoms (malaise, cough, weight loss) and a sputum analysis. It is not surprising that the disease was frequently misdiagnosed in the early stages as malaria, typhoid, or even a common cold. Even with a correct diagnosis, treatment was frequently far beyond the patient's means. The urban poor suffered most. Overcrowding was a way of life, as one Winnipeg housing inspector observed: "A house of ten rooms was found occupied by five families, also roomers – 20 adults and two children. Three of the families had only one room each. There were eight gas stoves, and none of these had hoods or pipes for carrying off the products of combustion and the odors of cooking. Two girl boarders occupied a portion of the cellar … There was one water closet, one sink, a bath and a wash basin. Two faucets had been fitted on the water-service pipe, and buckets placed under same in lieu of pipes."[78] How could such a patient sleep alone or afford eggs and milk? How could a "klondike bed" be made with only one blanket? Even something so seemingly simple as keeping the window open to allow "fresh air" in had its ramifications, as one writer bitterly pointed out to what he considered to be naive and idealistic slum workers: "It is far better that they are closed, and closed tight, for to open a window is to get a whiff of the gentle breeze from the slop box or neighboring stable, which fills the house with its intoxicating fragrance. Why come and repeat these same things to them – have they already not enough pangs? If you are going to help the people, you must know the fundamental cause and try to prevent its growing."[79]

### Notification: Identifying the Tuberculous

It was the issue of compulsory notification that demonstrated most clearly not only the conflict between individual rights and community protection but also how social reformers, with the best motives, could unwittingly persecute the urban poor. Under compulsory notification, private doctors, clinics, or individuals were required by law to report all known cases of tuberculosis to the department of health so that "appropriate" action could be taken. A prewar fascination with statistics and efficiency had become associated with a new emphasis on scientific organization and management. This had developed as an intellectual outgrowth of the new advances in science and engineering, strengthened by the increasing secularization of religion and the clear evidence of the concrete advantages of the application of engineering in sanitation, hydroelectricity, and industry.[80] It provided a philosophical justification and impetus for pursuing a "greater good" at the expense of individual rights.

Estimates of morbidity, based on a calculation of five to ten times a tenuous mortality rate, often seemed to depend on little more than the shock value and drama an individual wanted to inject into a speech. To determine the extent of the problem, anti-TB workers made compulsory notification a priority. But what use was compulsory notification if nothing could be done to aid the victim? Oliver Mowat, the premier of Ontario, had already made that harsh reality painfully clear in 1894 when he had been asked to pass an order-in-council instituting compulsory notification. "I recognize what is necessary to be done in these cases," he responded wearily; "you must not let them go near other people if they are infected, but will you tell me, Gentlemen, what are you going to do with them when you receive the notification?"[81]

As one doctor in Westmount, Quebec, bluntly pointed out, "A head of a family has tuberculosis, and if he reports it himself, he loses his employment ... if you are going to compel them to notify, you should

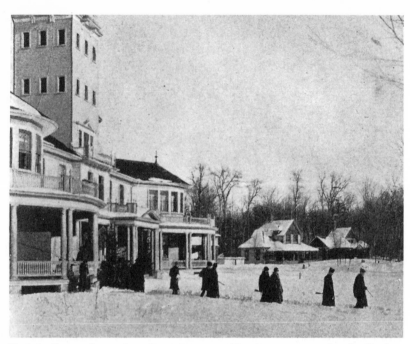

Muskoka Cottage Sanatorium, Gravenhurst, ON. Note large open porches for "fresh air" treatment. Reproduced from Knopf, *Tuberculosis*, 337.

also provide means for the family; because when people see starvation staring them in the face, they will not notify. They also ask the doctor not to do, and he has to choose between notifying and seeing the family starve."[82]

### The Role of the Sanatoria

Although of little value to the urban poor, the sanatorium was nevertheless the first and most popular means of implementing treatment. Many influential early pioneers in anti-TB work had personal experience with the disease and were staunch advocates of this method of treatment, sometimes having "taken the cure" themselves.[83] David Stewart, the superintendent of the Manitoba Sanitorium at Ninette, had been treated at Saranac Lake, while Sir Adam Beck, the leading force behind the London Health Association and the establishment of the Queen Alexandra Sanatorium, was the son-in-law of the president of the ladies' board of the Hamilton Health Association, which ran the Mountain Sanatorium.[84]

A sanatorium was, moreover, a concrete project around which anti-TB workers could rally. As early anti-TB workers were primarily volunteers and the funds they raised were often from personal donations and public subscriptions, a specific goal that would "do something" in the short term – treat patients – and yet be established in the long term as an institution was important.

Because the early sanatoria (other than the provincial sanatorium erected in Nova Scotia in 1904) were almost completely built with voluntarily raised funds, they were of necessity simple affairs – often literally a few shacks and tents to enable patients to take the fresh air. Besides, in keeping with social reform optimism, as one medical superintendent later remarked wryly, "tuberculosis was to be banished, bag and baggage, scrip and scrippage so soon, that it would be wasteful to build permanent buildings to care for it."[85]

The location of a site often proved to be an insurmountable obstacle to zealous canvassers, for they had educated an anxious public too well about the infectious nature of tuberculosis, and no neighborhood wanted a group of consumptives in its midst. "The result of all this discussion," said Dr Sheard, the Toronto medical health officer, in disgust in 1901, "is that matters at the present time are in a worse condition than they were ten years ago. The dissemination of the knowledge and the fear that the disease is communicable has had the effect of closing the doors of every hospital and home against the unhappy victim, and they are now literally left to die uncared for."[86] Practically, anti-TB advocates had little choice when they glorified the virtues of rural living. Public outcry had forced William Gage to build in Muskoka and there were many similar incidents across the country.[87]

In vain anti-TB workers pleaded for understanding and explained over and over again that careful consumptives (that is, those found in a sanatorium) were much safer than the ignorant sufferer with whom one came in daily contact. Testimonials from leading experts "proved" that towns with sanatoria were not only healthy but – what was possibly more important to economically minded businessmen – also more prosperous from increased business.[88]

It did little good. "Phthisiophobia" had struck, and the consumptive was ostracized unmercifully. Of thirty-four public hospitals in 1903, only thirteen had special accommodation for tuberculous patients, thirteen refused them, and eight accepted them only in a great emergency.[89] Some believed that the tuberculous were not only a physical danger but "mentally peculiar or something worse."[90] The irony of the situation was probably lost on the poor sufferer when the national association felt obliged to point out in 1902 that it was an anti-*tuberculosis* society, not an anti-*consumptive* society.[91] The sufferer probably saw little difference when it came to the results of its actions. Such public intransigency irritated sanatorium advocates. "In trying to educate the people as to the contagious nature of tuberculosis," observed a frustrated Elizabeth Shortt to the National Council of Women (NCW), "it is to be regretted that we have unfortunately created a sort of horror of sanataria ... It seems a paradox that people should get excited and go to all sorts of trouble and expense, if necessary, if a sanatarium is to be erected within a block of where they live, but are wholly indifferent to the danger of its prospective inmates going about carrying the bread or vegetables, or furniture of the public, or even working in their homes."[92]

Not only did they have to deal with a public fear they had a large part in creating, but anti-TB workers found some dissension even within their own ranks when the role of sanatoria was discussed. Should they treat only curable, early cases or advanced ones as well? Should they erect separate accommodation for advanced cases? And was the erection of sanatoria the most efficient use of funds? Perhaps education was a better answer – as Premier J.D. Hazen pointed out to a New Brunswick delegation, the Nova Scotia sanatorium "found that incipient cases did not care to come to the institution and the others came too late."[93]

This was a minority view. Most workers agreed that education was of primary importance but argued that it was an essential part of the sanatorium's "mission": it educated individuals, their families, and the general public, offered accommodation and possible cure, and protected the public by isolating an infectious case. A patient was educated, left, and proceeded to show others how to live. And from an economic point of view it was cheaper to care for impoverished tuberculosis victims in sanatoria, and cure a few, than have all dying in general hospitals at community expense.[94]

Providing free accommodation for those unable to pay and a time limit on treatment were two important and related problems of early sanatoria. There were only seventy-five sanatorium beds in Canada in 1901, and not one for the poor.[95] The National Sanitarium Association opened the forty-bed Muskoka Free Hospital for Consumptives adjacent to the Cottage Sanatorium in 1902, but this did not begin to come to grips with the problem. And whose responsibility was it – the responsibility of the federal government, the province, the municipality, or the voluntary associations?

To cope with the combined problems of a shortage of beds and a lack of funds to support patients, sanatoria initially limited the time a patient could stay – in some cases as little as four months. In Hamilton in 1907, some former patients whose six-month period of stay had elapsed were permitted to set up a tent colony to continue treatment; but no arrangements were made for their upkeep, and a dramatic newspaper account of their lack of food, clothing and, sanitary facilities led to the abandonment of the six-month rule.[96] More often, treatment was gradually extended, as long as the patient, or someone else, could pay.

The short treatment period reflected, as well, the doubt the public felt about the power of the sanatorium to cure the consumptive. "I knew Saranac Lake," said one sufferer, "I knew I had tuberculosis. I also remembered instantly that several relatives had died of it; that was the position I found myself in."[97] To counteract this problem, sanatoria attempted to adopt a policy in the early years of admitting only early cases. By this means they hoped to have a higher cure rate; patients would stay a shorter time, and they would not require the medical facilities a sanatorium neither had nor could afford. But time and time again sanatorium directors were confronted with the harsh reality that sufferers who were far advanced were too often the only ones willing to come – and they either had to be accepted or abandoned to die.[98]

### Outpatient Care: The Dispensary

Sanatoria did not touch the lives of the vast majority of tuberculosis victims: the urban poor. Even if accommodation had been available, they simply could not have afforded to leave home to stay in a distant institution. Montreal was a case in point. With no local sanatorium available for most of the decade, there were roughly two deaths reported every day (700 per year), while public health workers believed there were another 2,200 active cases in 1903 alone – probably a crude underestimate, but even these figures demonstrated the urgency of an alternative option.[99]

It was here in 1904 that the dispensary method was instituted as a cheaper, more effective way of treating large numbers of sufferers. Pioneered in Edinburgh and France as a clearing house for patients, it quickly became a comprehensive system of care, especially in Montreal, where funds for institutions were scarce. Patients received a thorough, free, clinical examination at the dispensary building, and then a visiting nurse or inspector examined their home environments, dispensed literature and cuspidors, and instructed both the patients and their families regarding their mode of life and proper care. The patients either periodically reported to the dispensary, or a visiting nurse travelled to their homes to check their progress. As a key part of the treatment, most dispensaries also supplied relief, including eggs, milk, and clothing.

A dispensary usually worked in conjunction with other agencies, such as the municipal or provincial laboratories (to have sputum examined), the Victorian Order of Nurses (VON, established in 1897), and charitable relief groups. Even the staunchest advocates of the dispensary realized it could not really cure but only improve the situation. With visiting nurses and inspectors, the high-risk areas (usually fairly obvious anyway) could be pinpointed and, they hoped, public opinion aroused. In a larger sense, it served the same purpose as notification.

Supervised by a visiting nurse, patients remained at home, returning to work when their symptoms ceased: their temperature normalized, their cough finished, they no longer suffered from night sweats, and their strength returned. The physiological state of their lungs was almost impossible to assess and therefore largely irrelevant. This quick return to a job would be condemned by experts in later years, but reformers saw little choice, as voluntary associations had no funds to provide the massive amount of money needed to support patients taking an extended convalescence, and governments were unwilling to accept the responsibility.[100]

The clinic or dispensary claimed not only to examine and educate both patients and their families but also to reach the greatest number at the cheapest cost. The salary of a visiting nurse paid for the supervision of hundreds of home patients, whereas the same amount of money looked after only one individual in a sanatorium. The appeal of a visiting nurse was therefore obvious, and local leagues were quick to use either the established VON (as in Montreal) or hire their own nurses. By 1906 nurses were employed in Montreal, Ottawa, Toronto, and Hamilton, so that by 1910 an organized, cooperative system was beginning to emerge whereby a professional (the nurse) was working under a voluntary body (the anti-TB league), with her salary paid for by the league or another volunteer group – an associated women's group, perhaps.[101]

By 1909 the Montreal league had established the most extensive dispensary system in the country. Members had erected a tuberculosis institute as a base to treat and aid consumptives, complete with nurses and the use of a city inspector, rooms for outdoor patients, classes, and verandas and a roof garden for day patients. However, they lacked beds for advanced cases and adequate sanatorium accommodation. By 1910 dispensaries had spread to Toronto, Hamilton, Ottawa, Winnipeg, Charlottetown and St John, New Brunswick.

Recognizing that sanatoria were beyond the means of most sufferers, and yet that their home conditions probably condemned them to death no matter what the nurse could do, reformers looked for cheaper institutional substitutes. Based originally on a German model, "camps" – day camps, night camps, and summer camps – were suggested, along with the "class method" (to be explained in a moment) as an inexpensive means of removing individuals from their environments.

A day camp was established on the dispensary porch for those who had no open-air facilities at home. Spending the day outside, patients usually received a milk and meat dinner at noon and were instructed to sleep alone at night with an open window. The tiring daily journey to the camp, the added expense of a supervising nurse and food, and the lack of employment were significant liabilities. A night camp enabled patients to sleep at the camp instead of at home, which not only afforded a certain protection to their families, but, more practically, permitted them to work during the day.[102]

The Boston-based class method initially aroused more enthusiasm. It not only required less space than the camps and sanatoria but was also cheaper: partial treatment at a sanatorium for three months cost $84, six months of day camp cost the same, but six months under the class method was estimated to be only $50. Analogous to a self-help or group-therapy session of today, it appealed strongly to reformers' middle class values, infused with a social gospel zeal. A church congregation assumed responsibility for ten to fifteen early cases, appointed a committee to handle financial arrangements, and worked with a doctor (who selected the cases) and sometimes a visiting nurse. Patients took the cure in the fresh air at home and when their fever abated, they met with the doctor, nurse, and other class members once a week in a room provided by the congregation, where they reported their progress. They were taught to take their pulse and temperature four times a day and were examined and weighed at the weekly meeting. Sometimes there was a "friendly visitor" to offer encouragement to patients at home. Although enthusiastically promoted, it failed to become widespread.[103]

## TB Legislation: Whose Responsibility?

In general, supporters of the prewar anti-TB crusade believed that the campaign required support in two areas to be successful: money for diagnosis and treatment and legislation to enforce their demands. There was a dispute, however, over which legislative body should be responsible for such a national problem. Clearly, municipal governments would be responsible for enforcing laws pertaining to the details of day-to-day living: inspection of milk, meat, and public dairies, for example. And the provinces should supervise and support the municipalities.[104]

Reformers differed, however, over the responsibility for public health under the British North America Act. Most seemed to agree it was a provincial duty, at least in part, to establish uniform legislation regarding notification, sanitary conditions, and food, factory, and school inspection, which the municipalities would then enforce. Moreover, it was this level of government that had more funds available and that could more easily establish local sanatoria, print instructions for tuberculosis victims on hygiene, and grant money to aid indigents.[105]

The jurisdiction of the federal government was more controversial. Since it controlled immigration and was considered wealthier and more powerful, some anti-TB workers demanded that it assume responsibility for eradicating the disease (a national problem). "A question affecting so vitally every living Canadian in the same manner," flatly stated A.J. Richer, a Montreal TB specialist, "should be dealt with in a national, not in a provincial spirit; in other words, federal measures should be applied."[106] Members of the federal government seemed to agree – both the Senate and the House of Commons passed resolutions in 1905 regarding tuberculosis, the latter expressing the opinion that "Parliament should take some active steps to lessen the widespread suffering and the great mortality among the people of Canada, caused by the various forms of tuberculosis."[107]

As a result, a joint committee of the Senate and House of Commons was appointed to investigate tuberculosis in Canada. It presented its report in the House on 13 July 1905, advising that "The work may be taken hold of by the Dominion government or by the provincial and municipal authorities with the aid of the Dominion government" and recommending in its seventh clause that the federal government contribute a yearly amount to the erection and maintenance of sanatoria, with the provinces, municipalities, individuals, and benevolent associations contributing the balance.

The report was adopted, but without this key clause. As a result, as R.L. Borden commented, "the report practically means nothing." Perhaps unsurprisingly, the federal resolution and the joint report were little more than a sop to public opinion. Despite this (or perhaps because of it) the national association, in conjunction with other health advocates, continually passed resolutions urging the federal government to establish a bureau of public health, under a minister, to deal with the problem of preventable disease.[108]

More often than not, there was a loose coalition between levels of government and voluntary associations, who worked almost as partners. Governments refused to spend money unless they were convinced of public interest in the matter – and this interest, it was agreed, was never more convincingly demonstrated than when the public contributed their own money through voluntary donations.[109]

Tuberculosis workers themselves believed in the necessary, even primary, role of volunteers. "Great philanthropists" were needed to contribute funds to the work, for no community by itself had enough money to deal with the disease, while the volunteer element increased the effectiveness of government action. Such volunteer reformers did not see themselves as pioneers with the ultimate goal of government taking over programs and institutions they established but as *partners* with the various levels of government, providing the manpower, organizational ability and human element, while government supplied funds, legislation, and officials to enforce it: "if the official bodies will unite with the philanthropic bodies with the main object in view of dealing delicately and considerately with the sick," pronounced A.J. Richer confidently, "the problem at once becomes easy to deal with."[110]

It was the Quebec Royal Commission on Tuberculosis (1909–10) that demonstrated most clearly the wide gap between reformers' desires and government action. The commissioners' recommendations included a wide-ranging list of social-reform era demands: strict enforcement of existing laws, hygiene instruction in the schools, popular education under the board of health, medical inspection of schools, shops, and factories, the establishment and maintenance of anti-TB dispensaries in the principal centres of the province, isolation of advanced cases among the poor, open-air schools for weak children, treating curable poor patients with the "class method," leaving the sanatoria for the rich or the rural patients who could not be treated otherwise, legislation to prohibit child labour, investigation and legislation regarding hours of work in factories, legislation against alcoholism, and meat inspection and the control of the sale of milk. For the long term, they suggested the gradual establishment of preventoriums, sanatoriums, agricultural and vacation schools, and better housing at reasonable rents for the working class. Above all, the commissioners maintained, it was the responsibility of the provincial board of health to direct the anti-TB fight in Quebec, and that board should be supplied with enough money and a competent staff to do it properly.[111]

Nowhere else is the comprehensive nature of anti-TB work as defined by the prewar social reformers so clearly demonstrated as in this report. And, in the aftermath, nowhere else is government failure to take the responsibility that was demanded of it so apparent. In 1910, the commission observed, the city's mortality rate was higher than that of any other large North American city. Twenty years later this would still be the case.[112]

In the rest of Canada the situation was not quite as bleak, for various levels of government were passing legislation and extending aid by the end of the decade, albeit in a patchwork fashion. Compulsory notification was enacted in Alberta, British Columbia, Quebec, and

Saskatchewan (though not strictly enforced). To a limited degree, British Columbia, Ontario, and Nova Scotia all contributed to the maintenance and capital costs of sanatoria.

### Education and Public Opinion

By the end of the decade, it had become clear to volunteer associations that to mobilize governments to become willing partners, more public education was needed. As one association demanded, "How can we create public opinion unless we give them information?"[113] So they attempted, with limited funds and a seemingly unquenchable optimism, to print pamphlets and newspaper articles, lecture church groups, and petition governments at all levels. In 1908 the national association obtained the federal electoral list, using it in combination with directories of some cities and towns that it did not include, and sent a copy of the leaflet "How to prevent Consumption" to every name on their list.[114]

Mass education was begun through tuberculosis exhibitions. The National Sanitarium Association had first borrowed a tuberculosis exhibit from the American National Tuberculosis Association in 1906 and brought it to Toronto for two weeks, where 13,000 people passed through it. Because of its evident popularity, public health workers were quick to exploit this new educational medium, and the secretary of the provincial board of health of Ontario organized a travelling Ontario government tuberculosis exhibit, complete with charts, literature, and lantern slides, to travel to towns, villages, and rural fairs.[115]

Fueled by both the reform era's fascination with statistics, the new themes of scientific management and efficiency, and a desire to move an apathetic public and indifferent government to action, anti-TB workers often argued in economic terms to drive home the meaning of the ravages of TB. Reformers insisted that employers could save money through increased worker efficiency and reduced absences due to illness by improving factory hygiene and sanitation. In 1903, A.J. Richer determined that tuberculosis deaths caused an annual loss of $8 million to the federal government, $4 million to the provincial governments, $4 million to the municipalities, and $32 million to the communities and families. In fact, if those 40,000 individuals estimated to be infected each year were included, there was a further annual loss of about $24 million, giving a total loss to Canada of a staggering $72 million annually.[116] However, such statistics, partly a product of reformers' zeal, were dubious, at best.

However, this period saw no comprehensive or systematic approach to education. As most of the work was left to local societies, efforts depended on the initiative and enthusiasm of local members. And although the major stated aim of the national association was education, it did not have a monopoly on the printing or distribution of literature – the federal and provincial departments of agriculture, provincial boards of health, and local associations were all involved. This lack of organization not only meant that some work was needlessly duplicated, but by 1910 was also causing jurisdictional problems – exactly whose responsibility was it? Solely that of the national association? Or should the local leagues do some printing and supplying? And what should be the role of each level of government?

### Relief Work

In addition to education and the establishment of sanatoria and dispensaries, the volunteer associations interested themselves chiefly in relief work. Not only did their limited funds frequently prohibit much else, but such an approach also tied in with prevailing social reform ideology and the methods – good food and healthy homes – touted to prevent and treat the disease. The secretary of the Montreal league, A.J. Richer, in a letter to all the doctors in the city, listed this work as the leagues' first function.[117]

Relief, like efforts in education, was organized on a local, patchwork basis, with the quantity and type dispensed again depending on the individual associations. Some, such as the Montreal and Ottawa groups, worked in conjunction with other charities, while others distributed food and clothing independently, or through their women's auxiliaries. The IODE was particularly active; each chapter even had a specific function – for example, the St Elizabeth chapter's sole duty was providing linen for Hamilton's Mountain Sanatorium – but again this depend very much on what local members desired to do. There was no clear-cut national policy or systematic approach until after the war.

In 1903, Dr T.G. Roddick, imbued with an unquenchable optimism born from only a dim understanding of the magnitude of the tuberculosis problem, could predict that "in twenty-five years, provided proper means are adopted, a case of consumption will be a curiosity."[118] It was a statement he himself would not make a decade later. As they investigated further and pushed for preventive legislation and adequate funds to attempt a cure, anti-TB workers came up against an almost insurmountable wall of public apathy, ignorance and fear, government indifference, and an economic system almost designed to perpetuate the human misery they were trying so hard to eliminate. By the start of World War 1 they could see all too clearly how entrenched tuberculosis was in Canadian society.

Ironically, the anti-TB movement had benefited a great deal from the ferment of intellectual, social, and economic changes occurring in Canada at the turn of the century. Darwinism may have helped create a crisis in religious thought that would ultimately lead to the secularization of Canadian society, but the anti-TB campaign profited from the social reform enthusiasm of the new liberal Christian theology and social gospel while it simultaneously exploited new advances in engineering and medical knowledge about the disease. The movement was linked to and drew strength from practically every aspect of social reform era thought – prohibition, social purity and venereal disease, eugenics, urban and industrial reform, scientific management, and organizational efficiency. With such broad-based support, the anti-TB campaign – in stark contrast to other more typical social reform causes – would be able to alter its focus and orientation yet maintain its momentum as Canadians confronted, first, a world war and then, reconstruction.

The first decade and a half of the twentieth century saw the establishment of the movement. The basic principles of "the cure" were laid down – fresh air, good food, and rest – and the institutional framework for carrying it out – the sanatoria, dispensaries, preventoria, camps, and open-air schools – was set up. Various governments were coming to a reluctant *awareness*, even if it was not transformed into much legislation, that they should accept some responsibility for Canadians' health. Reformers lacked funds and their efforts, as they were all to well aware, were merely band-aids on an open wound, but they were a start. It was the golden age of the amateur reformer, for even professionals knew little more than lay workers about the disease, and anyone could carry out the cure. No one was confined to one specialty – doctors, women's groups, businessmen, and clergy all interested themselves in a variety of interrelated urban social reforms. And in the following decade, new initiatives would develop from the principles this group of enthusiasts laid down.

# 2 Tuberculosis and the Great War

The war gave us a new social conscience, taught us a new standard of generosity and impressed upon us the practical value of individual and community health.

F. L. Schaffner, President, Canadian Association
for the Prevention of Tuberculosis (1921)

World War 1 not only brought home the tuberculosis problem to Canadians but also challenged in a dramatic and profound way the preconceptions they had of their country and the institutions that supported them. The care of diseased and disabled veterans would not only call into question but alter – in some cases almost unrecognizably – the diagnosis and treatment of the disease itself and, more generally, the role of volunteers and government. While 51,678 Canadian soldiers had been killed in action or died of war wounds, approximately the same number of Canadians had died at home from tuberculosis during the war period.[1]

The health of the recruits, however, took centre stage. Although only 3,825 members of the Canadian Expeditionary Force died from illness, at least three times as many men were hospitalized for sickness as for wounds, with TB rivaling venereal disease as the most severe medical problem. And both the sick and the wounded came to Canada to recuperate, straining an inexperienced Hospitals Commission, which hastily cobbled together whatever accommodation it could find. A decade and a half after the war had ended, 77,000 veterans still collected disability pensions.[2]

This problem was aggravated by the discovery that the "fittest and finest" were anything but: 35 to 40 percent of young volunteers were rejected when they first applied or were later found unfit for military service, while fully 50 percent of those drafted had some physical defect. Some passed the physical examination only to break down after enlistment – 35 percent of the tuberculous soldiers in 1917 had never been overseas. Their care, too, became a federal responsibility, at $1,200 to $1,300 a year each. England had discovered a similar state of affairs during the Boer War and had begun physical training and medical inspection of schools to correct it; now Canadians saw they would have to do the same.[3]

Proclaimed by order-in-council in June 1915, the Hospitals Commission was created to provide hospital accommodation and convalescent homes for soldiers invalided home from Europe. By October the commission was renamed the Military Hospitals and Convalescent Homes Commission (MHC), and its responsibilities had expanded to include retraining and rehabilitation, as well as care of patients who had yet to go overseas. Retraining, it was hoped, might prevent the messy "pension problem" the Americans had experienced after the Civil War.[4]

With the MHC soon overwhelmed by a physician shortage, inexperience, cramped and sometimes inappropriate hospital accommodation, and thousands of patients, dispute arose over whether the care of ill and injured soldiers should be supervised by the civilian-led commission or the military-run Canadian Army Medical Corps (CAMC). On 21 February 1918, the Department of Soldiers Civil Re-establishment (DSCR) was created, with most MHC hospitals transferred to the CAMC, while the MHC itself became the Invalided Soldiers' Commission, responsible for vocational training and the provision of artificial limbs. As the DSCR took over retraining, job-placement, and long-term or chronic care, the two organisations became largely indistinguishable.[5]

*The Military Patient*

Treatment of soldier patients differed from that of civilians. The MHC accepted full responsibility for the care of tuberculous soldiers and arranged with all principal Canadian sanatoria to receive them. Soldiers were paid while under treatment; and on discharge from a sanatorium the Board of Pension Commissioners, on the recommendations of the Advisory Committee on Tuberculosis, gave every tuberculous soldier a full disability pension for six months, after which he was examined again and his permanent disability determined.[6] As sanatoria became increasingly crowded, the commission hastily added new beds and buildings that not only stimulated local anti-TB work but became an important addition to postwar civilian accommodation.[7]

As tuberculosis workers soon discovered, soldier patients were far different from civilian patients. They had few financial worries, for they received their regular pay and allowances, but they often had a great deal of trouble adjusting to the discipline of treatment and the physical rest it entailed. Civilian doctors had no authority to discipline them. Ironically, civilians, with their personal and family obligations and financial sacrifice, had a stimulus to take the prescribed cure that the soldier lacked. The soldier found the medical routine unnecessary and tiresome, and sanatorium doctors frequently found the military patient disruptive and uncooperative. Even patients who were progressing might demand their discharge after six months and collect their pensions.[8] When soldiers rioted at the Mountain Sanatorium, the MHC appointed a military officer with authority to confiscate pay and allowances for misdemeanours.[9]

This step did not solve the underlying problem, for forcing soldiers to obey did not keep them interested in continuing treatment. (Interest was even a problem for civilian patients, because bed rest was continually extended for longer and longer periods.) In the first six months of 1916, 15 percent of the soldiers treated at Ste Agathe were discharged for drunkenness and insubordination, while 33 percent actually refused treatment and took their discharges by signing waivers. In desperation, the MHC set up a workshop, and "vocational training" began. Its primary objective was to provide the physical and mental stimulation of occupational therapy and to make "taking the cure" easier, while providing limited industrial re-education. Results were encouraging: with the vocational work in place, none refused treatment, only 0.5 percent were discharged as incorrigibles, and 7 percent actually asked to stay beyond their discharge to continue studying and training.[10]

Despite "rehabilitation," there appeared to be a growing number of unemployable tuberculous veterans: mandatory light work in sanitary, well-ventilated surroundings was difficult to find, particularly since the Canadian government, unlike the German government, for example, did not require industry to hire a certain percentage of disabled veterans, and coworkers were often fearful of associating with tuberculous convalescents. Therefore, in the mid-twenties, the Tuberculous Veterans' Association petitioned the Ralston Commission on Pensions and Re-establishment for sheltered workshops and an increase of one-third on any pension to meet additional food and shelter costs. The commission rejected the petition as "rank discrimination."[11]

*Diagnosis*

Wartime changes in tuberculosis work affected civilian patients almost as much as military patients. Both the war and the 1918 influenza epidemic stirred up nontuberculous conditions that made differential diagnosis more difficult. As a result, skill in diagnosis increased and the differences between tuberculous and nontuberculous respiratory diseases had to become more clearly defined.

While civilians often sought advice in the advanced stage of their disease, when it was all too obvious, an army recruit received a medical examination as soon as he was unable to march five miles carrying a rifle and a thirty-pound pack on his back. Incipient cases were discovered more frequently and required a more precise diagnosis – especially since 33 percent of the soldiers who were returned to Canada with suspected tuberculosis were found to be nontuberculous.[12] Their nontuberculous respiratory ailments still required treatment, however, so the scope of sanatorium care broadened.

With military patients suffering complications as a result of wounds, gas, frequent colds, excessive exposure, pneumonia, pleurisy with effusion, trench fever, dental infections, and even hysteria, in addition to tuberculosis, diagnosis was more difficult – and also more important, for the soldiers' disability pensions depended on the diagnosis. While prewar opinion had emphasized the number of tuberculosis cases diagnosed as other diseases, the war shifted the emphasis to the number of other conditions diagnosed as tuberculosis. Sputum examinations became correspondingly more important, and slight variations in chest sounds were discounted.

Partly as a result, sanatoria began to add x-ray departments and better laboratory facilities. In 1919 the DSCR, with the assistance of the research department of the University of Toronto (Connaught Laboratories) began research on pulmonary diseases.[13] "Pleurisy ten years ago," commented the superintendent of the Manitoba Sanatorium, "was Tuberculosis; pleurisy today is … pleurisy."[14]

*Sanatoria*

Independently of the war, sanatoria were undergoing profound changes. The optimistic assumption of the early years that good food and fresh air could cure the disease within months was being replaced with a more sober approach. Much, much more time was required, and tents and shacks would not serve the purpose. With the growing use of surgery and x-rays, sanatoria were slowly evolving into hospital-like institutions rather than summer camps or primitive rest homes; as a result, patients requiring the more specialized treatment began to transfer to larger, better-equipped sanatoria. Consequently, these institutions had a larger number of problem cases and a corresponding rise in their operating costs, and centralization and specialization was encouraged.

As a result of the war-time experience and new technology, medical supervision became essential, and nowhere could one receive constant medical supervision better than at a sanatorium. With the growing awareness that other aspects of a patient's health could affect recovery, sanatoria had begun, by the end of the war, to employ other specialists (gynecologists, surgeons, internists, and dentists) to correct related conditions. Treatment broadened as non-tuberculous health problems were corrected more thoroughly – as a result of repairing soldiers' teeth, sanatorium experts discovered the value of dental hygiene in aiding the cure by improving their overall health.[15] By 1920 the sanatorium had expanded its care to include not only advanced cases but nonpulmonary forms of TB and other respiratory conditions as well.

Before the war, tuberculosis workers had naively believed that all that was needed to deal successfully with tuberculous patients was unlimited financial resources and legislation, but the veterans proved this false. Individual education became essential, so that both the public and sufferers themselves understood the benefit of treatment and undertook it thoroughly and responsibly.[16] The war had accomplished for the soldiers what health reformers had urged for the whole population: hospitalization of nearly all cases. But hospitalization was almost worse than useless without proper education.

More visibly, the war affected the availability of institutional facilities. On the credit side, the federal government added beds, buildings, vocational workshops, and equipment, while on the debit side, sanatoria struggled against inflationary costs and staff shortages throughout the war period. The federal and provincial governments each gave $200,000 to build a sanatorium near Calgary, to be used later as a provincial institution for civilians, while the Saskatchewan Anti-Tuberculosis League, which had already raised $97,000 by public subscription, erected a sanatorium with both provincial and federal aid.[17] In all, the dominion government spent approximately $3 million on construction alone, with the stipulation that its contributions should be matched by the organization it assisted.[18] By 1919, largely as a result of federal government investment and its matching policy, sanatorium beds had increased from 1,840 to 3,860, with a corresponding expansion of all services, including x-ray and laboratory facilities and technicians, occupational therapists, and vocational workshops, dieticians, and medical specialists. The government also spent more than $8 million maintaining slightly more than ten thousand soldier patients. But despite this expenditure, by 1918, 96 to 98 percent of tuberculous Canadians were still treated at home.[19]

Tuberculosis workers still disputed whether a local sanatorium or a central one was more beneficial, but the pattern had already been established by the end of the war. A strong factor favouring the local sanatorium was the patients' proximity to home, so that they could stay longer and remain in touch with their friends and family, while if it was near a city it was easier for the sanatorium to obtain supplies and raise local charitable donations. On the other hand, it was easier to get competent medical staff in a larger, and thus central, institution. Ultimately, two factors determined the development of sanatoria: density of population and technical specialization. The regions with sparser populations – the West and the Maritimes – developed provincial sanatoria, while Quebec and Ontario developed local institutions. Even in the latter case, sanatoria were confined to major centres. With expensive equipment and specialized staff the cost was too prohibitive for small communities.[20]

Neither the federal government nor its deputy, the DSCR, had any wish to involve itself permanently in health care – it might erect tuberculosis facilities in an unparalleled building program, but it always arranged to hand them over to local or provincial authorities when the military had no further use for them. Ironically, the federal government thus provided equipment and facilities to strengthen provincial authority and responsibility, and helped push the provinces, by default, into organizing public health and caring for their citizens.

*Etiology and Pathogenesis: The Role of the Child*

As a result of both wartime experience and a realism engendered from over a decade spent struggling with the disease, anti-TB workers altered not only the focus of their diagnosis and treatment of the disease but also their concept of its etiology and pathogenesis. Discovery of the extent of childhood infection after the international conference in Washington in 1908 had shocked reformers, and they began to adopt the view that, although tuberculosis was not hereditary, many, if not most, adult victims were first infected as children, with lowered resistance causing them to break down with the disease years later.[21] Soldiers succumbing to what appeared to be reactivated disease supported this theory.

Along with wartime casualties, the child thus took on a new importance – "our greatest national asset" asserted the president of the Canadian Association for the Prevention of TB in 1919.[22] Although the proportion of tuberculous children under three was reputedly small, the infection in infants more often than not resulted in a fatal form of the disease. So babies had to be protected – first, isolated from the disease during the early years of life (which might mean separation from a diseased parent) and, second, fed only pasteurized milk. After the age of three, it was hypothesized, most children received small doses of infection (massive doses caused active disease), which built up immunity. During this period, when 90 percent of children were infected by the age of fifteen, it was more important to build up their resistance than to try futilely to isolate them from exposure to the disease.

With almost universal infection, experts were more concerned about the possible extension of an already existing focus of disease than new infection. Contact with a grossly careless consumptive should be avoided but, they serenely believed, there was little for an average adult to fear from ordinary contact. The physician-in-chief of the Toronto Free Hospital reflected this trend in thought when he observed in 1919: "It has been said that 'the careful consumptive is not a danger to anyone.' This might be modified to read 'the consumptive is a grave menace to infants, less dangerous to children, and no danger at all to adults if reasonable care is exercised.'"[23] As a result, anti-TB specialists began to differentiate between "primary" and "secondary" disease. The former attacked someone with no acquired resistance, while the more common secondary form resulted from an extension of a childhood infection. To prevent the secondary form, adults first had to build up their own resistance by avoiding overwork, poor housing and nutrition, dissipation, and other diseases, and they had to seek rest, sleep, good food, fresh air, and healthy living. Reinforced by the poor health uncovered in recruits, this approach gave a boost to the preventive and social reform side of anti-TB work.

### Treatment: Rest, Rest, Rest

Although the basic treatment of fresh air, rest, and nourishing food remained the same, emphasis was placed even more heavily on *rest*. The fad of forced feeding with milk and raw eggs was abandoned for a more common sense diet of regular balanced meals without extra lunches, and there was a declining emphasis on excessive weight gain as an index of the success of the cure.

It was the development of surgical techniques as a literal, anatomical application of the basic "rest" treatment that was significant now. The most popular was artificial pneumothorax. Air or gas was introduced into the pleural space between the lung and the chest wall, causing the diseased lung to collapse. Pioneered in Europe and the United States at the turn of the century, this operation became accepted treatment after 1910 in England and after 1912 in Canada; and even then only in very select patients – those possessing one lung healthy enough to take on the added work when the other was collapsed and a heart able to cope with the extra strain. Patients whose diseased lungs had adhered to the chest wall could not benefit.[24] Initially it was not considered for early cases but only when other, more traditional methods (the sanatorium regime, with or without exercise) had been tried and failed.[25]

Understandably, under these restrictions, suitable patients were hard to find. Once the lung was collapsed, refills (repeated injections of gas between the lung and the chest wall to maintain the lung collapse) were needed for up to three years before a "cure" was said to have occurred. x-rays were used to check that the lung had collapsed completely.[26] Successful collapse generally eliminated painful symptoms, reduced fever, stopped the cough and night sweats, and even decreased the amount of sputa. By 1920 this treatment was used only in 10 percent of the cases, but some experts optimistically believed it increased chances of improvement for these patients by 50 percent. Physicians began to experiment with other surgical techniques, still in their infancy, such as the removal of part of the chest wall for the purpose of collapse and operations to deal with intestinal tuberculosis.[27]

### Heliotherapy: Sunlight, the Natural Germicide

Although public health workers had known sunlight killed tubercle bacilli, heliotherapy – treatment with natural sunshine and ultraviolet (uv) light – became a popular, specific treatment only after Rollier, a Swiss, noted its effect on bone, joint, glandular, and abdominal tuberculosis in 1909. Although isolation, ventilation, and filtration would subsequently become the preeminent means of reducing environmental exposure to the bacilli and thus decreasing infection, recent studies have supported in a limited way this belief in the therapeutic properties of sunlight by demonstrating the germicidal properties of uv irradiation. It appears that uv light demonstrates greater efficiency than the more conventional methods not only in destroying tb organisms but also in reducing infection in guinea pigs exposed to ventilated air exhausted from a hospital tb ward. This, of course, does not support a claim that sunlight (or uv irradiation) can cure the disease.

Used first with children, who suffered most from the nonpulmonary forms of the disease, heliotherapy involved an almost absurdly simple treatment of gradually increasing exposure to sunlight, starting with the feet for ten minutes twice a day and working up to complete exposure for several hours (never burning). Too much exposure was believed to cause a relapse, and heliotherapy apparently had no effect at all on the most common type of tuberculosis, the pulmonary form.[28] But it, too, was seen as a useful addition to more traditional methods.

Thus, in keeping with the war-time emphasis on efficiency, organization, and specialization, Canadian physicians for the first time began to use specialized means of treating tuberculosis. Artificial pneumothorax and heliotherapy were both attempts, albeit only partially successful and with only a limited application, to deal with tuberculosis from a bacteriological perspective in a scientific and targeted fashion. This trend would intensify throughout the next few decades, with far-reaching consequences. Specialization, only just beginning, would develop among professionals. With the sanatoria forced to become more and more like hospitals to carry out this treatment, there would be an increased demand for more government support. And this, too, would be fostered by the war.

As sanatoria became entrenched as the pivotal focus of treatment, a novel method of evaluating tuberculosis services in a given locality came into existence: the number of available beds relative to the population, and later, the number of beds relative to each death. Since the lowest death rate was reputedly in the province with the most accommodation – Ontario – public health workers were tempted to view the situation in simple cause-and-effect terms: if enough beds were available, tuberculosis could be eradicated. To bolster their argument, they pointed out that Scotland had 1 bed for every 1,750 members of the population and the United States had 1 for every 2,857, while Canada made a miserable showing with only 1 for every 4,432 members of the population.[29] Even the war-time experience with recalcitrant military patients did little to shake the faith but only added the corollary that education might be necessary to enable patients to appreciate the value of sanatoria. It was an attitude that would have profound implications in postwar care.

### The Dispensary and the Clinic

Despite war-time construction, by 1919 only about 15 percent of the tuberculosis sufferers in Canada could be accommodated in sanatoria.[30] Alternatives were necessary. As a result, the clinic and visiting nurse played increasingly important, although changing, roles. The dispensary still supervised and cared for poor patients, but it was becoming more and more a consultation, diagnostic, and referral centre, not a welfare distributor – in the postwar era that role would be left to other charities and auxiliary associations. The dispensary analyzed sputa, examined and instructed patients, kept records, referred individuals for sanatorium treatment, supervised home cases with a visiting nurse, and in general became a link between the various tuberculosis agencies (sanatoria, preventoria, relief groups, and so on) and the patient. As with treatment methods, war-time experience encouraged specialization among institutions, linked together in an increasingly complex system. The clinic was evolving into a diagnostic and referral centre that coordinated sanatorium admissions, supervised home patients, and attempted to find early cases.

The clinic's new role as a diagnostic centre was promoted specifically by the war. The army referred dubious cases to the clinic specialists, for x-rays were too costly, inaccurate, and difficult to store, to be used as the sole criteria. An accurate chest examination, based on inspection, palpation, percussion, and auscultation depended largely on the experience and skill of the examiner, and the medical officers of the armed forces were not specially trained tuberculosis physicians.

### Public Health Nurses or TB Nurses?

If dispensaries were growing more medically specialized, the visiting nurses who operated out of them, ironically, were becoming less so. Early public health and visiting nurses had frequently been "tuberculosis nurses," hired as a fall-back measure because a local tuberculosis association lacked funds to build a sanatorium. Public health workers soon realized that a visiting nurse could do a more efficient and comprehensive job if she did not limit herself to one disease – so the "public health nurse" evolved. With a stigma attached to TB, patients were more receptive to a general visiting nurse, while it was easier to attract nurses if they would not be continuously exposed to a contagious disease.[31] Moreover, as the Toronto department of health soon discovered, having public health nurses instead of specialized tuberculosis and infant welfare nurses was more economical and efficient. They eliminated the duplication of work existing before the merger of the two functions in 1914, when two nurses might visit the same family; in fact, a public health nurse, paradoxically, discovered more tuberculosis cases in the process of visiting homes for other purposes.

The work of a public health nurse, according to Eunice Dyke, the Toronto superintendent of public health nurses, was to coordinate necessary medical and social facilities.[32] Just as the dispensary referred cases to different institutions, she referred individual patients to different social agencies, while caring for and educating them. Her job included running clinics, day nurseries, and civic investigations; providing tuberculosis, contagious-disease, and infant nursing; making arrangements for hospital admissions; and providing obstetrical and bedside nursing.[33] "The tuberculosis nurse," Dyke confidently predicted, "must ultimately develop into the public health nurse since the conditions which prevent tuberculosis are the conditions which maintain health. The public health nurse will remain when tuberculosis is a matter of history."[34]

The development of a public health nurse instead of a tuberculosis nurse also resulted from beginning government involvement in health care. A volunteer society concerned with one particular disease, such as tuberculosis, or one particular problem, such as infant welfare, would hire a nurse to deal specifically with that issue. As municipal, and later provincial, departments of health took over, they centralized operations. This pattern is most clearly evident in Toronto, which had over ninety public health nurses by 1917.[35]

Charles Hastings, a Presbyterian social activist, obstetrician, and founding member of the Canadian Public Health Association, had been appointed to head the Toronto health department in 1910. Based on principles of efficiency and scientific management, popularized in the prewar era and reinforced by the war, he transformed the department into a modern bureaucracy with an expanded staff organized into fifteen separate divisions. A diploma in public health was a prerequisite for employment for all medical officers after 1912. The social reformer was losing ground to the professional administrator, an expert who would run the department – and, by extension, public health – with minimal "interference" from politicians, uninformed laymen, or physicians.[36]

In 1916 Manitoba became the first province to employ public health nurses (with a third of their salary paid by the municipality), but others soon followed: British Columbia in 1917, Alberta in 1918, and Saskatchewan in 1919. With its sparse population, isolated settlements, and lack of medical facilities, the West, in particular, needed nurses organized on a provincial basis. By 1918, Manitoba had 25 district nurses – hardly an overwhelming number compared to 90 for the city of Toronto alone; but the whole country had only 423.[37] The number was increasing – visiting nurses were relatively cheap, versatile, and mobile – and thus essential when health facilities were at a premium.

## The War: Changing Concept of the Disease

Just as the war altered the institutional framework and concrete manner in which tuberculosis was diagnosed and treated, it also changed the philosophical attitudes underpinning the concept of the disease. Cherished tenets of social reform thought – the idealization of rural life, prohibition, eugenics and the dangers of foreign immigrants, the respective roles of the volunteers and the state – were explored and, in the light of wartime experience, either reinforced or rejected. More than the easily visible changes in sanatorium accommodation or the use of surgical techniques, this shift in focus would determine significant developments in the interwar campaign.

Urban social reformers' idealization of country life was beginning to wear thin even by 1914. If urban conditions were slowly improving, rural communities were virtually unaffected by any work done during the first ten years of the campaign. In 1913 it was reported that the incidence of tuberculosis may have been higher in the country than in the city, contradicting the notion that rural life offered salvation to the consumptive.[38] As public health departments were slowly established in Canadian cities – notably Toronto – and sanitation improved, rural communities often lacked the most rudimentary facilities: hospitals, nurses, a full-time medical health officer, and sanitary homes and schools. By the end of World War 1 the disillusionment with country life was almost complete.

The soldiers confirmed civilian experience – despite initial MHC and DSCR enthusiasm for agriculture and land settlement, it was clear that farming was hard work. In Ontario, although the government paid a third of the cost of sanatorium maintenance, rural patients rarely took advantage of it, for the municipality or township, always trying to save funds, only grudgingly paid the remainder, forcing patients to prove themselves indigent first – a humiliating experience. As a result, rural patients usually never went to a sanatorium until their disease had reached a hopeless stage. By the end of the war, anti-TB workers were reporting that the rural school child was actually 5 to 20 percent *unhealthier* than the urban one.[39]

### Immigration and Eugenics

Displaced veterans, resentful of the new "alien" workers, fueled the anti-immigrant feeling underlying much of the eugenics movement. Canada was still a "dumping ground": of seventy-six patients at the Mountain Sanatorium in 1914, only twenty-six were Canadian-born.[40] "We have imported at great expense," stated J.B. Black at the annual meeting of the Canadian Medical Association in 1917, "people from every misgoverned country in Europe – many of them unfit for Canadian citizenship, in order to swell our population, and at the same time we have left our own to die for want of intelligent care and protection."[41] "The men who have gone to the front," observed the Nova Scotia provincial health officer, "are those who, in theory at least, were best fitted to father a vigorous and virile generation – a generation which might flourish despite unfavorable conditions of environment. The loss by death and disablement must almost inevitably have an effect upon the birth-rate, and upon the stock quality of the next generation. The labours of world reconstruction must then devolve upon a depleted population, handicapped by a weak progenitorship."[42]

The increased importance of the child, the ravages of TB and venereal disease, and the underlying eugenics movement all blended together in a new Social Hygiene Movement in the immediate postwar period. Apparently first introduced by Havelock Ellis in 1912, it was largely an offshoot of the campaign against VD – theoretically, however, social hygiene was broader than any of its components: it was the "science of right living," intended "to create a finer, happier, nobler race." As interest in venereal diseases fell, interest in social hygiene as a general concept waned in the late twenties, and the organization finally changed its name to The Health League of Canada in 1935.[43] Its significance was that it, unlike social reform causes, focused on a more narrow definition of public health – an attitude that would play a key part in the anti-TB campaign, in particular, in the postwar period.

*The Limits of Education*

As we have seen, bitter experience with frustrating military patients had demonstrated both the essential nature and limitations of education. Tuberculous soldiers had proven that sanatorium care and freedom from financial worries alone were no guarantee of cooperation or an effective cure – a patient, and thus the community, had to be educated to see the value of the cure. On the other hand, all attempts at controlling venereal disease in the same patient population had confronted the intransigence of human nature in risking dangerous or unhealthy practices in spite of instruction. Moreover, from a pragmatic economic perspective, the public had to be educated to demand not only legislation but also financial support for facilities from various levels of government.

Anti-TB workers saw themselves as leaders and molders of public opinion. But it was very frustrating – as J.A. Jarry observed, even the 1910 Quebec Royal Commission on tuberculosis had recognized that "the anti-tuberculosis campaign relies on these three things: education, legislation, money." And it was a perennial cry that there was never enough money – for "with it we can educate both the people and the ruling classes, and then we shall easily obtain legislation."[44]

Money would also have a more practical use: building treatment facilities. For what good was finding cases, sanatorium advocates demanded, if they could not be treated? Yet the public seemed indifferent. "I would guarantee," stated C.H. Vrooman, medical superintendent of the Tranquille Sanatorium in exasperation, "if you were to announce in any city in Canada that there was a dozen cases of leprosy requiring segregation, accommodation would be provided in 24 hours; yet we all know that many advanced cases of tuberculosis are more infectious than the ordinary case of leprosy. Our business, then, is to sufficiently arouse the public conscience, and show the public the need."[45]

So education was to make the public understand and follow the cure, and then force governments to legislate and build facilities. Anti-TB workers discovered in dismay, however, that before the general public could be educated, they had to enlighten the professionals. Most general practitioners, specialists maintained sourly, were not taught to diagnose tuberculosis accurately, and many failed to recognize it even in its advanced stages. Based on the results of a questionnaire sent to sanatorium workers in Canada in 1914, A.F. Miller, the medical superintendent of the Nova Scotia Sanatorium, reported in disgust, "In the opinion of Canadian sanatorium physicians ... the Canadian practitioner is diagnosing the commonest disease in Canada in a manner that, were it any other disease, would stamp him as careless and inefficient."[46] Miller placed 40 percent of the blame for late diagnosis and late or incorrect treatment on the physician, but C.H. Vrooman of the Tranquille Sanatorium was harsher in his criticism. He estimated that fully 50 percent of the advanced cases he saw had reached that stage only because some general practitioner had either failed to make a correct diagnosis or had given improper advice, and he attributed this problem to a careless examination – the doctor did not take the trouble to expose the patient's chest, give a complete physical examination, and check the patient's sputum. Or, suspecting tuberculosis, he mistakenly deceived and sought to reassure the patient. Another critic blamed the medical men for not taking advantage of the provincial board of health laboratories.[47] Whatever the validity of the accusations, the survey itself and the physicians' responses clearly demonstrated the "town vs. gown" split that existed between specialists and public health advocates and the general medical profession.

Miller himself was more charitable, although no less elitist. He blamed poor medical education – because only one Canadian medical college required its students to spend time in a provincial sanatorium and hospital clinics were usually attended solely by patients who were far advanced, doctors rarely had an opportunity to familiarize themselves with the incipient form of the disease. The solution was obvious: tuberculosis should be studied in medical school, students should be forced to do a residency at a sanatorium, and practising doctors should visit clinics to improve their diagnostic and treatment techniques.

By the end of the war, Manitoba medical students did a stint of one week to six months at the provincial sanatorium, the Bruchesi Institute offered "perfecting courses" on tuberculosis for practising doctors, and a school of "phthisiotherapy" was opened at Laval University.[48] Shortly after the war some postgraduate public health nursing courses were offered at several universities, beginning with Dalhousie.

The methods of public education, however, had changed little from the previous decade and still depended on local initiative. But if the methods of educating were the same, the focus was shifting. Anti-TB workers began to attack personal apathy and ignorance, rather than poor environments and social conditions, as a cause of the disease. They now had a less idealized view of human nature, since they had seen federally supported soldiers still refuse treatment during the war, and they had come to realize that the lack of awareness that led the upper and middle classes to live unhealthily extended to the working class as well. "There are numerous factors which go to make up the large death rate of our slums," Charles Hastings stated in 1917, "of which ignorance is the most important."[49] Ten years earlier he would have faulted poor housing, low wages, and overcrowding. As George Porter, executive secretary of the Canadian Association for the Prevention of Tuberculosis bluntly put it, "We should have decent living wages and education as well."[50]

As with treatment, anti-TB workers recognized that legislation alone was of little use without public support – and therefore without education. Although Ontario law had made notification compulsory since 1912, only 40 percent of the tuberculosis cases resulting in death in 1913 had been reported to the authorities prior to death.[51] It was, again, another example of the differing attitudes of public health advocates and the average physician. Various solutions were suggested, from paying doctors for every case they reported to establishing provincial and municipal sanatoria and open-air schools to make the principle logical and practical. Wartime conditions in France brought home the point: tuberculosis ravaged that country, where it had never been a reportable disease. In fact, tuberculosis increased in all armies except the English army, which had had some public health and anti-TB work before 1914.[52] The lesson to be learned from that, public health advocates felt, was obvious.

*The Role of Volunteers*

Wartime experience in mobilizing and caring for the Canadian Expeditionary Force had shown firsthand the limits of voluntarism and the benefits of an efficient, professionally run enterprise. In the early years of the war, invalided soldiers had convalesced at the homes of wealthy Canadians, thrown open in a patriotic fervour. But unfortunately, results were lacklustre – kitchens and plumbing and heating systems needed improvement, and the wives and daughters, provided with courses from the St John's Ambulance voluntary aid committees, were ill-prepared for the drudgery of actual nursing. The MHC found it more efficient to borrow the naval hospital Esquimalt or the immigration hospital at Quebec, which was already adequately staffed and equipped. Moreover, as Morton and Wright observe, soldiers overseas had "developed little love for such private agencies as the Red Cross or the YMCA," and their wives had resented the Canadian Patriotic Fund's "affluent 'lady volunteers.'" Veterans resisted transferring what they perceived to be government responsibilities to charities. And – as disabled veterans demands for employment opportunities brought into glaring relief – what if voluntarism failed?[53] In a parallel development, with the extension and separation of municipal health departments, tentative government involvement was now occurring in public health. Reformers began to question, albeit in a limited way, the role of volunteer associations.

Some believed that a volunteer association was a trail-blazer and educator – a concept that would be more fully developed in the following decades. All agreed that it motivated the public to demand reforms from government, but there was a great deal of controversy over whether government or the association should take control and organize health. Who, in other words, should be an adjunct to whom? This question was especially crucial in the case of tuberculosis, which required both an extensive system of health care and a great deal of money to cope with the disease. The *Canadian Medical Association Journal* succinctly stated what appeared to be the prevailing opinion even in 1912: "Voluntary organizations are highly desirable for maintaining public interest in furthering education on the subject, but in those communities where most enthusiasm has already been shown in the fight, it is recognized that the control of tuberculosis is a task far beyond the resources of private philanthropy."[54]

Matters came to a head in 1912 when the Toronto league, deciding that anti-TB work could now be done by the city's comprehensive health department, gave up its charter.[55] Major Lorne Drum of Ottawa probably summed up majority opinion among the anti-TB workers when he observed, "Miss Dyke [Toronto superintendent of public health nurses] has said that the work of the official class is most important, but at the same time, it needs the aid of the voluntary class. In fact, it needs the aid of the voluntary class so much, that it could not do the work, unless it had these voluntary helpers."[56]

This attitude was encouraged, and yet limited, by the war. The MHC relied on voluntarily run dispensaries to examine soldiers for tuberculosis, used existing sanatoria for military patients, and had local dispensaries follow up soldiers discharged from sanatoria.[57] This cooperation extended to civilians as well. In Toronto the department of health worked closely with the IODE preventorium and the National Sanitarium Association, while in Hamilton, the Hamilton health association's Mountain Sanatorium provided the medical staff for a clinic, while the health department supplied the building and nursing services. Yet in all cases, professionals increasingly supervised the work and took charge. It was yet another expression of the philosophy of efficiency and scientific management that war work had emphasized.

Voluntary anti-TB agencies continued to do relief work, but here again there was a growth in specialization. Relief was delegated more often to women's auxiliaries or ladies' committees (as in Montreal and London) or to special groups established in conjunction with an anti-TB society solely for that purpose: groups such as the Samaritan Club, connected with the National Sanitarium Association in Toronto (1912). The belief was slowly growing that, although tuberculosis developed out of social conditions that had to be altered, volunteer tuberculosis groups should concern themselves with *tuberculosis* and leave welfare work to other charitable organizations or associated groups.

## The Role of Government

With the MHC and the DSCR setting an example with their comprehensive care of tuberculous soldiers, it did not take long for many Canadians to feel that, as the *Hamilton Times* wrote in an editorial, "with this effective organization of treatment for military consumptives before our eyes, it will be absolutely inexcusable if the country fails to organize an equally efficient campaign against the 'white plague' among our people as a whole."[58]

The Canadian Association for the Prevention of Tuberculosis (CAPT) moved a resolution in 1917 that the Department of Militia and Defence should extend its activities to training and protecting Canadian youth against tuberculosis (to ensure a healthy fighting force); the Calgary Anti-Tuberculosis Society, supported by the United Farmers of Alberta, United Farm Women, local councils of women, women's institutes, the WCTU, the Rural Municipalities Association and the Trades and Labour Council, demanded free treatment for all consumptives;[59] and the odd public health worker even suggested that a federal department of health could combine the after-care of discharged soldiers with care of "discharged" civilians. After all, as David

Stewart, the superintendent of the Manitoba Sanatorium, reasoned with impeccable logic, "If the wounded or tuberculous soldier be cared for until he is well, or helped indefinitely if he should not return to complete health, it is not difficult to argue that the soldier of commerce, of industry, or of agriculture, when disabled, should be cared for in the same way. If the man who fights abroad is to be provided for in illness, why not the woman whose work and child-bearing have broken her down at home; and why not the child, the worker, or if a stern need should arise, the fighter of the future?"[60]

Why not, indeed? This concept of state duty – this change in expectation – was probably the most important result of the war, more important than the more easily visible changes in diagnosis or treatment or the expansion of institutional facilities. The care of tuberculous and wounded soldiers had proved that the government could not only afford a public health program, but also run it efficiently if it so desired – there was no longer an excuse. Again, the veterans were instrumental in this profound change in attitude. Having risked their lives for their country, they resented and resisted the notion that their care and pensions should be extended to them as charity – instead, they demanded their benefits as a right.[61]

"A new responsibility has arisen," the Mount Sinai Sanatorium observed in its annual report: "What was an ennobling act of charity has become an unqualified necessity to the country. Conservation of life is the compelling force. The accelerated death rate has placed a premium on the living."[62]

Public health was no longer an activity that governments could dabble in at their own pleasure but a patriotic duty and a state responsibility. Echoing the veterans, what public health workers had requested in the prewar period, they now demanded as a justifiable debt owed Canadian citizens. "Every nation," Charles Hastings commented in the initially heady period of reconstruction, "has been expecting every man to do his duty, and now that the war is over, every man will expect every nation to do its duty. He will expect a democracy that will make possible the development of a sound mind in a sound body, both for himself and his offspring, and will make for him a clean pathway for merit, whatever it may be, and in which he will know that he has a chance to climb to the highest position. To this end a new democracy must rise."[63]

By 1920 not only the anti-TB campaign but public health work in general had been profoundly altered. No longer was the idealistic, amateur urban reformer in the vanguard – the professional had taken over and would now lead the crusade. Diagnostic and treatment techniques were becoming more specific, while institutional facilities had come a long way from the early shacks and tents – they included specialists and expensive equipment, more often than not provided at least partly by government. A system had been established whereby each institution (hospitals, dispensaries, and sanatoria) had clearly defined duties, instead of being a Jack-of-all-trades. With close to two decades of work behind them, in addition to surviving a war and a flu epidemic, anti-TB workers had, as mentioned, lost much of their naive idealism – but not their enthusiasm for or commitment to the cause. In fact, public health took on a new meaning. Anti-TB workers were no longer solely urban reformers – as we have seen, the war had demonstrated that soldiers from rural areas broke down as often as urban dwellers, while in some cases rural children were discovered to be actually less healthy than their urban counterparts.

The war demonstrated in a way that could not be ignored the appallingly poor health of Canadians, especially those reputed to be the fittest and, combined with the 1918 influenza epidemic, it placed a premium on human life. Governments were finally beginning to see the economic value of healthy citizens, while the federal government, by erecting a health care system for soldiers, established a precedent and demonstrated publicly to all that the state, if it so desired, could do the same for civilians.

The war had been fought to "make the world safe for democracy"; it was probably only natural, therefore, that public health workers in the postwar reconstruction period would demand a state-established health care system for all citizens. Canadians had sacrificed much in the war – if it was not to have been for nought, reformers believed, all levels of government now owed them a chance for a decent life – which included adequate health care. To be "well born" and healthy should no longer be for the privileged few, but the right of every citizen – especially the child. For in the child lay not only the potential for the eradication of tuberculosis but also the ultimate prosperity of the country.

# 3 The Interwar Years: A Medical Disease with a Social Aspect

I'm resting twenty hours a day.
I eat my meals and hit the hay
Till I get sick, when doctors say –
    It's Rest Hour.

And often times I think, with dread
That maybe someone, when I'm dead,
Will place these words above my head –
    It's Rest Hour
           Edna Grant, Queen Alexandra Sanatorium,
                    London, Ontario, 1932[1]

Aware of the shocking percentage of unfit military recruits, it was unsurprising in the initial, heady postwar period that many Canadians should enthusiastically adopt public health as "the true conception of reconstruction," and the "great duty of our generation"[2] – for, as one advocate predicted, "Following in the train of the war has come and is coming a social awakening, or, if you like, a social revolution, the basic idea of which is that if a democracy is to expand along sane lines it will be necessary for it to enact laws that will provide against this terrible waste."[3] If the world had been saved for democracy, each citizen had to be given an equal opportunity to achieve his or her full potential – and that meant a birthright of good health.

The federal government had involved itself deeply in the anti-TB campaign during the war, erecting sanatorium buildings, instituting vocational therapy and financial support for soldiers, and thus providing not only an example of state care but even an argument in favour of nationalizing medical services. With the close cooperation between the DSCR and Canadian sanatoria, as Howard Holbrook, medical superintendent of the Mountain sanatorium, noted, "it was only natural that the pioneer field in civilian Health Service would be that of tuberculosis."4 The benefits that accrued from adequate diagnosis and treatment seemed so evident that public opinion encouraged the provinces, which by 1925 had been forced to accept responsibility for the DSCR tuberculosis facilities, to involve themselves actively in the anti-TB campaign, and in public health generally.

By 1920, the anti-TB campaign appeared to be showing some results: the number of deaths, the executive secretary of the national association reported with satisfaction, was roughly equal to the number in 1901 (9,709), while the population had increased from about 5.4 million more than 8 million.5 The influenza epidemic, while aiding in lowering the tuberculosis death rate (many sufferers had died during the epidemic) revealed the inefficiency of many health departments, especially in the rural areas, which had been largely ignored during the prewar urban reform era. Osler had once said that to prevent disease, one needed "education, organization and cooperation."6 Together with specialization, these three key themes, an outgrowth of the war, became the watchwords of the postwar era.

The twenties and thirties in Canada were as disruptive and unsettling as the first two decades of the century had been. The percentage of urban population increased from 47.4 to 55.7 from 1921 to 1941, while a boom in the primary resource industries of pulp and paper, mining, and hydroelectric power changed the economic base of the country.7 While the urban frontier expanded to serve the new resource industries, and the suburbs of the large cities expanded, many small business, particularly those in smaller or outlying settlements, helplessly saw their markets eroded by the growth of department stores, such as Eaton's or Simpson's, with their aggressive mail order houses, and the competition from larger towns and cities now accessible with the improved road system. Civic boosterism failed to prevent more and more Canadians from going further afield to buy clothes and food, and gawk at the new consumer goods spinning off from the new technology: radios, refrigerators, electric ranges, washing machines.8

Partly as a result of the rise in importance of the new resources developed in tandem by the provincial governments and industry, the increased tax revenue the provinces received from gasoline and liquor, the limitation of federal regulations by the Judicial Committee of the Privy Council, and the more prominent role the provinces were forced to take in providing relief and social services after the federal government largely abdicated responsibility during the Depression, there was a profound change in balance of power between the federal and provincial governments, culminating in the Royal Commission on

Dominion-Provincial Relations. A new decentralized federalism developed in which, it seemed, provincial opinion and action was equal, not subordinate, to federal opinion and action. The number of managerial and administrative bureaucrats may have been growing in Ottawa, but it would not be until after the World War 2 that their attitudes would mold public policy in the creation of a welfare state.

### The Ascendancy of Science, Technology, and "Scientific Management"

Perhaps as important as the technological, political, and economic changes were the underlying philosophical influences. The interwar period would witness the preeminence and pervasive effects of *science*: not only literally, in the new resource industries such as hydroelectricity and consumer goods like the automobile and radio, but figuratively, with an emphasis in both business and society in general of the principles of "scientific management" – efficiency, organization, and administration.

Rooted in the prewar period as an optimistic application of engineering principles to solve society's problems, those values had been confirmed and promoted by wartime experience. Moreover, as Ramsay Cook has convincingly argued, efforts of late nineteenth- and early twentieth-century reformers to "regenerate" religion by linking it to social reform ideology ironically and inevitably culminated in a more marginal role for the established churches and increased secularization in Canadian society.[9] A vacuum was created – and in the interwar years, this vacuum would be filled by science.

All these changes, concrete and philosophical, would not only influence but be reflected in the anti-TB campaign. If medicine was both an art and a science, so was the anti-TB movement – and its very flexibility together with its indubitable technological and scientific links, allowed it not only to change but paradoxically to strengthen when the more rigid, moralistic social reforms foundered with the social gospel.

The most obvious and immediate consequence was a revision of Osler's dictum that TB was "a social disease with a medical aspect." David Stewart, superintendent of the Manitoba Sanatorium, went so far as to reverse the old social reform doctrine of "poverty breeds tuberculosis" – instead, "It is one of the greatest of all makers of poverty," he stated flatly in 1930, "and nothing is so wasteful as to treat poverty merely as poverty, to treat its symptoms rather than its causes. When a focus of tuberculosis is healed a focus of poverty is cleared up, and in the best way, by removing causes."[10] Prewar social reformers had tried to eradicate tuberculosis – a symptom of poverty – by improving living conditions in order to create healthy citizens. Anti-TB workers in the twenties and thirties attempted to prevent poverty – a symptom or result of tuberculosis – by making sure all Canadians were healthy enough to live and work. The prevention and cure of the disease using medically and bacteriologically oriented means (surgery, rest, heliotherapy, travelling clinics, and isolation of infectious cases) would ultimately lead to a more prosperous citizenry. Perhaps they were not abandoning old social reform ideals so much as shifting the emphasis – especially since some of the more pressing prewar demands had been satisfied.

## A Bacterial Disease and a Community Problem

Treatment of tuberculosis during the depression demonstrated with startling clarity how far anti-TB workers had come from prewar social reformer "cures" of better housing, sanitation, and a living wage. Many had been involved in the prewar campaign and were aware of the obvious connection between tuberculosis and poverty – but, as R.G. Ferguson, medical director of the Saskatchewan Anti-Tuberculosis League, pointed out bluntly, "this living standard method of combating tuberculosis has its limitations; it does not prevent infection."[11] It simply gave added protection to the more naturally resistant members of the community and prevented small infections from developing into disease. It was no help to the unresistant, or constantly exposed patient. Anti-TB workers left relief to local groups, social clubs, and relief organizations, and concentrated their energies on reducing infection. Most would have agreed with the straightforward logic of the medical superintendent of the Essex County Sanatorium in Ontario, who stated in 1934: "Tuberculosis comes from tuberculosis and not from coughs or colds or draughts or malnutrition or overcrowding, but from tubercle bacilli roaming round in the fields of lowered resistance. But the colds and malnutrition and overcrowding fertilize the soil where the bacillus loves to grow. Eliminate the bacillus and he cannot run amuck. Raise resistance and he finds the battle longer, harder, more expensive and the public pays. We must bottle up bacilli, kill them when we find them and put them out of business. That is our task."[12]

This focus on the role that bacteriological infection played in the development of the disease was symptomatic of the replacement of a social reform approach with a scientifically inspired ethos generally in Canadian society. Encouraging this development was another change in attitude that had grown out of wartime experience: the importance of the community rather than the individual, or the right of *public* health over *private* health. As David Stewart reflected in 1930, "Twenty years ago or more the first question was, *what* made this man tuberculous – dingy house, foul factory, late hours, dust, drink, bad environment generally? Now the first questions are likely to be: *who* made this man tuberculous? Where has he already scattered his disease? What circle of contacts is he infecting? Then we thought first and foremost of the diseased person, but now usually first and most of the infected community ... Cure for the sick man – compassion first – may make the stronger appeal, but cure for the infected community – safety first – pays the bigger dividends."[13] This was not as callous as it first appeared, for "the cure of the sick man is an essential part of the cure of the infected community." Nevertheless, if the two should clash, "the interest of the community is paramount."[14]

## Changing Conceptions of the Disease

Predictably, with such fundamental changes in Canadian society, the views of the nature of tuberculosis and the cause of infection, almost always in a state of flux, were modified yet again. Again influenced by wartime experience, the dogma that the disease was always a reactivation of childhood infection was altered to admit the possibility of new adult infection. The classification of the disease changed; with fewer children infected, authorities began to refer to the childhood type, or first infection, and the adult type, or re-infection, instead of childhood or adult tuberculosis, recognizing that many individuals now were first exposed to the disease only as young adults.[15] With open or infectious cases now considered a grave menace to both children and adults, the importance of isolation increased. Reflecting this new approach, J.H. Elliott estimated that while most individuals with pulmonary tuberculosis were first infected under 15 years of age, up to half of them had been further infected from another source as adults, and it was this second infection that determined the onset of disease.[16]

There was great dispute over what this new phenomenon meant: was a first infection desirable because of the limited immunity it produced (thus forcing the disease to follow a more chronic course), undesirable because it rendered the tissues sensitive (so that the individual would more easily fall prey to the disease when reinfected from an outside source), or simply the beginning of a progressive disease that was not influenced by exogenous reinfection?

As tuberculin-negative nurses and hospital employees fell ill, it was becoming increasingly apparent that the third option, once held so strongly by tuberculosis specialists, that all tuberculosis resulted from a breakdown from a previous childhood infection, was simply untrue. What became crucial was the importance specialists attributed to either of the first two theories, for this would determine the direction of the anti-TB campaign. Ultimately, the general conclusion was a compromise: an uninfected environment was optimum, but toward the end of the thirties the use of bacillus Calmette-Guérin (BCG), a controversial and only partially effective vaccine (discussed in more detail later in this chapter), was extended to particularly susceptible or exposed individuals. Uninfection, not increased resistance, became the goal. Practically, it was much easier to diagnose a person infected with tuberculosis in a community of tuberculin-negative individuals than to spot the same person under the old conditions of universal infection. And it was indisputable that someone who never became infected could never become sick. Work began to identify and supervise every positive case, theoretically eliminating all possible exposure.

Statistics seemed to support such efforts. The medical director of Saskatchewan's Fort Qu'Appelle Sanatorium and the president of the Canadian Tuberculosis Association (CTA), R.G. Ferguson, pointed out in 1936 that the rate of infection was dropping faster than the death rate, especially in those provinces able to isolate patients for treatment (that is, in sanatoria) during the previous fifteen years.[17]

The consequences were a mixed blessing. Specialists noted with dismay that uninfected children and young adults lacked even minimal resistance to the disease – and tuberculosis was still the leading cause of death of those between 15 and 45.[18] "A cynic might ask," commented the superintendent of the Manitoba Sanatorium in 1932, "if we are not doing more harm than good by clearing up so many foci of infection that young people can grow up thus uninfected and unprepared."[19] As a result, he added, halfway between the elimination of the disease and the partial resistance of universal infection, "any stray outside infection is a spark in dry grass, not a spark in the rather sodden grass of half or even a quarter of a century ago."[20] If individuals could not be "fire-proofed" with an effective vaccine, then it became the duty of tuberculosis workers to remove all centres of infection in all communities – and isolation would become a central plank of the anti-TB platform in the thirties.

In the past, tuberculosis workers had been inclined to accept complacently turn-of-the-century American expert E.L. Trudeau's dictum that there was less chance of an individual becoming infected in a well-run sanatorium than in day-to-day life. Although possibly true in Trudeau's era, when the disease was all-pervasive, North America had changed. With more and more young people uninfected, and thus unprotected, the danger of disease, or at least infection, was very real when they came in contact with patients in sanatoria or, even worse, general hospitals. Undiagnosed tuberculous patients admitted for other conditions unwittingly infected those they came in contact with – particularly vulnerable young nurses. The "antiseptic baby" had apparently grown up without acquiring any resistance to TB. A Saskatchewan study from 1930 to 1933 found, to the tuberculosis specialists' horror, that the number of nurses in training in general hospitals breaking down with tuberculosis was twelve times greater than the general population, and eight times greater than the number of normal school students (a group comparable in age and sex).[21] A New Brunswick study confirmed this finding. With more nurses breaking down in general hospitals than sanatoria, specialists were forced to believe that the source was undiagnosed disease.[22] In contrast to the experience of soldiers presumably reactivating their disease in the harsh environment of the World War 1 trenches, nurses in the interwar period gave almost irrefutable proof of the danger of *exogenous* infection. Evidence was accumulating that the tuberculin-positive reactors showing no visible infection when x-rayed were likely to fare better in a hospital setting than their negative counterparts. Since tuberculosis specialists had ensured that they were negative by shielding them from childhood infection, they could not now abandon them as young adults. If all nursing applicants were rejected who demonstrated a negative tuberculin reaction, it would mean rejecting 80 percent of the applicants in the Prairie Provinces and Ontario.[23] To remedy the situation, most agreed, required even more thorough identification and segregation of TB sufferers: x-ray examinations of all sanatoria and hospital staff and patients, a yearly check-up for the staff, and better instruction in how to avoid infection – as well as an improved standard of living for student nurses.

### Defining the Problem

To attack tuberculosis rationally and effectively as a bacteriological infection, the extent of the disease had to be determined. This required organization – first to locate cases (and thus, for the first time, establish some reliable statistics on the true extent of the problem) and then, as the problem with the nurses highlighted, to go one step further and attempt to limit exposure.

Only mortality rates were of any value, because doctors still failed to report cases. Even in Toronto, with its comprehensive health department, only 32 percent of those who died from tuberculosis in 1922 had previously been reported to the city as cases or suspects.[24] The prevalence of the disease could only be estimated from mortality rates and may have been from five to ten times greater than the mortality rates – no one was really sure. In fact, mortality rates themselves were debatable in the twenties, achieving consistency only in the decade before World War 2. Quebec changed its method of collecting and recording vital statistics when it cooperated with the Federal Bureau of Statistics in 1926, and aboriginal deaths were incorporated haphazardly into the general death rates throughout the decade, sometimes masking improvement.

With case-reporting unsatisfactory and morbidity data practically unavailable, and with local institutions failing to collect or organize information in a uniform manner, comparisons between ethnic or occupational groups or geographical regions were impossible. To run an efficient campaign, statistics on racial origin, occupation, the number of bacillary cases that were positive on admission and discharge, nonpulmonary tuberculosis, the extent of collapse therapy, the number of patients leaving sanatoria against advice, and the number of clinics were all crucial.[25] These statistics were again in keeping with an interwar emphasis on the increasingly important role of organization and the scientific management of business practices. In fact, although the correlation between poverty and tuberculosis had been asserted for decades, there was still no Canadian data adequate to prove it.[26] As a beginning, the CTA, with the help of the Dominion Bureau of Statistics, was attempting to get all institutions to use standard admission and discharge cards.[27]

With the rate of infection falling, it was becoming more difficult, without universal testing, to locate all sources of infection. "The days of the shotgun method of attack have passed," stated the secretary of the CTA in 1937, "and today we must substitute the rifle and carefully choose our targets."[28] Concerned not with universal infection but with "islands within" Canadian society, specialists focused their efforts on specific groups and geographic areas.[29] This focus too was a natural outgrowth of a trend dating from the early days of the campaign. In the prewar era, urban social reformers had concentrated on cleaning up slums as a focus of infection; as public health improved, anti-TB workers in the twenties naturally began to shift their gaze to the previously overlooked rural areas. In the thirties attention would shift again to specific occupational or racial groups that were particularly prone to infection – contacts, teachers, students, industrial workers (for example, miners), psychiatric patients, nurses, and aboriginals.

*Surveying the Population*

To gather reliable data on morbidity in order to gauge the extent of the problem, anti-TB workers realized they would have to examine supposedly healthy individuals. But to survey the whole country was as yet too imposing a task for their limited funds and technological expertise. With the value of child to Canadian society "proven" by the war, it was logical to turn first to the children they had examined so successfully en masse in the prewar period with school medical inspection.

A survey in Saskatchewan pioneered this strategy, with the Saskatchewan Anti-tuberculosis Commission's 1921 report to the government shocking not only provincial residents but experts across the country. Over 1,700 school children had been examined, their homes inspected, and the cows supplying their milk tuberculin tested. All indigent families receiving mothers' pensions were investigated. Aboriginal children were checked, hospitals and public health nursing services investigated, former sanatorium patients followed up, causes of delay of sanatorium treatment enumerated, and provincial statistics of tuberculosis deaths tabulated according to place of occurrence, age, nationality, and occupation.[30]

On the supposedly healthy prairies, 44 percent of the children were infected by the age of 6, 60 percent by 14, and 76 percent by 18. For aboriginal children the percentage was double this amount. On the Prairies, 0.84 percent of the children tested had active disease, while 18.3 percent of the cattle tested reacted positively to tuberculin in areas where raw milk was consumed – and milk infection, the commission reported, probably caused 25 percent of the cases of childhood tuberculosis. Thirteen percent of the mothers receiving aid under the Mothers' Pension Act were widows because of the disease. And there were not enough facilities to treat the sufferers – on 15 November 1921 the commission determined that 1,625 patients were receiving treatment at home, while of those patients who had actually gone to the sanatorium in the previous four years, 57.5 percent had left the institution for economic or other reasons before their disease had been arrested. Although former soldiers were followed up after discharge, there was no aftercare for civilians. Consequently, whatever improvement had been gained in the institution was often lost. Over 75 percent of the people who applied for treatment were unable to pay the cost themselves, and the vast majority refused to apply to the municipality for assistance until they were entirely incapacitated, not only lengthening the time and cost of treatment but too often condemning themselves to death.[31]

Like the recommendations of the 1910 Quebec commission before it, this commission's recommendations were comprehensive, flavoured with both old social reform concerns and the new, organized bacteriological focus. The commission advised constructing two more sanatoria, to be built in 1923 and 1924 near the centres of population;

providing for the care of children from homes with open cases of tuberculosis; improving the financing of treatment to reduce delay; improving and extending diagnostic facilities; extending the nursing service and providing follow-up work for all patients; testing all cows supplying milk to children and establishing accredited herd areas to encourage individual accredited herds; providing open-air rooms in graded schools; pressuring the federal government to make a complete survey of the aboriginal population; affiliating nurses' training schools with the sanatorium; and providing a travelling chest diagnostician to help physicians in outlying districts.[32]

The commission's recommendations provided a psychological jolt. Dramatic statistics of the past, usually based on vague estimations and tenuous data, were replaced with facts that confronted the province with a clearly defined situation for the first time. And defining the problem inevitably led not only to increased public awareness but to increased demands for more solutions. Somewhat less thoroughly, other provinces soon followed the Saskatchewan example.

As the Saskatchewan commission had pointed out, cases were still arriving at the sanatoria in far too advanced a stage – for the benefit of both individual and state, they had to be located earlier, before they had infected others and while they could still be "cured" at a minimum cost. Active cases had to be located, segregated, and treated – but the key in this era of community concern was to *prevent* the spread of infection to others. As one physician observed, "Perhaps more than any other disease, tuberculosis has forced humanity to look upon disease of all kinds, certainly all communicable diseases, from the national rather than from the individual aspect. Probably no other disease has so impressed man with the inadequacy of any attempt to control its direct manifestations and results, where no attempt had been made to guard others exposed to, but, as yet, not known to be possessed of the disease."[33]

A few industrial surveys were begun on a small scale, notably in Ontario in 1922 (among miners) and in Quebec in 1930, where five thousand workers in both dusty and hygienic trades were examined to determine the effect of dust on the respiratory system. There was also a general health survey in Montreal.

Surveys, then, were not only considered an effective means of tabulating the extent of disease and identifying individual sufferers but, more importantly, they also indicated to anti-TB workers those groups on which they should concentrate – and, equally important, those on which they should not. Two methods were employed: tuberculin testing, with x-rays taken of positive reactors (done most often with school children) and, more commonly in industry, where rates of infection were higher, bypassing the tuberculin-test screening and x-raying everyone from the start.

The limited industrial surveys in the twenties had demonstrated the tuberculosis rate to be higher in industry (particularly in industries involving silica dust), and the thirties saw a growing concern with this subset of the population.[34] In Quebec the provincial bureau of hygiene and the medical staff of McGill University cooperated to run the Quebec Industrial Health Survey, which had completed thirty-three hundred examinations by 1934 (out of an intended thirty-eight hundred).[35] The mining industry had long demonstrated a need for periodic examinations, and in British Columbia the New Metalliferous Mines Act of 1937 ensured that all miners there were examined annually by the travelling clinics of the tuberculosis division of the provincial government.[36] It was not pure altruism that motivated this legislation – individual companies had initiated surveys in the past to lower their compensation costs. Not only a cynic might see a connection between making silicosis a compensable disease in British Columbia in 1936 and the tuberculosis division assuming responsibility for examining all miners in 1937. Moreover, the cost of treating minimal tuberculosis was estimated to be at most one-third that of treating moderately advanced disease, while the chances of an individual being self-supporting again were ten times greater with minimal disease.[37] Prevention had always been more economical – now industry, beginning to assume a little of the economic burden, saw this fact in the light of self-interest.

Despite the depression, the numbers of surveys, although they were patchwork, expanded by the thirties to include psychiatric patients in Ontario, college and normal students, and school children; they were conducted in select Maritime counties, and even in some Quebec religious communities. By 1935 the CTA reported, six provinces were screening normal school students annually with tuberculin and x-ray examinations.[38] It was also ironically encouraging that the Western provinces, hardest hit in the "Dirty Thirties," were finding surveys of school children increasingly less valuable in unearthing unsuspected tuberculosis, as the rate of infection dropped. By the end of the decade the Saskatchewan Anti-tuberculosis League had ceased sponsoring general school surveys – only one active case for every thousand persons examined was being discovered – and had reserved its funds to check only those classes in which an active case had been identified. Manitoba and British Columbia agreed – the tuberculosis division in the latter province labelled tuberculin testing of school children "one of the least productive methods of case-finding," and continued it only as an aid in establishing an incidence of infection in a given community.[39]

In addition to surveys of select groups, specific geographic areas were now studied – notably the urban centres, long known to harbour pockets of infection, and in the rural areas "travelling clinics" were now exploiting the new automobile and road networks in several provinces.

## Diagnosis: More Precise, More Technical

If the surveys were necessary to determine the extent of the tuberculosis problem in Canada, accurate diagnosis of the disease in the *individual* patient became more bacteriological, technical, and expensive. And with the pulmonary complications of the war and the flu epidemic, diagnosis could be subtle.

By 1938 the CTA had outlined the steps, in order of importance, necessary in an adequate examination.[40] The first was the tuberculin test, increasingly valuable as a means of exclusion with the falling rate of infection. By 1936, only 14 percent of urban school children, 7 percent of rural school children, and 19 percent of young adults (normal school students) had a positive reaction in Saskatchewan. This eliminated the needless expense of x-raying uninfected individuals and focused attention on a much smaller group. That same year the Saskatchewan Anti-Tuberculosis League encouraged the medical profession to screen individuals suspected of having the disease before referring them to a clinic by providing tuberculin free.[41] However, the value of tuerculin was not considered universal. A New Brunswick district medical health officer pointed out that, although tuberculin might be useful in cities and towns, it was often impractical in remote areas where revisitation in forty-eight hours by the travelling diagnostician to interpret the test would be too time-consuming and expensive.[42] Nevertheless, in areas where the incidence of infection was plummeting, tuberculin became the cheapest way to isolate possible suspects.

Tuberculin's major liability was that it could not diagnose active disease. It was to x-rays – "the most reliable single diagnostic agent" – that specialists turned to discover the extent and progress of TB.[43] Moreover, when an examination had to be made in one sitting, either because the contact had travelled a great distance to the sanatorium or the travelling clinic was in the area for a limited time, x-rays were the only means of uncovering infection. Moreover, the switch from glass plates to the lighter, more flexible and convenient x-ray films, which took place in the interwar years, increased their popularity.[44]

Cost was sometimes a limiting factor – as the superintendent of the Nova Scotia Sanatorium observed in 1933, the price of chest films in an average general hospital was "practically prohibitive for the poor."[45]

With existing equipment and operating costs, it was still "manifestly useless" to propose routine x-ray examinations of all people.[46] Conversely, without x-rays it was impossible to find early tuberculosis. This problem would be resolved only when a cheap miniature film allowed the specialists to examine whole communities – even well individuals – in the forties.

In keeping with an organized bacteriological approach, the old standby, the sputum examination, took on a new importance. Although tuberculosis was certainly not ruled out by negative sputum examinations – only 58 percent of the patients at the Manitoba Sanatorium had positive sputum in 1932[47] – the presence of tubercle bacilli permitted a definite diagnosis of the disease (not always easy), and a person with consistently negative sputum or, better still, no sputum at all, was usually considered to be uninfectious. This was increasingly important in determining how long a patient was hospitalized, since tuberculosis workers concentrated their efforts on isolating all active cases to prevent spread of the disease. By the end of the decade, "No sputum, no tuberculosis" became for many the slogan of the tuberculosis control program, as more and more they attempted to "cure" the sick not simply for the sake of the sick themselves but to make them uninfectious and thus ensure the good health of the community.[48]

Although ancillary laboratory tests, together with the personal and family history, continued to be important, a physical examination, once the sole means of diagnosis, proved to be of diminishing significance as the thirties progressed. Now physicians were not only expected to pinpoint tuberculosis but to differentiate it from other, often deceptively similar, chest conditions. Bronchoscopy was added to x-rays as a diagnostic tool to determine nontuberculous conditions.

The sanatoria had a surprisingly high percentage of nontuberculous cases, sent for observation and diagnosis, occupying their short supply of beds. Over 29 percent of the patients discharged from the Queen Alexandra Sanatorium in London in 1933 had been treated for nontuberculous chest conditions.[49] This strained existing accommodation and was another factor forcing the sanatoria to become specialized hospitals.

Even in a straightforward case, diagnosis was still difficult and too often delayed, for tuberculosis was an insidious, chronic disease, demonstrating few symptoms until it was far advanced – of one hundred men over thirty-five studied at the Manitoba Sanatorium, eighty-seven were far advanced at the beginning of treatment, while the duration of the disease from the presumed onset to the time of diagnosis and treatment averaged a discouraging eight years.[50] As a result, proper diagnosis of an early case now required the aid of specialists: the radiologist, chest specialist, and laboratory technician. A conscientious but untrained general practitioner with a stethoscope was dangerously inadequate. And this added to the cost of tuberculosis control.

### Treatment: Bed Rest and Surgery

Treatment, like diagnosis, reflected the interwar emphasis on a bacteriological and technological approach organized and managed by specialized professionals. As the campaign became more entrenched, with the sanatoria evolving into hospitals from the prewar modified camps and resorts and with state support increasing, specialists came to regard rest as the paramount cure.

"I believe," wrote David Stewart in the late 1920s or early 1930s, "twice as much in rest and in twice as much rest for tuberculous patients as I did ten years ago."[51] He was not alone. All sanatoria reported an increase in bed patients and a longer treatment period. By 1928 the medical superintendent at the Laurentian Sanatorium maintained that it was impossible to obtain permanent results if the patient remained less than a year.[52]

Scientific knowledge of human physiology supported a rest treatment for tuberculosis. Autopsy findings had demonstrated that cavitation with necrosis occurred predominantly in the upper third of the lungs. This complication not only put the patient at increased risk of life-threatening hemorrhage – coughing up blood – but often reflected more significant, progressive disease. It was postulated that three mechanical factors prevented healing of such cavities: the surrounding lung's static elastic recoil maintaining traction on the cavity's walls and thus preventing collapse, dynamically increased traction from breathing, and upright posture leading to preferentially decreased apical blood and lymph flow. Bed rest worked on three fronts: it reduced functional residual capacity and thus static tension; it decreased ventilation and thus dynamic traction; and it improved apical perfusion by eliminating the pressure gradient promoted by upright posture.[53]

In North America, exercise was like arsenic: valuable in small, defined doses for certain patients under a doctor's close supervision but dangerously fatal to anyone else. No longer would advanced patients be advised to take brisk walks in the open air – now they were badgered to rest, rest, rest. As the superintendent of the Manitoba Sanatorium explained, "What a house on fire needs is the fire-fighter, not the carpenter. But when the fire is dead out, and the house must be made habitable, the carpenter is the man. At the first stage of

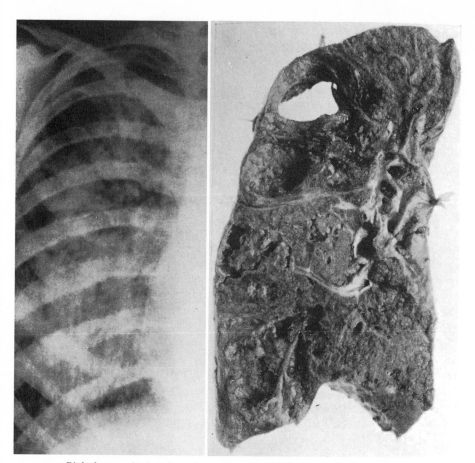

Right lung cavity in tuberculosis with corresponding x-ray findings. Reproduced from
Alexander, *Collapse Therapy of Pulmonary Tuberculosis*, 74–5

tuberculosis rest is the only treatment; at the repair stage, exercise
comes in. To keep on fire-fighting too long is much less dangerous
than to quit too soon."54

With a "cure" taking two to four years, it became practically and
financially impossible for most people to complete it in a sanatorium.
To deal with such pragmatic concerns, the CTA estimated that patients
should be free of active symptoms at least six months before thinking
of returning to work, and then they should devote all their leisure
time to the rest cure the first year back.55 For most, it was still a
daunting prospect. The rest the specialists advised included not only
bed rest but mental rest and, increasingly, rest of the diseased organ
by surgical means.

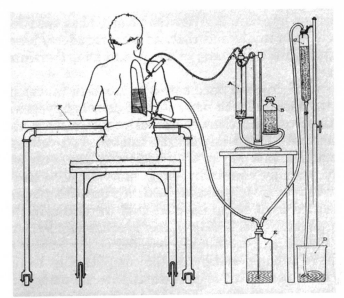

Artificial pneumothorax: two-needle technique for simultaneous removal of fluid and replacement with air. Positive or negative pressures in bottle A (and thus the pnemothorax cavity) are maintained by adjustments of the height of fluid level in B in relation to fluid level in A. Lower needle conducts fluid to aspiration bottle E. Vacuum in E is the same as that in the air chamber above the water level in C. Reproduced from Alexander, *Collapse Therapy of Pulmonary Tuberculosis,* 276

With their continued search for a specific, bacteriologically oriented treatment bolstered by improving medical technology, specialists began to place growing importance upon "collapse therapy," or surgically induced rest – especially pneumothorax (collapse of the lung) and extrapleural thoracoplasty (removal of several ribs to decrease the thoracic cavity and collapse the lung). The same physiological benefits attributed to bed rest – cavitary collapse, disease resolution, fibrosis, and healing – could theoretically be gained from surgical rest. James Carson of Liverpool had noted the benefits of open artifical pneumothorax in 1821; the Italian, Forlanini, promoted it in 1882 and began using it a decade later. Reassured by u.s. Civil War experience, which had demonstrated that over eleven thousand chest injuries had caused minimal symptoms, Murphy began publishing his experience with artificial pneumothorax induced by nitrogen injections in the Journal of the American Medical Association in 1898. Although it became generally accepted by the interwar years as one of the mainstays of treatment, its efficacy could never be formally established, since there were no adequately controlled trials. The first Canadian artificial pneumothorax was performed by J.M. Rogers of Ingersoll, Ontario, in 1898. Introduced into the Toronto Hospital for Tuberculosis during World War 1, it was attempted on 60 percent of admitted patients by the 1930s.[56]

Thoracoplasty was initially carried out in 1869 to treat empyema. Brauer, an internist, promoted it in 1907, advocating extensive rib resections to collapse the lung – a dangerous operation done under local anesthetic and associated with shock and circulatory collapse. Subsequent modifications, most notably by Sauerbruch and the American, John Alexander, led to staged operations, with partial rib resection. In the decade prior to the introduction of chemotherapy, thoracoplasty resulted in cavitary closure and negative sputum in up to 80 percent of patients.[57]

Less popular surgical techniques included unilateral phrenic nerve division for diaphragmatic paralysis, which resulted in more retained secretions and respiratory compromise than pneumothorax, pneumoperitoneum (injection of air into the abdominal cavity to theoretically elevate the diaphragm, which had minimal benefit), and extrapleural pneumothorax (injection of gas between the chest wall itself and the parietal pleura).

Although attempted before the chemotherapy era, pulmonary resection was too risky for general use. Results of a study reported at the 1940 annual meeting of the American Association for Thoracic Surgery showed 40.2 percent and 20.5 percent mortality rates for pneumonectomies and lobectomies respectively, which were usually associated with disease spread, bronchial fistulae, empyema, and toxic pleuritis. These results were not surprising, since most resections were performed with tourniquet technique and ligation. "Either the patient suddenly turned blue and died because the bronchial stump had blown," reported one veteran nurse, "or the patient suddenly turned white and died when the artery had blown." From the late thirties to the early fifties roughly one-third of the patients with pulmonary tuberculosis had some form of collapse therapy.[58]

The development and increasing use of x-rays, surgical instruments and techniques, and anaesthetic agents, and the availability of blood transfusions and facilities for supplying adequate oxygen made surgery more practical and successful. An endotracheal tube with a cuff to prevent catastrophic aspiration and subsequent life-threatening pneumonia was introduced in the late thirties, while Griffin and Johnson began using the relaxing agent curare in Montreal in 1942, so that intravenous anesthesia became available in addition to the expanding number of inhalational agents.[59] The emphasis on noninfection, the

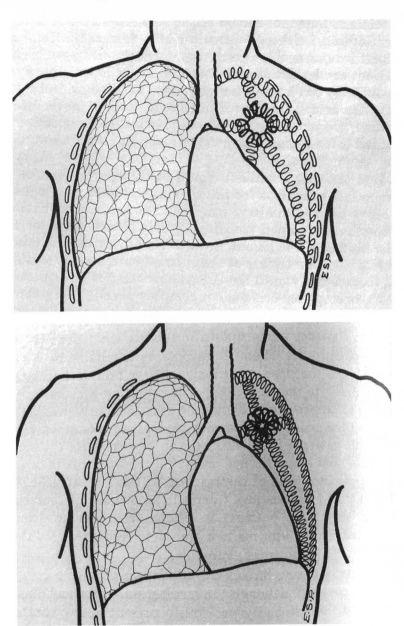

Physiological rationale of thoracoplasty. *Top*, rigid thoracic walls surrounding the lung prevent cavitary closure – coils represent shrinking fibrous tissue. The diaphragm is pulled up, ribs and mediastinum shift towards the diseased side, and the cavity remains open. *Bottom*, ribs are resected, and the soft thoracic wall is free to yield to the pull of the contracting fibrous tissue, permitting collapse and cavitary closure. Reproduced from Alexander, *Collapse Therapy of Pulmonary Tuberculosis*, 428

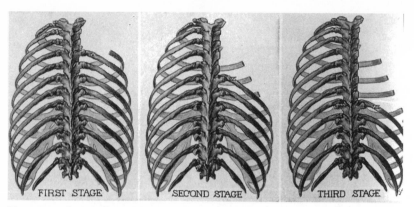

Three-stage thoracoplasty: (1) resect all of first rib and cartilage, part of transverse process of vertebra, posterolateral portion of second and third ribs, and all second and third transverse processes; (2) resect remaining posterolateral portion of third rib and portions of posterolateral fourth and fifth ribs and the transverse processes; (3) resect posterior and parts of lateral sixth and seventh ribs and transverse processes. Reproduced from Alexander, *Collapse Therapy of Pulmonary Tuberculosis*, 452

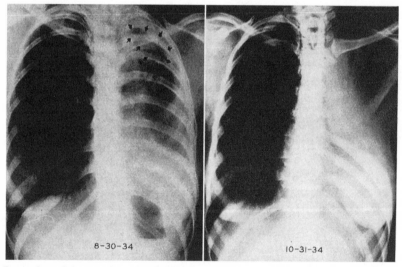

Posterolateral thoracoplasty. *Left*, left-sided cavity (with arrows); *right*, after three-stage, seven ribs posterolateral thoracoplasty. Scapula is not resting on any ribs and has fallen forward. Cavities are closed. Reproduced from Alexander, *Collapse Therapy of Pulmonary Tuberculosis*, 453

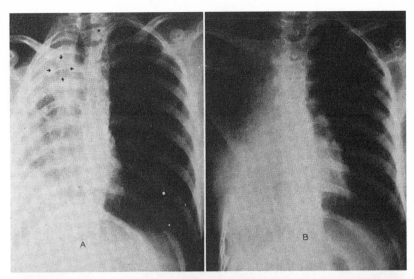

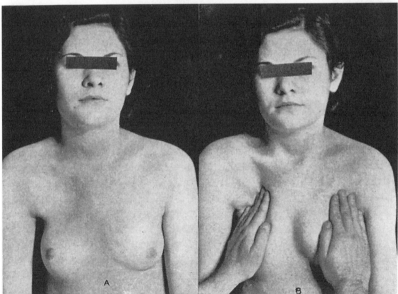

Collapse therapy with thoracoplasty. *Above left*, productive TB with cavitation; *right*, collapse after thoracoplasty with up to ten ribs removed; *below*, photograph of patient, whose x-ray is above, with a posterior and anterior resection and hands showing position of anterior portions of ribs. Reproduced from Alexander, *Collapse Therapy of Pulmonary Tuberculosis*, 556

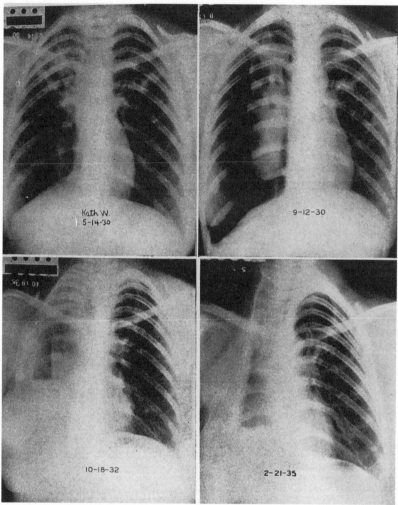

Staged surgery for persistent tuberculosis: pneumothorax thoracoplasty, and phrenic paralysis. *Upper left*, x-ray three months after sanatorium admission, nine years after onset of TB. Far advanced TB with large right lung cavities, small left lung cavity. *Upper right*, right-sided pneumothorax induced May 1930. Adhesions prevented cavitary closure. Temporary left phrenic paralysis in August 1930 to close left-sided cavity and aid healing preliminary to thoracoplasty. *Lower left*, persistent large right cavity with pyopneumothorax. *Lower right*, staged, seven-rib right-sided thoracoplasty in Nov.-Dec. 1932, with right permanent phrenic paralysis in Jan. 1933. Cavities closed, empyema obliterated. Sputum disappeared June 1933. Patient discharged Feb. 1934 as "arrested case." Reproduced from Alexander, *Collapse Therapy of Pulmonary Tuberculosis*, 126

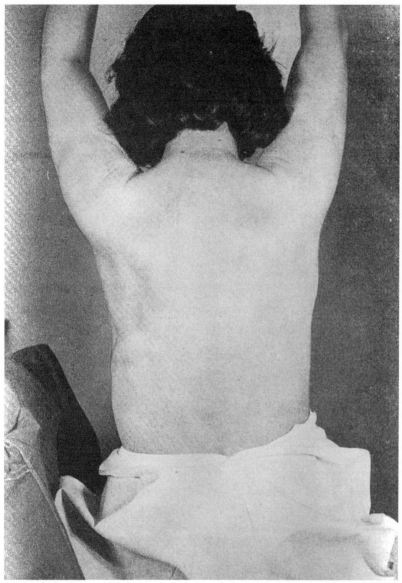

Patient after thoracoplasty, to show "minimal" deformity. Reproduced from Hatfield, *Handbook on Tuberculosis*, 71

high cost of sanatorium accommodation, and the shortage of beds all encouraged a more extensive application of surgical treatment. Follow-up studies of former sanatorium patients demonstrated that 60 to 70 percent of those patients with an open cavity and positive sputum would be dead within three years, and 80 to 90 percent within five. Of those who survived, most remained chronic invalids.[60] Collapse therapy, on the other hand, while not a cure-all, offered a speedier recovery, usually stopped hemorrhaging, and rendered at least 50 percent of successful cases sputum negative.[61] A study of 460 former patients of the Kentville, Nova Scotia, sanatorium showed 58 percent of the moderately advanced cases and 25 percent of the advanced cases who had received artificial pneumothorax were well and working, while only 22 percent and 5 percent respectively of those who had not received the treatment were well.[62]

There were also economic considerations for the individual, which Norman Bethune, then a Montreal chest surgeon pleading for early collapse therapy, enumerated in 1932: "Compression saves time, saves money, and saves life. The patient with early tuberculosis who, through economic pressure, can afford to spend less than two or three years in a sanatorium must have mechanical pressure. Lack of time and money kills more cases of pulmonary tuberculosis than lack of resistance to that disease. The poor man dies because he cannot afford to live. Here the economist and sociologist meet the compressionist on common ground."[63] Twenty years earlier anti-TB workers would have plied poor patients with food and clothing in an attempt to "cure" their disease. Now, specialists collapsed their lungs.

### Sanatoria and Collapse Therapy

The extension of pneumothorax to more hopeful cases permitted sanatoria to discharge patients earlier and give them refills (reinjections of gas into the pleural space to maintain lung collapse) as outpatients instead (for artificial pneumothorax still took two to five years). Sanatoria could extend their services to a greater number of patients – the Royal Ottawa Sanatorium reported in 1936 that it cared in this fashion for almost 50 percent more patients than its adult bed capacity would have permitted.[64] To cope with this growing number of former patients who still needed refills, local practitioners were sometimes trained to give artificial pneumothorax in order to remove some of the strain on the specialists – by 1935, for example, the medical superintendent of the Queen Alexandra Sanatorium in London reported that one staff member spent four afternoons a week doing nothing but giving out-patients refills. Demand grew for local

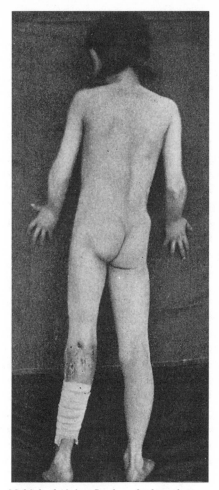

Multiple draining fistulae of tubercular
knee in childhood bone and joint
tuberculosis. Reproduced from Klebs,
*Tuberculosis,* 747

centres where this could be done cheaply and efficiently; the Ontario
department of health, after a 1937 survey of tuberculosis control in
that province, established some eighty refill centres, while the staff at
the St John Tuberculosis Hospital in New Brunswick built pneumothorax outfits to sell at cost ($6.50) to local doctors.[65]

Not all localities used collapse therapy extensively – Montreal,
despite its world-renowned thoracic surgeons, was a notable example.
The tuberculosis committee of the Montreal Medical Society pointed

out that in that city diagnosis was often made too late for the treatment
to be of value, the serious lack of beds prevented patients from being
institutionalized early enough to begin effective treatment even if they
did receive it, many were not well enough to travel to the various
clinics for refills, and there were no facilities for administering it in a
patient's home.[66] Collapse therapy, to be effective, could not be carried out in isolation but needed the support of the other adjuncts to
the Canadian tuberculosis control program: sanatorium accommodation and sufficient beds, clinics, and public health nurses. Where these
adjuncts were available however, it was quickly becoming, after rest,
*the* specific treatment for tuberculosis. Artificial pneumothorax was
attempted with 60 percent of all patients admitted to the Toronto
Hospital for Consumptives in the 1930s, with 55 percent of the
patients at the Queen Alexandra Sanatorium by 1936, 52.8 percent
at Tranquille by 1938, and over 80 percent of the pulmonary patients
at the Manitoba Sanatorium in 1936.[67]

Heliotherapy continued to be used with bone, joint, glandular, and
intestinal tuberculosis. By 1926 half the patients treated by the
Saskatchewan Anti-Tuberculosis League received some form of light
therapy.[68] More developed technology also permitted specialized medical procedures and equipment to deal with less common forms of the
disease, including intravenous injections of calcium chloride in cases
of intestinal complications and electrocautery to reduce the complication of laryngeal tuberculosis. One writer estimated that 10 percent
of tuberculous patients had kidney involvement, and by 1927 the
Canadian Medical Association was advising that every pulmonary
patient be routinely given a barium meal to catch the intestinal form
early.[69] Diagnosis of nonpulmonary cases was made at a late, almost
hopeless stage; and with the percentage of sufferers treated at sanatoria increasing, the problem became more obvious. In Saskatchewan
non pulmonary cases rose from 1.1 percent of all cases in 1920 to
18.94 percent in 1925.[70]

*TB and Other Diseases*

Ironically in the midst of a depression, specialists began to study the
association of tuberculosis with other diseases, notably diabetes, cancer, and silicosis, rather than investigating links with social conditions.
The Ontario Board of Health (in cooperation with the Division of
Industrial Hygiene) examined gold miners and quarry-men in 1925
and discovered a higher incidence of tuberculosis in those exposed to
silica dust. Quebec ran an industrial health survey of five thousand

employees in 1930 to find out if organic, inorganic, or metallic dust predisposed individuals to tuberculosis.[71]

This interest reflected the increasingly emphasized medical or bacteriological approach to tuberculosis, as well as a more general concern with industrial hygiene. While child welfare work ensured that infants and school children did not succumb to the disease, industrial hygiene was supposed to follow up this initial investment in workers' health to prevent them breaking down as adults. This approach was only common sense, as Sir Arthur Currie pointed out in 1926, harking back once again to more general interwar themes: "A good health service in an industrial concern is a good investment, for good health among the employees means ... greater efficiency, larger production, and higher dividends."[72]

The relationship between cancer and tuberculosis stimulated new questions. As the tuberculosis rate fell, specialists noted with dismay a rise in the cancer rate. Was this increase a direct result – and if so, why? Did tuberculosis actually prevent an individual from becoming cancerous, or were there certain conditions favourable to one disease and unfavourable to the other? Or was it simply that as tuberculosis took a diminishing toll of the youth, more adults survived to fall prey to cancer? These questions mark the beginning of a concern with adult mortality that would increase as, one by one, the causes of preventable infant deaths were eliminated. Instead of people living longer, public health workers would find, frustratingly enough, an increasing number of deaths due to conditions and diseases of middle age – notably cancer and heart disease.[73]

The DSCR had pioneered occupational therapy to keep recalcitrant soldiers occupied and willing to follow the rest treatment, and by 1920 this therapy had been extended to most civilian patients. As time required for rest treatment lengthened, tuberculosis workers discovered that patients needed something to occupy their minds while they took the cure, or they became glum, fretful, and hard to handle.

As an expected corollary to the emphasis on months, sometimes years, of treatment devoted primarily to rest, patients' depression and boredom began to undercut the value of the cure. But if technology, in the form of collapse therapy and the more complex hospital-like sanatoria, had promoted the emphasis on rest, it was also technology that provided a partial solution: radio. As Stuart Houston chronicles in his biography of R.G. Ferguson, two patients owning the only radio sets at the Fort Qu'Appelle Sanatorium in 1923 ingeniously rigged up an extension to bring radio programs to each bed in the sanatorium. Sanatoria across Canada adopted similar set-ups. As one of the patients explained in the in-house *Valley Echo*, "Our sanatorium physicians feel that radio is one of their strongest allies. Otherwise restless patients will lie quietly for hours listening to their favorite programs ... their diseased lungs are given that much better opportunity to heal."[74]

### Follow-up and Prevention of Relapse

With rehabilitation more an ideal than a reality, sanatorium physicians were seeing a growing number of patients as readmissions. Their disease arrested, they had left the institution and as a result of over-work, overplay, inadequate rest treatment, or simply poor living conditions, they had relapsed. Not only was it discouraging for the individual sufferer, but, sanatorium experts maintained, it was poor economics for society to spend money and effort curing patients once and then allowing them to fall ill a second time.

Unsurprisingly, it was the DSCR that pioneered follow-up work by a visiting nurse, for it had a sizable investment in each tuberculous soldier, both in his cure and the pension he could collect if allowed to become completely disabled. This method, too, filtered into the civilian community. Public health nurses and local anti-TB societies began including follow-up care more often as one of their duties. A study at the Fort Qu'Appelle Sanatorium of 1,747 discharged patients emphasized the economic gains to be made: 10 percent had relapsed, with 8 percent readmitted for treatment, at a cost of $24 thousand a year. An undue proportion of relapses occurred among those return-ing to heavy jobs – the percentage of labourers who relapsed was twice the average, while that of farmers was three times the average.[75] It was a final statistical blow, if any were needed, to the social reform era's notion that farming was a suitable occupation for the tuberculous.

Aftercare might protect those who returned to the regular work force from recurrent disease, but it did not solve the problem of those who were incapable of holding down a full-time job. If employment could not be found for them in regular businesses – and it was becoming increasingly evident that it could not – then a life on the dole or in some form of sheltered employment was the only solution. Since most employers preferred to make a financial donation rather than set up special working conditions for handicapped employees, some sort of agency-run workshops were considered to be the only practical solution. In the case of the soldiers, workshops had to be set up quickly – as J.H. Holbrook, medical superintendent of Hamilton's Mountain Sanatorium bluntly pointed out, "Ex-service tuberculous men are dying sufficiently fast to do away with the need if they are not assisted at once."[76]

From 1919 to 1922 the DSCR established special workshops in Toronto, Hamilton, London, Brantford and Kingston, and the Red

Cross aided in setting up one in Montreal.[77] By the thirties, rehabilitation remained a much-discussed, but neglected, field. Most agreed it was necessary, especially when jobs were so scarce – but only the Samaritan clubs of Hamilton and Toronto and various volunteer groups in Vancouver and Victoria attempted some sort of sheltered employment or reestablishment of former patients in industry. As a result, patients were institutionalized longer than necessary, due to the reluctance of those in charge to see their illness recur on their return home.

Associated with both convalescent care and rehabilitation was follow-up. On a superficial level, keeping track of discharged patients enabled a sanatorium to evaluate long-term success and aid others in estimating the value of sanatorium treatment – goals in keeping with the interwar emphasis on scientific management and efficient administration. A study of 3,569 patients discharged from Saskatchewan sanatoria from 1917 to 1934 found 53.9 percent well and working, 7.9 percent working with symptoms, 10.4 percent unable to work, and 23 percent dead.[78] On a more practical level, follow-up was important in ensuring that the initial government-funded treatment – and investment – was protected. "We too often find," commented the Vancouver Survey Committee in 1934, "patients on whom the province and municipalities have spent thousands of dollars [in treatment], coming back broken down again due to the lack of being followed up. Not only do patients come back, but bring with them others whom they have infected. Money spent in this way is wasted. It is analogous to pouring water into a barrel and allowing it to run out at the other end. It does not appear reasonable, human or businesslike."[79]

With collapse therapy rendering patients sputum-negative more quickly, there was a greater need for effective follow-up work. It was considered especially critical in the first four years, when most relapses occurred. As a result, as follow-up intensified, its purpose expanded. In the twenties and early thirties, the major emphasis had been on "recovery of function" – the disappearance of symptoms and the ability of patients to resume work. As the thirties wound down, the focus shifted to the community and thus to the *infectivity* of the patient – and so, paradoxically, follow-up became yet one more prong in the tuberculosis campaign of *prevention*.[80]

*BCG*

BCG (Bacillus Calmette-Guérin) was an attenuated live TB vaccine developed over two decades at the Pasteur Institute in Lille, France, by Albert Calmette, the medical director, and his associate, Camille Guérin, a veterinary surgeon. In 1921 they began human infant vaccination trials that seemed to demonstrate its efficacy; that same year, Canadian testing began and was ultimately conducted under the auspices of the Associate Committee on Tuberculosis Research (ACTR) established by the National Research Council of Canada in 1923.

Vaccination trials in Canadian infants commenced with Dr J.A. Baudoin at the Université de Montréal in 1925, under the supervision of a member of the Pasteur Institute. Baudoin was a Rockefeller Foundation fellow who had studied at Johns Hopkins University in the United States and had personal and professional ties to Calmette. Supported by annual grants of $2,000 from the National Research Council, by 1934 he had 5,126 infants enrolled in his trials, with data supposedly demonstrating that the mortality rate in the 1-to-12-month-old and 1-to-7-year-old vaccinated groups was, respectively, one-quarter and one-third the rate of comparable unvaccinated controls. By 1941, 44,734 infants had been vaccinated with a 61 percent decrease in mortality in children 15 years old and younger. Convinced by his data, the Quebec government had begun BCG vaccinations among school children by 1949.[81]

In the rest of Canada, and particularly in the United States, BCG was greeted with more skepticism. Georgina Feldberg has attributed this at least partially to a nascent scientific nationalism of Americans, who wished to do their own testing and set their own standards, but as Feldberg has also documented, there were significant problems both with Calmette's original data and his theoretical rationale for the vaccine that caused concern. Not only were many leery of his argument that an orally digested bovine form of the disease could transform into the human form, but many also questioned his contention that the transformed bovine bacillus, which no longer produced active disease yet conferred immunity, could be relied upon never to alter again – that its decreased virulence was hereditary.[82] Moreover, although Calmette had vaccinated 43,283 children by 1927, he had comparative data available only for 1,050 and had used the general population as his controls. And he had separated the vaccinated infants but not the "controls," from their infected environment. Finally, he had included TB deaths in the first ten days in the controls but not in the vaccinated subjects.[83]

Not only had some researchers noted a change in the virulence of strains of BCG, but the tragedy in Lübeck, Germany, in which 71 of 250 children vaccinated had died by 1930, seemed to support a cautious, if not hostile, approach. J.G. Fitzgerald, director of the Connaught Research Laboratory at the University of Toronto, called for more studies. Although it would ultimately prove to be 80 percent effective, many probably agreed with the physician-in-chief of the Toronto Hospital for Consumptives, who suggested that BCG be altered to BGC – Better Go Cautiously.[84]

Although BCG was pioneered in Quebec, probably the only attempt at well-controlled trials was carried out under the auspices of the NRC committee on tuberculosis by R.G. Ferguson, who worked from 1933 to 1943 with the aboriginals of Fort Qu'Appelle, Saskatchewan. Ten times more likely than Caucasians to fall prey to TB, Canadian aboriginals in the twenties and thirties were a high-risk group. By 1947 it was clear that the incidence of TB was five times greater in the unvaccinated group and that the disease, when it occurred, was more extensive and severe.

Ferguson began with the oral vaccine but soon switched to an intracutaneous form. His trials were more scientifically rigorous than either Calmette's or Baudoin's. He paired families as controls – and, unlike the French and Quebec data, by 1938 his data demonstrated that while the general death rate in each matched group was the same, BCG decreased tuberculosis mortality in native children in an infectious environment by 75 percent. Its protection, he concluded, was not "absolute" but "considerable."[85]

By 1959 the British Medical Research Council, with its own studies, would support his view, concluding that BCG was 80 percent effective. By that point, however, isoniazid had been discovered, which not only provided prophylaxis against disease in an exposed population but, as Feldberg points out, could be incorporated more easily into a sanatorium or hospital regime.[86] In the interwar and immediate postwar period, however, BCG was extended to all tuberculin-negative student nurses and sanatorium and mental hospital employees in Saskatchewan – individuals known to be high-risk.

In addition to its incomplete coverage, other liabilities precluded wide adoption of BCG. With a fast-declining rate of infection, it confounded easy identification of exposure to TB, for it could result in a positive tuberculin test, not to mention scarring from ulcerated lymph nodes.[87] Determining those most likely to succumb to the disease was increasingly valuable, so specialists were reluctant to relinquish the utility of tuberculin as a screening tool for a somewhat dubious means of prevention. For those continually exposed, the advantages of BCG were beginning to outweigh the liabilities – especially in areas where the tuberculosis campaign had lagged or in groups particularly infected or at risk – in other words, aboriginals, hospital employees, and francophone inhabitants of Quebec.

*Case-Finding*

With surveys delineating the extent of the disease in Canadian society and diagnosis and treatment becoming more scientific, it appeared to specialists such as David Stewart that case-finding – identifying the individual sufferers – was often "medieval."[88] It was left to individual initiative – frequently the patient's – to determine if someone was sick enough to consult a doctor. "The doctor is called," he noted, "not when the man begins to be sick, but when he has begun to despair of getting well," and he outlined a new aggressive attitude that, he asserted dogmatically and with more than a hint of intellectual arrogance, specialists must adopt if the tuberculosis problem was to be attacked properly: "If the disease has to be let go until unexpert, untrained, ignorant, backward, reluctant, remote, scared, wrong-headed people come to a point at which they can stand it no longer, then not much can be done in the way of cure of tuberculosis. If we are to get disease under treatment at a stage amenable to treatment and with any prospect of cure, we must go and hunt for it."[89]

To find cases, tuberculosis workers used established sources – family doctors, clinics, sanatorium applicants and former patients, tuberculosis death notices, school medical examinations, and public health nurses – and they developed new sources: travelling diagnosticians, extension clinics, and, most important of all, examination of contacts. "Prevention," decreed Stewart, reflecting the attitude of many tuberculosis experts, "must begin *when* infection begins – that is usually in early childhood; and prevention must begin *where* infection begins – that is usually in the home."[90] To diagnose tuberculosis at an early stage, they had the paradoxical problem of identifying cases *before* obvious symptoms developed – and this meant, in practical terms, before sufferers even suspected they were sick. Lacking the technology and social will to examine all Canadians, tuberculosis specialists began to select specific groups: children, (who were easier to deal with through a school inspection system that was already set up), surveys of students and industrial workers, contacts (because the home was now thought to be the chief source of disease), and residents of rural areas.

## Travelling Clinics

Before the war, public health workers had concentrated almost exclusively on urban health; in the twenties, they turned their attention to rural areas. Programs instituted in the first two decades had left much of the countryside unaffected. The war had shown that the incidence of tuberculosis was as great among country-bred soldiers as urban dwellers, but the sanatoria and dispensaries that had so laboriously been set up to serve the cities were almost completely lacking in rural townships. The population was often sparse and difficult to organize, and rural municipalities seldom evinced any interest in either erecting sanatoria or even paying for the accommodation of their residents in established institutions. Few had a milk bylaw or inspector, so that, ironically, people were safer buying milk in the city than in the country. As urban conditions improved, the sanatorium medical superintendents noted with dismay that their rural patients were still generally hopelessly advanced by the time they were admitted.

More cynically, rural areas were not only a source of infection but an economic burden on the better-organized urban centres – by 1927 the Mountain Sanatorium in Hamilton had more patients from the surrounding areas than from the city itself. Since Ontario sanatoria were forced by law to accept any patients sent, under penalty of forfeiting the provincial allowance of 75 cents per day per patient, urban centres complained that they were unfairly burdened with a responsibility that rural municipalities were unjustifiably evading.[91]

There were two solutions. Since rural municipalities were generally small and sparsely populated, they could not organize locally the way their urban counterparts, particularly in Ontario, had done. Thus some form of county or, better yet, provincial organization, was necessary. Secondly, to diagnose cases early, travelling clinics, either government- or sanatorium-run and funded at least partially by voluntary funds, were established to examine select rural patients before their disease was found to be untreatable. Like advances in other aspects of the anti-TB campaign, this step too was predicated on the extension of new technological breakthroughs in Canadian society in general – in this case, reliable automobiles and an extensive, interconnected road system.

The Red Cross pioneered the first travelling clinic in Nova Scotia in 1920 and, through the CTA, it established extension clinics out of the sanatoria in Hamilton, London, Gravenhurst, and Kingston. Not only was it a fruitful method of unearthing TB sufferers (out of 473 individuals examined in Ontario in 1923, 207 were diagnosed positive), but it also demonstrated a need for a comprehensive examination of all rural suspects. In 1923 the Ontario and British Columbia governments appointed travelling tuberculosis specialists. By 1925 Saskatchewan, New Brunswick, and Nova Scotia had been added to the list,[92] and by the end of the decade all provinces except Prince Edward Island had some form of travelling diagnostician or clinic.

Despite these variations, clinics were remarkably similar. First, doctors in a given area were contacted, told of the planned clinic and of its goals, and asked to refer patients. No patients were seen unless they were referred by their own physician or public health or school nurse. The diagnostician, the diagnostician's nurse, and, occasionally, an x-ray technician set up the clinic in a hospital, school, hotel, or any other available public building. It was held for two to six days, with each patient receiving a tuberculin test, x-ray, and physical examination. Films were developed and evaluated when the specialist returned to headquarters, and the results were sent to the doctor, health officers, and health departments concerned, not to the patients themselves.

For this selective examination to function efficiently, clinics needed the support of general practitioners, and by operating in this manner, specialists felt they were allaying local physicians' fears that they were either trying to undercut the physicians' authority or steal patients. Often the patients examined were contacts – Stewart reported 50 to 75 percent were in Manitoba – but advanced cases were assessed too, in case they needed artificial pneumothorax, had to be removed to a sanatorium, or were a source of infection.[93]

By arriving with much fanfare, organizers of such clinics also hoped to educate both general practitioners and the public about the symptoms of early disease and methods of prevention, in addition to diagnosis; and by catching cases early, they would theoretically reduce foci of infection in the community and lessen the resultant expenses of the local and provincial authorities. Perhaps not surprisingly, these clinics also discovered a significant amount of nontuberculous disease and disability in otherwise well Canadians.

By the late thirties in Saskatchewan, with its plummeting rate of infection, there was an encouraging sign: travelling consultants had outlived their greatest usefulness. By 1937 only one operated, in the southern part of the province, where the depression, it was felt, made a consultation service imperative. Instead of examining suspects and contacts, the consultant's primary objective was to demonstrate tuberculin testing, thus teaching local doctors an inexpensive technique to rule out suspects and ease the burden on the sanatorium of unnecessary examinations. Case-finding was carried out through the general practitioner together with the stationary clinics (there were eight outside the sanatoria by 1937), where the league x-rayed all contacts, suspects, and former patients for free. Improved communication and transportation had extended the influence of the sanatorium and the stationary clinic into the countryside, minimizing the need for the travelling clinic. Just as Canadians could drive to nearby centres to shop instead of relying on local retailers, so they could travel to the nearby TB institution.

Clinics – the urban stationary type and the newer, rural extension or travelling variety – were evolving into institutions whose function was to find early cases and thus ensure a constant flow of patients to the sanatoria. The clinic became a link between the sanatoria and the general public: it continued to screen and refer cases (50 percent of the cases diagnosed at the Royal Edward Institute were nontuberculous),94 educate patients and their families, and supervise them if they received home treatment; and it did follow-up work, with the aid of public health nurses, when they were discharged from an institution. Like sanatoria, clinics were becoming more specialized, almost hospital-like, in their approach, with specialized outpatient departments, tuberculin tests, x-ray examinations, and even heliotherapy and artificial pneumothorax. Where the municipality did not supply them, they ran summer camps and open-air schools – for example, in Montreal. In that city the Bruchesi and Royal Edward Institutes also cooperated in BCG vaccination and family placement work. There had even been a suggestion that the dispensary, like the new central clinic in Winnipeg, should be the central agency to gather all tuberculosis data and to coordinate the different agencies. Auxiliaries of some form (often women's auxiliaries) were still associated to supply relief, but relief was now only a minor, associated part of tuberculosis clinic work. The clinic's emphasis, like that of the sanatorium, was bacteriological and technological.

Stationary clinics became increasingly popular in the thirties, as a result of improved communication, the prevailing hard times, and a growing public awareness of the advantages of early diagnosis. Maintaining the services established in the twenties (diagnosis through specialized clinics and examination of contacts), they also established follow-up of former sanatorium patients and provision of pneumothorax refills. As collapse therapy was used more frequently and earlier, sanatoria began to discharge patients with suitable homes during the course of their treatment, rather than at its completion, and these patients continued to receive their refills from and have their progress monitored by the clinics. Consequently, these institutions were changing from simple diagnostic centres to out-patient treatment centres for noninfectious cases.

*Registration and Notification*

Fundamental to all case-finding was an adequate system of case registration. It was impossible to ensure that all contacts had been examined and all arrested cases followed up without some system of reporting. Notification to the local health officer, even at this late date, was often irregular and generally came from the sanatorium after the patient was admitted.95 Conditions varied, of course – Toronto reported in 1935 that 18 percent of the total tuberculosis deaths were of people who had not previously been reported, while the estimated figure for

Montreal for the same offence as late as 1939 was 60 percent. Despite the social dislocations of the thirties, the overall situation improved, however. In 1935 the CTA noted with some satisfaction that statistics were no longer showing more deaths reported than cases, and it tentatively estimated that annually there were probably three cases for each death in any given community.[96]

In rural areas, in particular, efficient case registration and the effectiveness of the anti-TB campaign rested squarely on the shoulders of the family doctor. Despite the specialists' sometimes disgruntled view of general practitioners, in Alberta over three times as many cases were referred by the medical profession at large as were referred by the clinics, while half of all tuberculosis cases discovered in Saskatchewan were definitely diagnosed solely by the family doctor, and over half the remainder were suspected and referred by the family doctor to the league.[97] TB specialists acknowledged that unless the family doctor notified the health department of all new cases, there could be no comprehensive follow-up or examination of suspects and consequently no decrease in the rate of infection. If the specialists opined sourly that poor notification was due too often to ignorance in diagnosing or laziness in reporting, the general practitioner complained, in turn, that there was no reason to bother reporting diagnosed cases when the local medical health officer showed no interest, took no action, and offered no help.[98] It was a problem that had existed at the turn of the century but that the depression brought again to the fore. What could the family doctor do if the patient was penniless, the municipality refused to pay, the local board of health or medical health officer was apathetic, and the district lacked sanatorium accommodation? To most specialists, the solution was obvious: central direction, under a provincial tuberculosis division, and free treatment.

In keeping with the shifting emphasis to prevention and safeguarding the *community* rather than the individual, general practitioners were exhorted to take a more aggressive approach to the disease. Since they were responsible for finding most of the cases, tuberculosis specialists insisted they had a duty to detect infection early, using all the machinery at their disposal – and this included not just using the diagnostic tools of tuberculin testing, sputum analysis, x-raying, and a personal history and physical examination, but using the general practitioner's office as a referral base or clearing house to the specialist, sanatorium, diagnostic clinic, anti-TB association, and welfare agency. General practitioners were even expected, in some cases, to give artificial pneumothorax refills. They were to be new and improved Good Samaritans of the interwar period: "The man who can deal effectively with tuberculosis," decreed Stewart, "is the militant type of practitioner who gets a description of the thieves even while he tends the wounds, then rides out forthwith to arrest them."[99] For most general practitioners, it was an imposing, if not daunting, task.

Although the general practitioner might be the basis on which case-finding activities of the tuberculosis campaign rested, travelling diagnosticians, like sanatorium physicians, were of paramount importance as consultants: but, as they were careful to state, *always* consultants – patients had to be referred through their family doctor. This was a tactical attempt by the specialists to win the goodwill and support they needed from the general practitioner if they were to run an effective campaign.

The percentage of active TB the clinics uncovered was determined by the selectivity of referring doctors and the rate of infection in a given area. For example, Quebec reported finding 3.81 percent of those examined by clinicians to be new positive cases, while Manitoba found 7.6 percent.[100] This was not because Manitoba had a higher incidence of the disease – the opposite was true – but because potential suspects were screened more effectively before being referred. Such percentages were important only in the light of cost and whether clinics were bringing enough new cases to light to reduce disease. Manitoba reported with satisfaction that newly diagnosed tuberculosis patients were becoming fewer in those districts visited year after year by the travelling clinic, although the clinic was held responsible as well for the increase in the number of sanatorium patients and the total burden of sanatorium maintenance costs.

As a source of infection, tuberculosis workers pinpointed the most fruitful group of all in the twenties: contacts. With more milk being pasteurized, exposure to active human cases generally became the main source of individual infection. Fully 95 percent of infected Canadian children, it was estimated in 1933, had become infected by an adult, while a study at Montreal's Royal Edward Institute revealed that 3 percent of the contacts examined had active tuberculosis, and another 3 percent inactive tuberculosis.[101] According to the CTA, there were three objectives in contact examination: discovering the original source of infection in the home, detecting cases of early tuberculosis, and initiating measures to render contacts less liable to contract tuberculosis. Every contact had to be tuberculin tested and those who were sensitive x-rayed. Certain contacts had to be supervised for three to seven years – notably tuberculin positive children and young adults and individuals exposed to continual infection.[102]

*The Role of the Sanatoria*

With more municipal and provincial tuberculosis divisions established as the decade progressed, the tuberculosis control program became more organized on both government levels, and the tracking down and supervision of all those exposed became more systematic and, as a result, more comprehensive. By 1933 in Ontario, 1935 in British Columbia, and 1937 in Manitoba, all tuberculosis cases were reported to a central office, and contacts were followed up by the family doctor, the clinic (stationary or travelling), and a public health nurse, when available.[103] In Saskatchewan they were examined by the city health department and the Saskatchewan Anti-Tuberculosis League (at the league's clinic).

If rest had become the fundamental treatment, sanatoria were the bedrock of the campaign. Home treatment, even when administered through the most comprehensive, well-regulated dispensaries, had never been completely satisfactory – the Bruchesi Institute reported a fall-off in attendance during bad weather, while workers at the dispensary operated by the Hamilton Health Association complained that even moderately advanced cases, upon feeling better after a few days rest, disregarded instruction. With the emphasis on complete rest, together with surgical and technical procedures to effect a cure, it was obvious that home treatment was not only too limiting in what it could offer but presented too many tempting distractions to a patient who felt fit and yet was obliged to remain in bed.

With reasonably complete statistics collected for the first time, those interested in the tuberculosis problem also saw a direct correlation between the tuberculosis death rate and the number of available sanatorium beds. Although it may have been a case of "seeing what you look for," this pattern reinforced the importance of sanatoria – especially when it was linked with the number of indigent cases treated. Robert Wodehouse, secretary of the Canadian Tuberculosis Association, blamed the high death rates in Nova Scotia, New Brunswick, and Quebec on the lethal combination of an insufficient number of beds and inadequate care of poor patients.[104] With travelling clinics uncovering cases daily, the situation became more critical. "What is the use of finding sick and infective people," an exasperated David Stewart inquired, "if we can just wish them well and leave them as we find them?"[105] It was the same problem the issue of notification had raised in the prewar period. Paradoxically, an increase in preventive work (that is, case-finding) meant an increased demand for treatment – and treatment for all cases, advanced as well as early. For by isolating advanced cases, tuberculosis workers felt they were reducing infection of the contacts and ultimately forwarding again the work of prevention. Sanatoria, it was argued, were thus an essential part of the campaign to *prevent* the disease.

By 1925 all DSCR facilities had been returned to the provinces or voluntary associations owning the original buildings. Now every properly equipped sanatorium had laboratory, x-ray, dental, surgical, and heliotherapy facilities administered under separate departments, and they were staffed by surgeons, pathologists, radiologists, ear, eye, nose, and throat specialists, dentists, and technicians, as well as chest physicians and nurses. Since most patients were confined to their beds (95 percent at Muskoka in 1924), sanatoria were now more properly hospitals. They had observation areas to evaluate and test patients before assigning them to a ward. The Lake Edward Sanatorium in Quebec even had a movie theatre.[106]

Sanatorium architecture changed to reflect this altered role. Beginning with Gravenhurst, infirmaries were constructed with beds not facing the light but parallel to it; this arrangement enabled patients to study more comfortably (which was important with increasing emphasis on occupational therapy), and set-back verandahs were built at the Mountain Sanatorium to take advantage of the summer sunshine, so important in heliotherapy.

The sanatorium was, however, more than a nursing home or hospital for tuberculous patients – it was a referral centre as well. General practitioners began to send doubtful or complex cases there for diagnosis, while the sanatorium staff, seeing the benefits of this early diagnosis and recognizing the need for an active case-finding program to unearth rural patients, ran sanatorium-based extension clinics, which increased their diagnostic work yet again. The Saskatchewan Sanatorium took 2,043 x-ray films in 1920 and 5,238 in 1924 – a rough indication of such a shift in emphasis. This increased by 28 percent again in 1927 in that province alone.[107] Cost was minimal: roughly a dollar for each person examined.[108] As a result of extension clinics, sanatorium follow-up work increased, not only to aid in evaluating the success of the sanatorium treatment but more pragmatically to prevent relapses.

The sanatorium's most important role, many sanatorium workers rather idealistically believed, was as a teaching centre. The superintendent of the Manitoba Sanatorium ranked that institution's work, in order of descending importance, as teaching, diagnosis, and treatment. Theoretically, it taught patients about hygienic living and taking the cure, doctors about differential diagnosis, nurses about care, and the public about the disease in general. It was to be "the University of Tuberculosis in the community it serves, a place for research, for study, for instruction."[109] In this way sanatorium directors allied themselves not with the general practitioners or community physicians caring for individual patients but with the administrators, bureaucrats, and academics increasingly directing public health in Canada.

Since most sanatorium workers were now viewing the sanatorium as an instrument not only of treatment but also of prevention, this attitude became increasingly popular; for one of the primary tools of preventive medicine was education. And since the sanatoria had the knowledgeable specialists, it was obviously their duty, through affiliations with nursing and medical schools and with extension clinics and public lectures, to spread this knowledge to all. "To diagnose is good," commented Stewart, reflecting this anointed role as professional manager, "but to teach diagnosis is better. To treat and to cure are good, but still better is to teach the principles of treatment cure. To check disease in a few earlier cases is good; but to spread widely abroad a knowledge of prevention of disease and of the laws of health – that is better."[110]

## The Paradox of Prevention and Bed Shortages

The emphasis on prevention created a paradoxical problem by the end of the decade: an acute bed shortage. When the soldiers had vacated the sanatoria in the immediate postwar period, many had found themselves with excess beds, but the emphasis on rest along with aggressive case-finding, including travelling and extension clinics and examination of contacts, soon filled them and left long waiting lists. Viewed in a cynical sense, then, the emphasis on rest may, initially, have been unconsciously self-serving. The construction programs could not keep pace – a new hundred-bed building erected by the Tranquille Sanatorium, supposed to prevent overcrowding for years, was soon occupied and a waiting list again started so that cases originally diagnosed as early were moderately advanced on admission.[111]

The superintendent maintained that this problem was also due to an increased readiness on the part of the public to go the sanatorium – by 1930, he rarely encountered individuals who refused treatment, a common occurrence at the beginning of the decade. Beds available in general hospitals did little to alleviate the problem. It was discouraging and frustrating for the tuberculosis workers, for beds were the key: "beds for treatment, observation, for segregation; even beds to die in, so that family and friends may not suffer from the last fatal seed scattering from the tuberculous deathbed." Beds, in other words, for everyone: suspect, active, and hopeless. "Our worst problems," Stewart lamented, "are really the problems of trying to struggle along without beds."[112]

Like their industrial counterparts in the interwar period, sanatoria had become "big business." The federal government had expanded their facilities in a fashion undreamt of before the war and had set the pace for provincially and voluntarily raised capital investment throughout the twenties. The Royal Ottawa Sanatorium was worth

$600,000 by 1926,[113] while the new laundry building alone built that same year at the Mountain Sanatorium cost $98,000.[114] The new sanatorium built by the Saskatchewan government at Prince Albert in 1930 had 206 beds and cost an impressive $1.5 million. In 1927 the estimated replacement value of institutions to treat pulmonary tuberculosis in Canada was approximately $14.5 million.[115]

The per capita cost fell gradually throughout the twenties. At the Tranquille Sanatorium, for example, the total gross per capita cost (with slight fluctuations) went from $1,429.85 in 1921–22 to $1,364.24 in 1927–28;[116] while the average stay for each patient increased as one moved west: in 1927 it was 300 days at Laval Hospital in Quebec, 321 at Muskoka, 347 in Manitoba, 374 in Saskatoon, and 438 in British Columbia.[117] This pattern suggested either a greater number of advanced and incurable cases or better financial support. The provinces and municipalities were paying more of the cost of accommodation: Robert Wodehouse, CTA executive secretary, reported in 1928 that while the Nova Scotia Sanatorium had a discouraging 75 percent of its patients treated at their own or friends' expense and that while New Brunswick's Jordan Memorial Sanatorium had 52 percent, Quebec's Laurentian Sanatorium 38 percent, and the St John County Hospital 30 percent, every other Canadian institution had only 21 percent or fewer. In other words, at least 80 percent of the patients in most Canadian sanatoria were funded by provincial and municipal governments and voluntary donations by 1930.[118]

There seemed to be a direct correlation between the number of available beds, the number of indigents treated, and the tuberculosis death rate. Saskatchewan, with the lowest death rate in the country, cared for 78 percent of patients at the expense of the province and municipalities by 1929. The number of patients treated for every 1,000 advanced cases was even more striking: Quebec had the lowest number with 114.6, while Saskatchewan had 1,177.6[119] To the tuberculosis specialists, these statistics were irrefutable proof that an effective campaign needed an adequate supply of beds maintained at public expense.

Sanatorium management itself caused controversy. Three provinces – Alberta, British Columbia, and Nova Scotia – operated their sanatoria directly under a government department; three others – New Brunswick, Saskatchewan, and Manitoba (and, eventually, Prince Edward Island) – operated under a lay committee or commission partly appointed by the government and partly by other representative means; while the remaining institutions, including those of Victoria, Vancouver, Halifax, Winnipeg, and St John, operated under city or separate voluntary boards. The question was: which method was more effective? Although Nova Scotia ran a provincial institution, 75 percent of the patients supported themselves or were supported by their friends, which defeated the purpose and, Wodehouse believed, was a prime cause of that province's dismal death rate, for indigents with their many contacts went untreated. To add insult to injury, the Nova Scotia government actually spent more than most sanatoria on a per capita basis – roughly $1,000 a bed each year, in addition to all the patients' fees collected. Finally, in defiance of the efficiency and organizational principles promoted generally in the period, anti-TB staff in that province were not even coordinated under the same minister: the nurses' work and education were supervised by the Nova Scotia Tuberculosis Commission, while the diagnosticians were under the health department.

In keeping with scientific management ideals infused with a healthy dose of voluntarism, Wodehouse, like many, believed a sanatorium management committee was the most efficient form of organization. As Saskatchewan and Manitoba demonstrated, such a committee could run an institution, conduct travelling clinics, and coordinate nurses' activities; and it could use the same personnel for follow-up work, case-finding, home supervision, and educational work, making the tuberculosis control program cohesive and comprehensive. It did not conflict with government, since it carried out government policy and reported yearly to the minister of health. Based on an overriding philosophy of organization, professionalism, and specialization, the secretary of the CTA maintained that health departments were not organized to administer institutions – they were instead the "sanitary police to enforce observance of Health Acts and formulate new statutes to meet new and changing conditions and carry on education."[120]

A more mercenary consideration was that the public rarely made bequests to government projects. A committee, then, would "humanize" the program and treatment of patients and, to attract public support, keep its activities in the public eye by pioneering new programs. The role of a voluntary committee, then, according to one of the more influential anti-TB fighters, was that of a manager. Funded by a province and under its control, it exercised authority through its lay and professional volunteers and independent professional staff, *not* public officials; it controlled first an institution and, by extension, the anti-TB campaign in general.

## A Medical, Not a Social, Disease

By the thirties, with the technical, specialized methods now in vogue to arrest the disease, the social reform home treatment with its emphasis on "milk, eggs, and the back verandah" was considered dangerously obsolete. Technology, especially surgery, had increased to such an extent that, ironically, the superintendent of the Mountain Sanatorium even advised that a separate medical service be established in every large sanatorium to bring the different departments into contact with one another and to manage cases that were neglected because they were no one person's responsibility.[121] Thus, burgeoning accommodation began to create a problem early anti-TB campaigners would never have thought to consider: keeping close personal contact with the patients. With sanatoria now departmentalized for greater efficiency and accommodating hundreds of patients each, a few specialists were beginning to worry that the patients were getting lost in the shuffle. Increased specialization and the use of surgery led, in turn, to a demand for more staff, which increased costs. By 1937, with 8,500 beds in the country, roughly $7 million a year was spent on sanatorium maintenance alone, most of it from public funds.[122]

"There is one specific for tuberculosis and only one – prevention," insisted the medical superintendent of the Essex County Sanatorium in 1934, reflecting the views of most of his associates, "and the most powerful weapon in the battle against infection is *segregation*."[123] Ferguson noted that the rate of infection fell faster than mortality in communities having a large proportion of active cases institutionalized, which seemed to indicate that the value of sanatoria lay not so much in lowering the death rate by their cures as in lowering the infection rate by segregation and isolation.[124] It was logical, specialists reasoned now, as well as humanitarian, to give those with the worst disease (the most infectious) first preference. This attitude was a complete about-face from the prewar period, when sanatorium superintendents had concentrated on trying to accommodate early cases and excluding others. Now all cases had to be treated in an institution – the early cases because such treatment benefitted the individual and cost the state less, and the advanced cases because it protected the community. In addition to its role as a hospital, the sanatorium served the same function as a leprosarium: for tuberculosis, like leprosy, would eventually be eradicated by the isolation and control of infection.[125]

Pressure on available accommodation and the expense of hospitalizing patients in sanatoria brought another problem to the attention of the specialists – that of dealing with the chronic, incurable patient who did not need anything other than board and lodging and the noninfectious patient who, while recovering, required only convalescent care. The depression aggravated the situation, and sanatorium superintendents complained bitterly that they were forced to keep these "maximum benefit" cases tying up beds, at needless expense, because they had nowhere else to go. In 1931 the Royal Ottawa Sanatorium reported a turnover barely exceeding one patient per year, due to advanced admissions and the gradual accumulation of chronic incurables. This problem was made more acute in Ontario, where the payment of mothers' allowance was often contingent on isolation and institutional treatment.

To move patients out of the sanatoria more quickly, artificial pneumothorax to make patients noninfectious was emphasized, together with the establishment of refill centres and the training of general practitioners to give these refills. Again, there were unexpected consequences. Since provincial and municipal governments were together paying for most maintenance costs by the thirties, most were reluctant to risk the added responsibility and expense of caring for noninfectious patients. In fact, exploiting the preventive no-infection rhetoric, some tried to dodge the problem completely – in 1939 the tuberculosis division of the British Columbia government announced that the only patients to be admitted for treatment were those for whom an element of tuberculosis control existed. Nonpulmonary patients were abandoned as a result of this ruling. It was an inhuman result of concern for the community, made at the expense of the individual.

*The Depression*

The depression brought the general issue of health and welfare to a head in the thirties, but considering the social upheaval and inadequate social services, it had less of an effect on the sanatoria than might have been expected. Existing services were largely maintained, rather than cut back wholesale – although there was some decrease, notably in Manitoba, where the public health nursing service was drastically reduced.[126] There was, understandably, a greater demand for public beds and free clinics, and the sanatoria who depended on paying patients for their revenue obviously suffered most. In 1933, the Calydor Sanatorium (a private institution) reported a third fewer patients than the year before, while the Laurentian Sanatorium reported a 30 percent drop in revenue in 1931, and then again in 1932.[127] Provincially funded institutions found the growing number of indigent patients a burden. However, the falling price of commodities lessened the effects of the depression on the sanatoria. This decline, combined with staff reductions and a stringent control of expenses, enabled most sanatoria to continue operating at the same level or, occasionally, with lower costs and increasing government support, to extend their services. Only Quebec complained in 1932 that it was impossible to increase the number of beds due to the Depression.[128]

The depression, in a more general way, served to highlight how far the specialists now directing the tuberculosis campaign had come from the concerns of the prewar social reformers. They were fully aware of the implications of widespread poverty and unemployment – yet they left the problem of relief and social reform to other pressure groups and organizations. Instead of involving themselves *as a group* in large-scale relief work to prevent disease, they concentrated their energies on eliminating sources of infection by isolation, segregation, and collapse therapy. The medical superintendent of the Central Alberta Sanatorium unconsciously reflected this preoccupation when he observed in 1931 that "presumably the present economic depression is having its effect on the health of many. Just as the deaths increase, so will the source of infection to the balance of our population, and it would appear reasonable to expect a greater need of sanatorium beds."[129] Beds and surgery – they were the two specifics. More and more, specialists left social service and relief work to professional social workers, volunteers, and the state. Although concerned as individuals, the depression demonstrated very clearly that, as a group, they did not consider this work part of their job.

### Education: Lay and Professional

The lay public still had to be educated to take full advantage of the new scientific knowledge, and the public, specialists were now well aware, learned slowly. The futility of passing a law such as an antispitting ordinance or notification if the majority did not understand the motive for it or the importance of obeying it they had learned first hand in the prewar era. Science had advanced so rapidly that, as the superintendent of the Mountain Sanatorium pointed out, it was no wonder people took "short cuts to health" with patent medicines.[130]

To promote tuberculosis education, the standard methods continued to be used, with material frequently borrowed from the American national TB association. (This approach also reflected the more general influence of American trade and culture in the interwar period.) By 1928, the Canadian association seemed to be papering the country: it was sending out 9 million posterettes annually, one set for every student in every school in every province, with each set to be used as a subject for a health lesson by the teacher and a composition by the pupil. By 1929 this number had increased to 16 million.[131]

The professionals also had to be educated about the disease. By the end of the decade, most Canadian medical schools recognized that their students needed more practical experience than they were acquiring in the general hospitals, and they sent them to either local clinics or sanatoria for a few weeks or even a few months. The travelling clinics theoretically helped train the general practitioners, for reports of the diagnostician's examinations and conclusion were sent to the patient's physician, who was encouraged to examine the patient again to verify the specialist's findings. This practice offered informal "postgraduate studies in tuberculosis," as the superintendent of the Mountain Sanatorium hopefully termed it.[132]

Like doctors, nurses also needed practical training in tuberculosis; as R.G. Ferguson observed in 1925, "At present, unfortunately, the graduate nurses of general hospitals know merely enough of tuberculosis to be mortally afraid of it and to want to keep away from it. The principal result emanating from instruction of these schools is phthisophobia. A few months experience in a sanatorium would dissipate this traditional fear."[133] In response, general hospitals slowly began sending their student nurses for training periods of several months at the sanatoria, and public health nursing courses were organized in the universities, so that by 1930, 36 percent of the 1,521 nurses engaged in public health work in Canada had taken at least a one-year postgraduate course in public health nursing at a recognized university.[134] Along with the physicians, nurses were becoming more specialized.

What were the results of all these years of education? The results were difficult, if not impossible, to assess. It was rather discouraging, for example, that after years of antispitting bylaws, the tuberculosis division of the Greater Vancouver Health League was still harping on the problem, while the city health department obligingly stenciled prohibitions on the pavement.[135] It was yet one more example of the uselessness of legislation when it was not supported by public opinion; and Grant Fleming probably came closest to the truth when he observed rather cynically in a Canadian medical booklet that "Spitting is an unpleasant habit. Spitting will continue until such time as it is forbidden by social custom. People do not put their knives in their mouths any longer because such a method of eating is frowned upon."[136] Others were more optimistic. The Quebec Committee reported that nine thousand more consultations and ten thousand more x-rays were done in 1939 and attributed this fact solely to the educational campaign.[137]

The only formal survey of public awareness was a 1939 American Gallup Poll published in the CTA Bulletin that revealed a fair amount of confusion among the general public: 76 percent of those polled believed tuberculosis to be "contagious," and 52 percent thought it was inherited – but only 18 percent believed germs to be the principal cause of the disease. "How else than by germs, demand a baffled *Bulletin* writer, "does the remaining 58 percent think a disease can be 'caught'?"[138] Although taken in the United States, Canadian specialists, interestingly, saw the poll as a valuable guide to Canadian public attitudes.

*From a Social Disease with a Medical Aspect*
*to a Medical Disease with a Social Aspect*

The twenties have been much maligned as a conservative, self-seeking decade, one in which " Canadians searched for normality rather than novelty," and one that "witnessed the general decline of the progressive spirit which had previously buoyed up many a reform movement."[139] Although this dictum might be true of some aspects of urban reform, it would be a mistake to apply it wholesale to all spheres of prewar social reform activity – for it was certainly not true in the field of tuberculosis or, most likely, in public health in general. The objectives and underpinnings of the anti-TB campaign differed in a crucial way from those of other social reform causes – most notably prohibition and women's suffrage. Inspired by the social gospel, their ultimate purpose had been to create a better society, with crime, disease, and social injustice eliminated. When such a utopian society did not occur and specific social reforms failed to be universal panaceas, disillusionment set in; the reforms were discredited and the social gospel experienced a profound crisis by 1928.[140] This crisis, as Ramsay Cook argues convincingly, may have ultimately resulted, in turn, from the manner in which prewar intellectuals had confronted the challenge of Darwinian science and "regenerated" their religion by focusing on God's Kingdom on Earth. Although stemming the crisis in the short term, such a solution led inevitably to further secularization in Canadian Society.[141]

The anti-TB workers had supported various social reform causes to improve society, but their ultimate objective was the creation of a healthy, disease-free nation. Thus, the expected *result* of most social reform demands – a better society – was only a means to an end and would lead to a *further* result: the eradication of tuberculosis and perfect health for Canadians. For those involved in the anti-TB crusade, this goal was included in the definition of a better society, but it was also a result or an extension of it. Therefore, when the utopian society the prewar social reformers envisioned failed to materialize and the moral fervour of the social gospel dissipated, those interested in the anti-TB cause simply turned to other means – clinics, travelling diagnosticians, surgery, x-rays, increasing isolation of patients – and, using a technological and community-oriented approach, concentrated specifically on the germ to achieve *the same goal*: eliminating the disease and promoting good health.

Nor did the anti-TB movement experience the opposition within the community (from veterans, the working class, and residents of the cities) that helped defeat prohibition.[142] It was difficult, after all, to oppose something that worked to rid the country of a debilitating disease that had caused so much suffering and human misery. Moreover, there was no alternative to dealing with the problem of disease analogous to government control of the sale of liquor, which dealt with the abuses of alcohol. The prohibitory measures that prewar reformers had demanded, notably antispitting measures and notification, were but a minor part of the campaign in the twenties, which instead concentrated on discovering the disease, protecting the community, and treating the individual. The anti-TB movement was therefore more positive in its approach and less restrictive of individual action, and it lacked the somewhat oppressive morality of prohibition. In fact, because the anti-TB campaign did not succeed in eradicating the disease in the way the prohibition movement and women's suffrage succeeded in obtaining their demands, it did not have the problem of continuing to defend and enforce much prohibitory legislation or of maintaining the zeal of its members. Finally, the veterans, who had helped defeat prohibition, aided the anti-TB cause – not only by causing the federal government to add to existing facilities for their treatment but by setting an example for civilian care.

As a result, while other social reform causes were undergoing a profound crisis in the twenties, public health in general and the anti-TB movement in particular retained much of the urgency and sense of purpose inspired in the prewar period by the social gospel, and they were given, in addition, a new impetus by the war and the influenza epidemic, which heightened Canadians' awareness of the value of health. Paradoxically, the decline in the influence of traditional religion and the failure of the social gospel to continue its momentum may actually have strengthened the anti-TB campaign. A vacuum had been created with the secularization of Canadian society – and it was science, in all its figurative and literal, and philosophical and technical manifestations that filled the gap. Fighting an indubitably bacteriological disease with progressively more scientific methods, the anti-TB movement was simultaneously altered and supported by the changing intellectual climate.

By 1928, when, Richard Allen maintains, "crisis had overtaken all major phases of the social gospel,"[143] a federal department of health had been created; the insurance companies were supporting educational demonstrations in the Maritimes and Quebec; Saskatchewan municipalities were demanding the extension of free treatment to all residents; health units were being established in rural areas; travelling diagnosticians were uncovering more cases of tuberculosis; and lay volunteers, through the growing number of service clubs, were supporting the anti-TB cause through the Christmas Seal sale, which had just been organized on a national basis the year before. Unlike other social reform causes, the anti-TB crusade was able, therefore, to change and adapt its methods and sometimes shift its focus but to retain its ultimate goal and deal with the new Canada anti-TB workers and other social reformers had done a large part in creating.

The decline of the anti-urban bias, for example, which affected prohibition, failed to harm the anti-TB cause. Tuberculosis specialists instead concentrated their energies in a new and relatively undeveloped field: the rural areas. The cities, by and large, had achieved a modicum of sanitation and improved standards of living, while in contrast the rural areas still lacked even the most rudimentary health services. The war had elevated the concept of state responsibility for its citizens' health from a benefit to a right in the minds of health workers, and this concept, combined with the inability and disinclination of rural municipalities to finance or run a comprehensive scheme of health care, forced the provinces to act.

Mirroring developments elsewhere in Canadian society, notably in the new resource-based industries, the interwar period witnessed increasing provincial involvement, both in supervision and financial support, and a corresponding relinquishing of authority by the federal government. The provinces, once they found themselves paying, at least in part, for maintenance of tuberculosis patients in sanatoria, realized that to prevent costs from rising uncontrollably, they would have to ensure isolation of infectious cases, as well as adequate diagnosis and prevention. The most natural place to start was the disorganized, unhealthy rural areas – so county health units and travelling clinics were established.

With the decline of the social gospel, the twenties also witnessed, as we have seen, a more bacteriological approach to the disease (focusing on the germ as the primary cause), along with the growth in technology and specialized methods of treatment and the takeover of the direction of the campaign by the specialists. They were generally sanatorium physicians or employees of one of the voluntary agencies, educational demonstrations, commissions, or committees, and they began to determine policy, direct initiative, and even apportion funds. As a result, amateur lay volunteers now started to funnel their energies through the service clubs, and a division of labour was established that would hold for the next two decades. The local Rotary and Kiwanis clubs would run the Christmas Seal sale and raise funds, which they would turn over to specialists – often a sanatorium superintendent or travelling diagnostician – to use for a specific purpose. Their role, though critical, became submerged by the government and para-official agencies assuming authority. This development, too, was merely a reflection of the underlying principles of efficient scientific management and organization.

It is misleading to say that reform died – in tuberculosis work it became organized, specialized, and businesslike, but hardly moribund. Many of the prewar goals – local pasteurization, antispitting laws, and the erection of sanatoria – had been achieved. Now tuberculosis workers, with government help, systematically surveyed the field and began to attack the problem where it was worst – in rural areas – and where the disease was most often found – among contacts. Meanwhile sanatoria and clinics regularly increased their facilities and extended their influence. The federal government had funded the expansion of sanatoria during the war – now the insurance companies, the Rockefeller Foundation, and the Red Cross pumped money into prevention and educational demonstrations to encourage the people to demand a comprehensive state-run health program as a right.

It was a period of education, organization, specialization, and cooperation, although it lacked the heady enthusiasm and idealism of the social reform era – after all, Canadians had come through not only a world war but a world-wide influenza epidemic. Anti-TB workers consolidated the gains they had made in the prewar period and, with persistent determination, began altering an "incoherent, isolated and individualistic" campaign, that subsequently developed into "a rounded-out plan for the application of conscious, systematic health control."[144] They were doing more work – but their very organization, ironically enough, tended to mask it. This was especially true of volunteer efforts – when only volunteers had been in the field, they had been much more noticeable, even though their work might have been isolated and sketchy. Now, with increasing government involvement, volunteer efforts were almost easy to overlook.

The thirties began with a depression and ended with a world war. Despite the fears of many tuberculosis specialists, much was achieved during that troubled decade, while the patterns begun in the twenties were more firmly established. The depression brought the problem of an inadequate maintenance system relying on municipal support to a head, and with the example of Saskatchewan to follow, ironically enough, others slowly began to extend free treatment to their residents, so that by 1939 tuberculosis treatment was virtually free in Ontario, Alberta, British Columbia, and Manitoba. The federal government was left to assume the responsibility for aboriginal health care and for extending the grants-in-aid that the provinces were demanding, but it would have no real authority over health care policy, which remained a provincial prerogative.

Eliminating infection became the focus of the campaign, and, with increasing state support, tuberculosis workers concentrated on the individual as *a member of the community*, not an isolated victim. "More beds" was still the unceasing cry, but for a somewhat different purpose – no longer were sanatoria erected or extended solely because they were the most effective means of curing an individual but because they isolated a source of infection. As a result, techniques such as artificial pneumothorax and examinations of contacts, which reduced infection, achieved a new importance.

Even more important was the shift in attitude that had begun ten years before and was highlighted by the depression. David Stewart's dictum that to "cure poverty, we must first cure disease" reflected the outlook of many of his associates.[145] The specialists energetically attacked the disease throughout this decade at what they perceived to be its fundamental source: the germ. They left the problem of social and living conditions to other relief organizations, interested individuals, and professional social workers. By the thirties tuberculosis, which Osler had once deemed a social disease with a medical aspect had become a medical disease with a social aspect.

A stock-taking at the end of the decade found results generally encouraging. Although the problem of accommodation and financing treatment still had to be solved in the Maritimes and particularly Quebec, Saskatchewan not only had enough beds but was finding fewer active cases. There were over ten thousand sanatorium beds – almost two for every annual death – in the country;[146] the problem of childhood tuberculosis had been reduced to a minor concern; bovine tuberculosis was gradually being eliminated; the rate of infection in adolescents was falling; more cases were discovered earlier; and individuals were beginning to fall prey to the disease at a later age. By 1938, 48 percent of the new cases discovered in Saskatchewan were incipient.[147] But there was a new concern: unprotected youths, such as nurses, with no resistance, who were unwittingly exposed to disease. The issue of rehabilitation still had to be dealt with. Moreover, the optimistic predictions of public health workers that the elimination of tuberculosis, the scourge of youth, would increase the average lifespan was not being borne out by the facts: although the expectation of life at birth had increased over the past generation, the expectation of life for those over forty had not.[148] Cancer and heart disease were killing increasing numbers of people. It was, as one discouraged authority observed, "somewhat of an anti-climax," rather like a game in which "we pile up encouraging points in the first period, only to lose them before the onslaught of our adversary in the last period."[149]

By the end of the decade, the anti-TB campaigners believed they had much to be proud of, and still more to do. The tuberculosis death rate was falling, and the provinces and municipalities were shouldering, albeit sometimes reluctantly, an increasing amount of the burden. And responsibilities had been defined and a pattern established that would hold for the following decades. David Stewart nicely summed up the pragmatic attitude of cautious optimism, determination, and realism with which the anti-TB campaigners sailed into the forties: "We have not won our war; we have just been skirmishing for position. We are not done; we are just nicely ready to begin. We have not solved the problem; we have just tried a few experiments. We have spent millions in patching. Now we are about ready to begin preventing ... we have succoured damaged travellers with food and sun and maintained them at the inn, but now it is time to get out and police the road from Jerusalem to Jericho."[150]

As the country mobilized for World War 2, another technological breakthrough was occurring in South America that would revolutionize the preventive campaign in Canada: the development of a cheap, miniature x-ray film. The result was that while the campaign in the thirties had concentrated on selected suspects to eliminate disease, the forties would witness mass surveys of the whole population.

# 4 The Interwar Years:
## The Changing Role of Volunteers

I gradually developed and introduced into all his charities the principles of scientific giving, and he found himself in no long time laying aside retail giving almost wholly, and entering safely and pleasurably into the field of wholesale philanthropy.

Frederick T. Gates, advisor to John D. Rockefeller

[M]an comes to see that the science of business is the science of human service. He comes to see that he profits most who serves his fellows best.

Arthur F. Sheldon,
addressing the Association of Rotary Clubs, 1910

With increasing government support for and involvement in health care, it was only natural that attention would continue to focus on the role of volunteer societies. In the prewar period volunteer health work had been "of necessity incoherent, isolated and individualistic";[1] the twenties found volunteer societies becoming more organized, more specialized, and better funded. They were also criticized – especially the lay volunteers themselves. With the tuberculosis campaign directed more and more by specialists such as sanatorium and department of health physicians, lay workers were sometimes faulted for inadequate knowledge and overlapping work, and they were accused of expending funds unnecessarily. For many public health advocates, government control was necessary to obtain the organized administration, expert advice, provision, and care that were beyond the scope of the private citizen; and the Montreal Anti-Tuberculosis and General Health League probably reflected prevailing opinion when it observed in 1925 that "the function of a voluntary health agency such as ours is to assist in developing a public opinion which will first create a demand for, and second, enable the municipal authorities to undertake a reasonable health program; for it is our understanding that

Health is a responsibility of the State, and, therefore, a voluntary-health agency has a place in assisting, but not in relieving the State of its health responsibilities."[2]

Volunteer agencies, as Peter Dobkin Hall has pointed out, were privately organized to act in the public sphere and were "concerned with assertions of moral power, the discovery of arguments most fitted to act upon the majority, and hopes of drawing over the majority to their own side ... They are, in sum, the sources of moral authority that govern the direction of public life."[3] Volunteers were the "free irregulars, formerly so common in war," according to the chief medical officer of New Brunswick, while the government authorities were "the mobilized and disciplined force whose only business it [was] to combat the onset of disease and the habits of improper living."[4]

"It is with the laity," the New Brunswick minister of health had stated in 1924, "that the success of any public health movement rests";[5] but as the governor-general, Byng of Vimy, commented that same year, with specialists directing anti-TB efforts, it was sometimes difficult to know "what an ordinary, mere layman can do."[6] To say, as the one-time secretary of the CTA did, that government needed the moral support of volunteer agencies and educated public opinion was all very well, but what precisely did that statement mean in concrete terms? What were laymen to do?

The old prewar style of voluntarism still operated: the IODE maintained preventoria, and various anti-TB leagues, and women's auxiliaries provided relief and supported summer camps, dental work, visiting nurses, and open-air classrooms. But relief work was done more often by specialized relief groups, and the plethora of small, local anti-TB associations seemed to be thinning out. There was the odd complaint that "reform was dead" and an occasional plea to revive the old local groups – but as the secretary of the CTA, George Porter, pointed out at the association's annual meeting in 1924, the situation was not as bleak as it superficially appeared. Admittedly, out of one hundred societies organized in Canada, only twenty-five were still reporting progress. But another twenty-five percent had been transformed from tuberculosis societies into dispensaries, hospitals, and sanatoria, while others had simply changed their names. Some had merged together, like the various societies in Toronto that had become the Associated Dispensaries of that city. A full 40 percent had been organized only for a specific purpose – usually to establish a sanatorium – and had disbanded when that purpose was realized. In Saskatchewan, 20 percent of the societies had been formed to choose delegates to send to Regina to organize a provincial association and erect a sanatorium. The same was true of Alberta, while in British

Columbia, societies had been organized to assist the Tranquille Sanatorium with grants of money. The rationale for their existence disappeared when the provincial government took over the institution.[7]

The volunteer societies that had evolved during the social reform era and World War 1 would undergo profound changes in the interwar period. Like Canadian society in general, and probably influenced by it, they would manifest many of the same themes that were rooted in the prewar period and now flowering in the political and economic spheres: specialization, scientific management, and efficient administration and organization. Three types of voluntary organizations took centre stage in postwar Canada, each in its own way an outgrowth of the prewar urban reform movement, yet each reflecting a particular focus and expertise: the philanthropic foundation, most significantly the Rockefeller Foundation; the large-scale voluntary association, such as the Canadian Tuberculosis Association; and the service clubs – the Rotary clubs, the Kiwanis, and the Kinsmen. In both synergistic and conflicting ways, all would alter the anti-TB campaign.

*Philanthropic Foundations*

As described by F. Emerson Andrews, a philanthropic foundation is a nongovernmental and nonprofit foundation; it has a principal fund of its own, is managed by its own trustees and directors, and is established to maintain or aid social, educational, charitable, religious, or other activities serving the common welfare.[8] Since the Rockefeller Foundation became the most prominent and influential example of such an institution in public health, both in Canada and the United States, it deserves discussion in detail. Its origins and development reflect many of the social and political changes current in North America and account for its successful influence in Canada after the war.

The founder of Standard Oil, John D. Rockefeller, Sr (1839–1937), has been simultaneously vilified as the most rapacious, cruel, and corrupt of the great nineteenth century robber barons and lauded as a great philanthropist. Raised a strict Baptist, he gave a portion of his income monthly to charity, with his gifts increasing as his wealth accumulated. In the 1870s and 1880s his gift-giving was haphazard, much of it related to church activities. In 1892, however, impressed with the organizational ability, energy, and shrewd business sense of a Baptist minister, Frederick T. Gates, he hired him to become his principal advisor in both business and philanthropy. Over the next two decades Gates, who, as Rockefeller himself later noted, had the social gospel "passion to accomplish some great and far-reaching benefits to mankind,"[9] combined with the reform era's belief in efficiency and organization, formulated a policy based "on the principles of scientific giving" whereby the old-fashioned "retail charity," whose purpose was to ameliorate a specific problem, was abandoned for a new institutionalized "wholesale charity", in which suffering was to be prevented rather than ameliorated. Among the new, institutionalized charities, the Institute for Medical Research was established in 1901, followed in 1903 by the General Education Board, the Sanitary Commission in 1909 (to eradicate hookworm in the southern states), and the Rockefeller Foundation in 1913, with gifts totalling about $447 million.[10]

Jerome D. Greene, the secretary of the Rockefeller Foundation, outlined to a congressional commission in the United States the informal guidelines that determined funding decisions. Again, in keeping with political and economic developments in the interwar period, the guidelines emphasized centralization, efficiency, specialization, and organized management.

1  Individual charity and relief are to be excluded except as an indirect result of giving aid to other institutions.
2  Purely local institutions or enterprises are to be excluded, unless they serve as a model to others and are part of a general plan for improvement of similar institutions.
3  No gift or agency can render a permanent service unless the gift or the agency "offers the means or the occasion for evoking from the community its own recognition of the need to be met, its own will to meet that need, and its own resources, both material and spiritual, wherewith to meet it."
4  When giving, to make the community responsible, the Foundation will assume less than half the cost of expenditures.
5  The Foundation will avoid gifts in perpetuity.
6  "As between objects which are of an immediately remedial or alleviatory nature, such as asylums for the orphan, blind or cripples, and those which go to the root of individual or social ill-being and misery, the latter objects are preferred – not that the former are unworthy, but because the latter are more far-reaching in their effects."[11]

Such thinking clearly would inspire unrelated philanthropic organizations in the interwar Canadian anti-TB campaign – particularly the Canadian Life Insurance Officers Association.

Between 1917 and 1928 the Rockefeller Foundation spent $40 million in grants to improve and promote medical education and science in Europe, Canada, and the United States, $10 million for hygiene and public health schools in the United States, and $3.7 million on research fellowships.[12] Beginning in 1916, as "a partner, but not a patron,"[13] the Rockefeller Foundation's International Health Board, under Wycliffe Rose, a philosophy professor, not an MD, undertook the development and support of county health organizations in the United States – work that would be extended to Canada in the twenties. Not content to eliminate a particular disease such as TB, Rose's goal was to convince states and nations to erect a permanent infrastructure to take care of all public health. Previous study had shown the local county generally to be the most effective unit of organization to provide health protection to rural residents. Therefore, each county demonstration unit was provided with a full-time minimum staff of a physician as health officer, a sanitary inspector, a public health nurse, and an office assistant. The county paid 50 percent of the cost, and the balance was provided by the state board of health and the International Health Board, with the foundation withdrawing its support once the unit had proven itself successful. "Demonstrations in which the authorities do not participate to a substantial degree from the inception of the project," Rose observed, "are not likely to be successful. The county must be sufficiently interested to risk something, to follow the plan critically, to take over the cost of the work gradually but steadily, and within a reasonable period to assume the entire burden of direction and expense."[14]

In 1917 the International Health Board accepted an invitation from the French government to help stem the alarming wartime increase in tuberculosis. Basing its approach on a successful campaign against hookworm, a preliminary statistical survey was made to determine the prevalence of the disease, dispensaries were established, and popular and professional education was carried out. Revealingly, this was "not an impertinent importation of scientific knowledge into the land of Louis Pasteur" but a "demonstration of method" and "organized teamplay."[15] And beginning in 1928 the foundation began a broad international investigation of the epidemiology of TB using both tuberculin testing and mobile x-ray units in rural and urban surveys.[16]

### The Rockefeller Foundation and Quebec

Funded by the Rockefeller Foundation, Quebec began in 1926 to attack the rural health problem with a system that would be adopted by three other provinces by 1930: the county health unit. As in the United States, counties or townships were organized into health units under provincial supervision, each with its own full-time medical director, public health nurses, sanitary inspector, and clerk. The doctor's duties included public lectures, educational talks to mothers, control of infectious diseases, and school inspection; the nurses examined school children, instructed teachers about hygiene, and visited homes, while the sanitary inspector helped enforce the laws regarding water supplies, sewage, and quarantine.[17] After 1928 – the same year the foundation began specific TB surveys in the United States – Quebec began incorporating travelling tuberculosis diagnosticians (with follow-up work done by the district nurse) into this system, with twenty-three units operating by 1930. These units, which included four full-time and six part-time tuberculosis clinicians, covered nearly half the rural population and cost $291,000 annually.[18] In keeping with Rose's ideology, the system was a general, comprehensive attack on rural health problems whose goal was to educate people to improve living conditions, protect infants and children, aid in eliminating preventable diseases, and lower the tuberculosis rate.

It was discouraging work for Quebec diagnosticians. By 1930 clinics were often indifferently advertised and poorly attended by lung patients, since tuberculosis was still considered a shameful disease in rural Quebec. Most visitors attended the clinic out of curiosity and to obtain a free x-ray examination, and, under the pretext of education, clinicians had to examine all visitors, sometimes late into the evening, risking harmful doses of radiation from their rudimentary x-ray machines. It was ironic that Quebec, with a sorry public health record in its largest urban centre, should be the pioneer in this aspect of rural health.[19] By 1929 British Columbia had four clinics in operation, and Saskatchewan had just established one, while Alberta instituted a travelling clinic that included a surgeon, dentist, and two nurses. Ontario and New Brunswick, although they had no units, per se, had health districts under full-time health officers.

Such units were not cheap. Alphonse Lessard, the director of the provincial bureau of health, reported that Quebec spent $12,000 on each one, of which half was provincial money and half was collected from the local municipalities; while F.C. Middleton, the deputy minister of the Saskatchewan department of public health, estimated that it would cost that province $14,000, with half that sum paid by the municipalities.[20] The clinics thus not only marked the first serious commitment to rural health on the part of the provinces but symbolized more generally provincial assumption of responsibility for Canadians' health. The municipal contribution ensured that rate-payers supported and valued the unit system, while provincial funding was recognition that a rural population, despite its needs, lacked the means to organize or finance such a system alone. This was very much an extension of the philosophy of the Rockefeller Foundation, which had helped finance the first units in Quebec, British Columbia, and Saskatchewan and had volunteered to fund two districts in Alberta in 1931. The foundation contributed 25 percent for a limited time (one to three years) if the province contributed 25 to 50 percent and the municipality contributed the balance.[21] And this, in turn, again increased provincial authority in health matters.

## Demonstrations and County Health Units

The work of the Rockefeller Foundation's commission for the prevention of tuberculosis in France had shown that some kind of organization (at least a health centre or dispensary) was necessary immediately following publicity work to make that work at all effective,[22] while the foundation's work establishing county health units and an educational demonstration at Framingham, Massachusetts (financed by a $100,000 grant from the Metropolitan Life Insurance Company), demonstrated to all what could be done with proper organization and adequate funding – the latter study noted a 67 percent reduction in the tuberculosis death rate over a five-year period (1918 to 1922).[23]

As the Rockefeller Foundation had outlined, the object of a demonstration was ostensibly twofold: first, to show that a reasonable budget, properly spent, combined with extensive and constant public health work would improve health and lower the tuberculosis rate; and secondly, to educate people in the demonstration area and surrounding district about preventive medicine and hygiene. As the director of the Quebec Provincial Bureau of Health observed in connection with the Three Rivers demonstration, "What we are entitled to expect during the first years is a thorough knowledge of the situation, the tracking of nearly all cases, and education of the people for the safeguarding of their health against contagion."[24]

Following a pattern that was similar in many respects to the work of the Rockefeller Foundation with the county health units, demonstrations were established in Quebec (Three Rivers and Montreal) and in the Maritimes during the decade,[25] since the Eastern provinces had the most dismal showing in the anti-TB crusade. Earlier surveys of school children had, in a limited way, been a stock-taking of the situation – the demonstrations would include a more comprehensive survey in a defined geographic area, with various different health measures, staff, and facilities (physicians, nurses, clinics, and so on) employed for a limited time. The long-term objective was to educate people to demand this health machinery on a permanent basis. Demonstration areas were chosen specifically because they had high infant mortality rates and high tuberculosis death rates and could thus serve as impressive examples of what could be achieved with adequate organization and funding. Public health workers had realized in the prewar period that people had to be educated to demand state support, but in the twenties they began to use concrete examples of what should be done, instead of verbal exhortation, to make their point.

These demonstrations, or committees, also exhibited the postwar attitudes of cooperation and organization, combined with large-scale foundation-style financing. They were theoretically voluntary agencies, but they were semiofficial in character, in that they were efficiently organized and run by hired specialists in close cooperation with and partially funded by provincial departments of health. What differentiated them from the latter was private funding,[26] the fact that they ran for only a limited time (usually five years), and their purpose: to demonstrate, as already mentioned, the positive results of a public health program, in order to create public demand for it on a permanent basis and thus force the government to step in. This was the principle on which the Rockefeller Foundation worked so effectively.[27]

### The Red Cross

The postwar Canadian Red Cross was a rudimentary version of the foundation-style voluntary society, and it did much to establish the idea that voluntary agencies *supplemented* and inspired, but did not replace, government. With the end of the war, the Red Cross had a substantial amount of money remaining and amended its act of incorporation in Parliament in 1919 in order to aid in the prevention of disease and improve public health. One of the diseases it concentrated on was tuberculosis.

First, in an effort to organize voluntary agencies and prevent overlapping, it created an advisory and consultative committee that met with representatives of provincial departments of health and voluntary associations to define their positions and relationships to each other.[28] To demonstrate a need and create a demand for a particular service, it established departments of public health nursing for a three-year period at the universities of Toronto, British Columbia, and Dalhousie, funded extension clinics from Ontario sanatoria into twelve surrounding rural areas (for which the Ontario Red Cross gave $2,500 a year), and helped finance surveys of school children at a cost of $1,000 each across the country. Other activities included support for travelling clinics, public health nursing, and funding x-rays, sometimes, as in Prince Edward Island, in conjunction with the provincial government.[29]

The Red Cross also funded educational tuberculosis work: it provided lantern shows, awarded prizes of $250 each for clinical and laboratory research in a sanatorium, helped pay the travelling expenses of a visiting British tuberculosis expert touring Canada in 1924, as we saw earlier, and financed the printing of five anti-TB publications. By 1925, when the grants ended, the *Canadian Medical Association Journal* estimated that the Canadian Red Cross Society had put nearly $90,000 into direct financial assistance for tuberculosis work in Canada.[30]

## The Three Rivers Demonstration

The first demonstration formally labelled as such was established at Three Rivers, Quebec, in 1923, for a five-year period. A pulp, paper, and textile city of under thirty thousand, it had burgeoned recently and suffered the predictable problems of overcrowding and poor sanitation. With no available tuberculosis accommodation and no tuberculosis cases diagnosed before death, it was considered to be an ideal place for a tuberculosis demonstration.[31] Demonstrating cooperation between state and voluntary agencies, and demonstrating, as well, Rockefeller Foundation guidelines for funding, it was financed by an annual contribution of $12,500 from the provincial board, $5,000 from the Canadian Red Cross Society, $5,000 from the federal government, and $2,500 from the Sun Life Assurance Company (the last three contributions were administered through the CTA). It was run by a six-member committee presided over by the director of the Provincial Hygiene Service. Roughly one-third of the people in the Three Rivers and Cap de la Madeleine area were examined by the dispensary by 1927, including factory workers and all school children. It included tuberculosis and infant and child welfare work, and it centred around a completely outfitted dispensary under a full-time medical director with two visiting nurses. Everyone who came to the dispensary was examined free, and those with lung trouble were referred to their family doctor. Indigents were treated without charge.

Again, results seemed obvious: by 1925 the ratio of known cases to reported annual deaths had risen to 8 to 1, while the tuberculosis mortality for the five-year period before the demonstration was 124.8 per 100,000 and 97.9 after.[32] It was suggested that this could have been even lower had an adequate number of sanatoria beds been provided – and as a result the new 150-bed Cooke Sanatorium was opened in June 1930. It was this educational aspect, TB workers believed, that made the demonstration so successful – it showed the citizens and local government the value of adequate expenditures on health. The health budget of the city of Three Rivers trebled from 1923 to 1925, while it spent $60,000 on the demonstration itself, passed pasteurization and tuberculin testing laws, and erected a $300,000 filtration plant.[33]

### The Insurance Companies and Public Health

With almost identical goals and methods as the Rockefeller Foundation, another influential, organized, and wealthy group entered the Canadian public health field in the twenties: the insurance companies. In the prewar era, they had shown only a lukewarm interest by sending health literature to policyholders, but the spectacular results of the Framingham demonstration in the United States (funded, as mentioned earlier in this chapter, by the Metropolitan Life Insurance Company) and the decreasing death rate in any area that instituted a comprehensive public health program encouraged them to act with a vengeance – after all, as the *Public Health Journal* drily noted, "a lowering of the community death rate makes for the financial stability of life insurance companies."[34] Robert Wodehouse, secretary of the CTA, was blunter still when he wrote to V.R. Smith of the Canadian Life Insurance Officers Association in 1926. "It is a fact," he pointed out with irrefutable logic, "that the four provinces east of Ontario have the highest provincial death rate from tuberculosis in Canada, and twice that of Ontario, and it is true that they have at the same time the highest sickness rate from the same disease in Canada. Both these factors spell *great loss of effort* on the part of the people, *great loss to the* individual households, and great loss to insurance *companies* carrying *Health* and *Death* risk policies."[35]

### Organizing the Maritimes

As a consequence of the high rates of death from tuberculosis in the eastern provinces the Canadian Life Insurance Officers Association (CLIOA), through the CTA, began to finance demonstrations in the unhealthiest areas, and the Maritime Tuberculosis Educational Committee and the Nova Scotia Tuberculosis Commission were formed for that purpose. The companies did not stop there. Sun Life (through the CTA) gave thirty scholarships of $500 each to send salaried tuberculosis workers to Britain, France, and Italy in 1928 for postgraduate studies, and they organized a North American study tour for fifty British doctors, aided in the employment of trained, full-time travelling chest diagnosticians in Quebec, and helped finance the Three Rivers demonstration. By 1930 some companies were paying for complete and confidential examinations of their policyholders in an effort to catch disease and correct a condition early on,[36] while CLIOA, through its health committee, had become so involved in upgrading maritime health programs that it voted $75,000 to be administered through the CTA over a five-year period to create a full-time health service in Prince Edward Island.[37]

With such striking results in Quebec and with the Massachusetts-Halifax Health Commission,[38] tuberculosis workers next turned their attention more fully to the Maritimes, an area that seemed to lag behind the rest of the country in dealing with the ravages of the disease. A 1925 conference of tuberculosis workers held at Kentville, Nova Scotia, had recommended that provincially and municipally supported treatment for indigents be provided, possibly financed by the pool system, that the work of travelling diagnosticians and public health nurses be extended, and that a campaign drive for funds and educational work be carried out. In 1926 the CTA formed the Maritime Tuberculosis Educational Committee, financed by CLIOA, with $10,000 a year provided for two provinces to carry out a three-year educational program (to be extended another two years if warranted).[39] New Brunswick and Prince Edward Island were organized under a medical director with a central office at Moncton. This physician conducted chest clinics twice a year on Prince Edward Island in cooperation with the provincial Red Cross nurses, which so stimulated demand for a provincial health service that a full-time provincial health officer and chest diagnostician was appointed, a board of health formed, and a sanatorium built. CLIOA agreed to help finance this project for another five-year period. By 1931 everything except the Junior Red Cross and crippled children's work was under the supervision of the newly established provincial board of health.

In New Brunswick, a travelling chest diagnostician worked in the eastern half of the province, while the western area was covered by another diagnostician from the department of health. In 1928 the tuberculosis committee granted money to maintain both diagnosticians, and a further grant was made to finance a third operating out of the Jordan Sanatorium. These regular clinics found cases earlier and more often and, combined with the educational work of the committee, encouraged the municipalities and counties to assume more financial obligations and support more indigents. The demand for increased facilities to accommodate the newly discovered cases grew, and a children's building was added to the St John Tuberculosis Hospital, while the Jordan Sanatorium was renovated and a new infirmary with 140 beds added. The provincial government raised its per diem grant to the St John Tuberculosis Hospital to $1.00, while plans were completed for a new institution in the northern part of the province. As in Three Rivers, results were promising: in New Brunswick, the death rate from tuberculosis fell from 96.6 per 100,000 in 1926 to 84.2 in 1930.[40]

The CTA had pushed for a central, united program operating out of Moncton, but Nova Scotia refused to go along with the scheme, and instead set up its own tuberculosis commission with $10,000 provided by the provincial government and a $5,000 grant from CLIOA (administered by the CTA).[41] The commission carried out most of the anti-TB work in the province. It campaigned vigorously for more hospital accommodation for advanced cases and municipal responsibility for indigents, while the department of health directed the work of two travelling diagnosticians and, in cooperation with three commission and four county public health nurses, did the follow-up work. Sidney, Yarmouth, and Glace Bay all voted money to build tuberculosis accommodation, so that more needy cases were being supported by the municipalities in the Kentville Sanatorium by 1929. Although the $5,000 CLIOA grant ceased in 1930, anti-TB work continued. The nursing services and clinics were run under the newly formed ministry of health, and the provincial government voted $400,000 to increase bed accommodation throughout the province (including 100 extra beds at the Nova Scotia Sanatorium at Kentville).[42]

Nevertheless, the CTA was less pleased with the results in Nova Scotia than in the other two provinces. Ironically, there was still the problem of accommodating indigents in the provincial sanatorium and, in general, the results in Nova Scotia had not, the CTA executive secretary, Wodehouse, felt, justified the expenditure. Such a dour view may be partly due to political tensions over who would have ultimate control – the professional-style voluntary association or the local leaders. Wodehouse traced the reason back to the commission. As he reported somewhat righteously in 1930, "we have been disappointed with Nova Scotia. They started well but they soon became political, as we expected they would, and tried to avoid the same by having united central control. They appointed the provincial Conservative organizer for two elections to be the medical head of the Tuberculosis Commission. The Commissioner also had other handicaps besides his previous political occupation." As a result, he concluded, "we have never been able to get a sufficient number of poor cases cared for in the Provincial Sanatorium."[43]

## The TB Problem in Montreal

Montreal had spent roughly half a decade under either a tuberculosis demonstration or a survey and yet still continued to fail to deal with the disease. By 1930, according to an outside report commissioned by the Royal Edward Institute, the health department still did not take any direct part in supplying the services to control tuberculosis, but subsidized private agencies instead – which meant essentially the Bruchesi and Royal Edward Institutes.[44] The state of health of Montreal residents continued to be appalling. When Montreal's tuberculosis death rate was 152.2 per 100,000, the infant death rate was 148.9 per 1,000 living births, and the number of annual deaths for persons under two years of age from diarrhoea and enteritis was 1,249, the comparable figures for Toronto were 65, 71.9, and 87 respectively. It was irrefutable proof, as health workers constantly preached, that "health was purchasable" – for Toronto spent $835,000 ($1.60 per capita) on its health department in a year, while Montreal spent a mere $272,000 (42 cents per capita) for the same purpose.[45] And to the dismay of tuberculosis workers this expenditure was actually decreasing: from 42 cents in 1923 to 41 cents in 1924 to 40 cents in 1925.[46] The moral could hardly be clearer.

Despite the prominent example of American foundations – the Rockefeller, Carnegie, and Russell Sage foundations – funded with gilded-age fortunes, interwar Canada never saw the development of native-born equivalents: individual Canadians using their personal fortunes to establish independent philanthropies. The American examples may have been due to a unique and peculiar set of circumstances – economic, industrial, religious, and political – existing in late nineteenth-century America that permitted the acquisition of vast wealth, yet infused society and the new industrialists with a complex mix of progressive ideology supporting scientific management and the social gospel. In any event, the new industrialists in Canada, such as Adam Beck or William Gage, tended to fund specific causes directly – for example, the London Health Association and the National Sanitarium Association.

This tradition continued in Montreal in the twenties, influenced by the benefits of surveys and demonstrations established elsewhere. The Montreal Anti-Tuberculosis and General Health League was conceived in 1924 and backed financially by Lord Atholstan. It was English-dominated and English-run, although it operated in both language communities, setting up English and French demonstration areas complete with surveys, clinics, public health nurses, vaccinations, and classes in hygiene and health. By 1928 funds were running out and the demonstration was coming to a close.[47] Like the Quebec Royal Commission before it, the league had formulated a set of demands that were essential if Montreal was to have anything approaching an efficient health service.

In 1927 the league's directors met the executive committee of Montreal city council, which promised another $50,000 for the health department to implement some of the league's suggestions. By June

1928, thirty members were added to the department staff, including nine milk inspectors, public health nurses, and a bacteriologist.[48] Buoyed by this success and with the city sensitive to public health issues, since it was just recovering from a typhoid epidemic, league members believed the time was opportune to get the public interested in a health survey. So it offered the use of its staff, the committee on administrative practice of the American Public Health Association was called in as consultants, and the Metropolitan Life Insurance Company published the report in 1928.

Of a possible 100 points, the report gave Montreal only a meagre 55 for the tuberculosis services provided.[49] Reporting was unsatisfactory – fewer than two cases of tuberculosis were reported for each death; only a little over half the required number of home visits were made by public health nurses (due to a lack of nurses); only three-fifths of the patients who should have been institutionalized were in sanatoria, which had far too low a percentage of incipient cases admitted and no organized follow-up of ex-patients; and there were no open-air classes or preventoria for predisposed children. Only clinic attendance was up to par. "The skeleton of good service is locally present," the survey committee concluded with polite restraint, but all agencies had to be coordinated and funds and personnel supplied to extend the nursing, medical, sanatorium, and hospital facilities.

As a result, the city council created a new board of health in 1929, arranged for diphtheria immunization to begin throughout the city, and planned grants for destitute mothers before, during, and after childbirth.[50] Although far too much of the burden was still being carried by the voluntary societies, particularly in tuberculosis work, it was a beginning.

### The New Importance of the CTA

When local tuberculosis societies or associations had first affiliated with the national organization, the CTA had adopted a hands-off fund-raising policy, relying on donations, particularly the federal government grant, to promote education and leaving local societies to raise their own funds for their own local projects. As a result, the influence of the dominion association was necessarily limited.

In the twenties, it moved into national prominence as an intermediary: the Sun Life Company, the Red Cross, and CLIOA all funnelled their grants to the various committees, commissions, and surveys through the CTA, which organized and coordinated activities and allocated funds. This was particularly true in Prince Edward Island, where CLIOA, in combination with the executive secretary of the CTA and, to a lesser extent, the local Red Cross, organized the new provincial health service. The functions of the CTA – "to educate, agitate, stimulate, co-ordinate and co-operate," as the president explained in 1924[51] – took on a new meaning when it arranged half the financing of the Three Rivers demonstration (at a cost of $31,000 annually), and it had expended an impressive $363,860 under its authority by 1929. Association receipts rose from around $14,000 in 1921 to $51,000 by 1927.[52] Along with its increased financial clout, the CTA had, by 1925, representatives on the executive boards of the Ontario division of the Red Cross, the Dominion executive of the St John Ambulance Association, and the health committee of the Ontario Medical Association.

Questions raised in the United States about possible conflicts of interest created by interlocking directorships between philanthropic foundations and large corporations began to appear to be pertinent in Canada as well. By 1930, backed by the insurance companies, the CTA was becoming a force to be reckoned with in the public health field. The interrelationships between CLIOA, the CTA, and the provincial governments in the Maritimes, particularly in Prince Edward Island, demonstrated just how influential as a pressure group voluntary forces had become, especially the national organization. All three players worked in close cooperation – but both CTA executive secretary Wodehouse and the insurance executives had definite ideas concerning the most efficient handling of the tuberculosis problem, and they were not above manipulating governments when attempting to obtain a desired result. Together they functioned like a large corporation or chain store moving into and efficiently taking over a small-town market – a familiar experience for many Canadians, particularly small businessmen, in the twenties.

In Nova Scotia, the Tuberculosis Commission had continued to operate after the Maritime Tuberculosis Committee finished up in 1931, and CLIOA agreed in a letter to the commissioner, Joseph Hayes, to contribute $1,500, contingent on the provincial government matching the grant.[53] It was a tactic the Rockefeller Foundation had used since its inception to encourage a reluctant or dubious government to fund public health.[54] Wodehouse, too, was involved in the political machinations. "I will try my best," he wrote to E.E. Reid of CLIOA in 1931, "to get the Government of Nova Scotia to give this extra $1,500. We will certainly never get it if we give the money first and I think I had better lead them to believe that they will not get it unless the Government gives the money. If, after the session, they still have not come across, in so far as the Government is concerned, to the Commission, possibly we had better consider assisting the Commission with the grant. We cannot very well afford to tell the Minister that Colonel Hayes actually asked you to give the money in order that he might induce the Government to assist them, but I am certain that this was the case."[55]

The government saw the case differently. They had just finished setting up a provincial organization under a department of public health which, as G.H. Murphy, the minister of public health, pointed out to Wodehouse, was "capable of spending to the very best advantage every dollar the province can afford for public health purposes. It seems then on the face of it to be poor business for us to hand over to the Tuberculosis Commission money that we can spend, to say the least, as effectively as they can."[56]

It was in Prince Edward Island, however, that Wodehouse and the insurance executives really made their financial influence felt. In 1930 the expenditure on public health on the island was roughly $18,700, consisting of $11,800 from the Canadian Red Cross, $4,500 from the Maritime Tuberculosis Educational Committee, and a mere $2,400 from the government.[57] Since the turn of the century, those interested in the tuberculosis campaign had been agitating for a health department, but to no avail; and until the Maritime Tuberculosis Educational Committee was established, most of the public health work was carried out by three Red Cross nurses. The committee had stimulated public awareness and government interest to the point that the government built a fifty-bed sanatorium and appointed a diagnostician and chief health officer in 1928, but it was obvious that public health work would be limited without a health department. CLIOA agreed to contribute $15,000 a year over a five-year period to aid the province in setting up a department of health, and an advisory committee consisting of E.E. Reid (London Life), V.R. Smith (Confederation Life), and R.E. Wodehouse was established to work in conjunction with P.A. Creelman, then the chief health officer of the provincial board of health.[58]

It was a case of he who pays the piper calls the tune, and the "advisors" soon became the overseers and administrators, making decisions and determining the manner of reorganization. Charlottetown had wanted to remain separate and control its own share ($2,000) of the donation, but Wodehouse quickly squelched that notion. It was "continued decentralization," he said, adding that "We are bringing $75,000 for hoped for permanent centralization. Under the above suggestion we would create a similar situation to Nova Scotia and the Maritime Committee."[59] And that was a mistake, he felt, not to be repeated. For the Nova Scotia campaign had become mired in parochial politics and, he believed, had consequently become less efficient than the others. His and the insurance men's authority seemed absolute.

The chief health officer asked the CTA executive secretary's approval before he hired a new nurse;[60] while Mona Wilson, one of the Red Cross nurses transferred from the society to the new department, complained several times about Wodehouse's high-handedness. They clashed first over his order that the nurses take their holidays in June before starting work for the department of health in July – they would, she pointed out, be forced to cancel school inspections;[61] and then they clashed again when he decided to purchase roadsters for the nurses instead of closed cars – the weather in Prince Edward Island, she commented rather sarcastically, was hardly suited to driving around without a roof.[62]

It was astounding just how much interest Wodehouse and the insurance executives took in what seemed to be relatively minor considerations in the organization of a complete health department, such as the problem of the nurses' cars.[63] The fact that it was Wodehouse, in conjunction with CLIOA businessmen – not the chief health officer – who decided what should be done indicated not only how deeply involved he was in every detail of the establishment of the new department but how far his authority extended. From 1931 to 1937 (the duration of the grant),[64] the chief health officer was in the peculiar position of being little more than a figurehead in his own department. The first minister of health had called Wodehouse "the real sponsor" of the new public health program, while Reid paid him the accolade of being not only a medical man but a businessman.[65] Just as John D. Rockefeller had discovered Frederick T. Gates, as a minister with shrewd business sense, to be the ideal deputy and advisor to his foundation, so the life insurance executives placed their trust and money with Robert Wodehouse. Noting the good results (the tuberculosis death rate had fallen from 100.7 per 100,000 for the five-year period prior to 1931 to 82.6 for the same period following) the CTA felt confident in asking CLIOA for $30,000 to conduct a three-year campaign in Quebec.[66]

## Provincial Voluntary Associations

The CTA did not confine its activities to those initiated with CLIOA. It was still the national centre for the collection of data on the Canadian tuberculosis problem; it still printed and distributed the *Bulletin* and roughly one and a half million pamphlets. In addition, it functioned as an advisor to local groups, both voluntary and governmental.

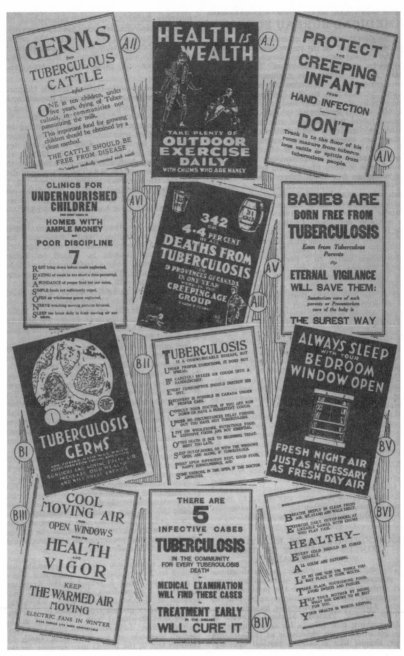

Posters distributed by the Canadian Tuberculosis Association. Reproduced from the Canadian Tuberculosis Association, *Bulletin*, 2 (Mar. 1924), 8

More importantly, the CTA promoted the establishment of provincial voluntary organizations paralleling the provincial tuberculosis divisions, in an effort to establish a more efficient and comprehensive campaign. Two reasons influenced this strategy. When education was left to local associations to manage, even with the national organization supplying advice and literature, it was often sporadic and inefficient, and too often it did not reach whole sections of a province. A well-run provincial campaign would include the whole province in its scope. The Christmas Seal campaign, organized nationally by the CTA in 1927, as we have seen, gave added impetus to this movement for centralization, for the specialists now considered it not only the most effective means of education available but also an important source of funds. To exploit it properly, the CTA executive insisted that it should be organized uniformly on a provincial basis.

The Nova Scotia Tuberculosis Commission, established in conjunction with the Maritime Tuberculosis Educational Committee, had represented the first effort at forming a provincial educational organization. With the loss of CLIOA funding, it had folded by 1934. The New Brunswick Tuberculosis Association was therefore the first committee organized provincially for this purpose in 1932,[67] and it (like subsequent associations) was financed by Christmas Seals, cooperating with local committees to run the sale and handling areas not otherwise covered. Other provinces soon followed its example. By the end of the decade, all Canadian provinces except Ontario, the bastion of local voluntarism, and Nova Scotia had some form of provincially organized voluntary tuberculosis association to parallel the government association.[68]

*Service Clubs*

With tuberculosis work controlled more and more by specialists, lay workers began, as was mentioned in chapter 3, to work through the service clubs – the Kiwanis clubs, Rotary clubs, the Associated Travellers', and the Kinsmen – and women's groups such as the old standby, the IODE. Like the philanthropic foundations, the service clubs had their roots in turn-of-the-century America and were molded by much of the same middle-class progressive-era ideology, stressing cooperation, efficiency, organization, and social responsibility. If the foundations were a reflection and outgrowth of the new larger corporations and monopolies, however, the service clubs were the representatives and voices of small businessmen and independent professions banding together to resist both their loss of influence in society and the economic threat to their livelihood from the department, catalogue, and chain stores and the new resource-based industries and monopolies. As occupation became less meaningful as a guide to social standing, they promoted the concept of service – perhaps partially as a result of the pervasive influence of the growing number of women's clubs – as a way of reasserting their influence and incorporating older, traditional ideas of community loyalty and local obligation into their energetic boosterism.[69]

Canada in the period following World War 1 was ideally suited to the service club movement. Friends of a Chicago Rotary Club member formed the seventeenth Rotary Club in Winnipeg in 1909, and close business and family connections promoted northern expansion.[70] Both Kiwanis and Lions established Canadian clubs shortly after their founding, and all experienced explosive growth in the twenties. World War 1 had emphasized cooperation and organization and a rhetoric of service, while the displaced veteran returning to Canada, often lonely, found himself in a strange city or town in a new job and yearned for the fellowship and camaraderie he had had in Europe. With service club policy restricting membership to one or two individuals from each profession or business establishment, the expansion of a variety of clubs was almost guaranteed.

In an increasingly secular Canada, club spokesmen adopted the language of the social gospel and promoted the themes of cooperation, responsibility, service, and ethical business practices with an almost religious zeal – a stark contrast to the pragmatic corporate and foundation ideology of efficiency, organization, and rational scientific management.[71] With retailers, small manufacturers, independent professionals, and some mid-level corporate employees who were trying to promote local business ventures as the membership base, the majority of clubs in the interwar years were formed in towns with a population of under 10,000 – again they were well suited to both the new resource-based towns in the hinterland and the struggling, more established centres threatened by urban expansion.[72] Service clubs, which were straining to find an independent middle ground between the unrestrained individualism of the monopolistic resource industries and chain and department stores, on the one hand, and government regulation, on the other, and whose expansion was paradoxically encouraged both by the growth of a branch-plant economy in Canada and by a small-town resistance to corporate culture, were ideally suited to Canadian society.

Club members were ridiculed and satirized as Babbitts by the intellectuals of the period, whose opinions have too often been unquestioningly adopted by subsequent historians, and it is ironic, as Jeffrey

Charles points out, that both the club members and their scornful critics were reacting to the same twentieth-century dilemma – "how to preserve a sense of individual significance in mass society." Yet while the critics' modernism rejected both Victorian sentimentalism and the standardization and materialism of the emerging corporate business society, the service clubs were proud of their business achievements and staunch fans of the mass culture as represented by the sentimental Rotarian poet Edgar Guest, whose doggerel verses were frequently quoted by admiring members to add an inspirational note to their speeches.[73] This situation was aggravated in Canada, where resentful concern about the pernicious influence of the new American mass culture – magazines and films – was raised again and again.[74]

If the Rockefeller Foundation was premised on "wholesale" philanthropy, the service clubs were still very much "retail" in their outlook. Charity was in most cases local, sporadic, piecemeal, and unsystematic. Typical projects included relief work, establishing or benefitting a local institution, and buying and donating equipment[75] – even when the work was done for the benefit of a national charity such as the Salvation Army or the CTA, their focus was almost invariably local. As such, their influence, although pervasive throughout Canadian society, was disjointed and easy to overlook.

Like the old tuberculosis leagues and social reform groups of the prewar era, the service clubs were local organizations, working independently, raising money for local projects. With the tuberculosis campaign increasingly managed by professionals from the top, these service clubs became the one means by which amateur volunteers could influence the direction of the campaign. The Rotary clubs or the Kiwanis saw a local need – a new sanatorium wing to be built or furnished, a clinic to be established, a visiting nurse to be supported – organized locally, campaigned for funds, and then had the satisfaction of seeing concrete results that benefitted their immediate neighbourhood.

The importance of these groups increased after the Christmas Seal sale was organized on a national basis by the CTA in 1927, for the service clubs invariably ran the sale and raised the funds that supported local tuberculosis activities. Ironically, their importance was often masked by the fact that another agency – either a sanatorium, department of health, or quasi-official committee – administered these funds and received the publicity, but it was the service clubs that supported the campaign on the grassroots level. Like the anti-TB leagues of twenty years earlier, they were sometimes stubborn, individualistic, disconnected, and parochial. But more and more the specialists were coming to rely on them not only for local fund-raising but for public awareness as well.

The establishment of the new voluntary provincial organizations under the aegis of the CTA in the 1930s did not spell the end of the local associations or service clubs in the campaign. Provincial associations might have been formed to run a more efficient and comprehensive educational campaign and Christmas Seal sale, but local groups and service clubs were still its basis. In Prince Edward Island and Alberta, for example, it was the local associations themselves who decided to join together and form a provincial organization, but they continued to run the Christmas Seal sale locally, using the profits for surveys, x-rays, and nurses salaries. In British Columbia the volunteer groups were not only essential members of the Vancouver Survey Committee but continued to play an important part in the campaign even after the government organized the tuberculosis division – occupational therapy, for example, was left solely in the hands of the Junior League, and the Rotary Club which built the laboratory in the new Vancouver Unit. Even Saskatchewan, with its record of provincial responsibility, ran the Christmas Seal sale largely through the Associated Canadian Travellers, while in Ontario voluntary associations continued to run even the sanatoria.

*The Christmas Seal Campaign:*
*More Funds, More Organization*

The organization of the Christmas Seal campaign in 1927, using methods already proven successful in the United States, was probably one of the most influential developments of the interwar period. Local associations had sold stamps in the past, but in 1927 the CTA began to centralize operations by printing and supplying Christmas Seals to local groups, who in turn ran the campaign and used the proceeds (less 10 percent for the national association's expenses) in any way they saw fit.

The total amount raised increased from about $83,000 in 1927 to $151,000 in 1930.[76] Christmas seal profits gave volunteer associations the necessary money to achieve the CTA's general goal of stimulating public demand by pioneering in new health fields and adding to already established programs. The money was used in all areas of anti-TB work.

The way in which Christmas Seal money was administered also revealed the cooperation between government agencies or officials and voluntary associations, and it reinforced the growing belief in Canada that voluntarily funded tuberculosis programs supported, but did not replace, state ones. For example, the salary of the travelling diagnostician in Alberta was paid for by the provincial tuberculosis association, but the health department paid all the other expenses connected with diagnostic and follow-up work. The travelling medical health officer in British Columbia was a health department employee, but the Tranquille Publishing Society, through Christmas Seal funds, paid for a nurse to assist him and bought a portable x-ray machine.

By the 1930s, the Christmas Seal sale had become important not only for its obvious profits and educational value but as a factor in religiously guarded local autonomy. Local committees arranged their own program, ordered their own supplies, prepared their own mailing lists, wrote and printed their own letter of appeal, arranged local publicity, took care of the contributions, sent a report to the central office, and then turned over the net returns from the campaign to the local tuberculosis association for preventive work: supporting clinics, public health nurses, x-rays, welfare work, educational work, rehabilitation schemes, and summer camps.

The CTA had its own responsibilities, with a full-time staff member devoted to Christmas Seal work. It acted as a coordinator and consultant, selecting a design, then printing and distributing the Christmas Seals along with the cards, billboard posters, letterheads, envelopes, and theatre trailers that were sent to local committees; arranging national advertising; holding meetings (from 1935 on) for Christmas Seal committee representatives; and sending out a newsletter and a field worker to visit the local groups to help standardize and improve their methods.

This system had several important results. As the Christmas Seal sale grew more popular, the responsibility of the local groups increased, and it became critical that some sort of standards and pattern of organization be established so that the greatest profit, in both money and education, was derived from the seals. Some local groups were suspicious of suggestions from those in authority, whether department of health employees or CTA staff. The defining of roles that had begun in the twenties was clear-cut now. Service clubs and voluntary associations fully accepted the principle of the specialists directing the anti-TB campaign – although they were sometimes reluctant to turn over, without question, the funds they had raised to the specialists who would decide whether it should be used for preventive work or an additional piece of equipment. *They* were responsible for running their own Christmas Seal sale, and they resented interference from above. The specialists could advise, but not dictate. In Vancouver, for example, where the IODE and Kinsmen together ran the sale, they took a dim view of the attempt by the tuberculosis division of the Greater Vancouver Health League to form a large Vancouver committee in which their respective identities would be lost.

Having a particular service club associated with the sale possibly made it less universal,[77] while the club, which had various interests, could not always afford the time needed to wage an all-out effort.[89] In Montreal, where local autonomy was, the CTA executive consistently complained, carried to inefficient and ridiculous lengths, the Kiwanis Club agreed that personal solicitation and an organized follow-up system would probably increase the returns, but with 13,000 special letters and 35,000 general ones sent each year, they just did not have time.[78]

Turning proceeds over to the specialists to use for their specified purposes served to mask the importance of this grassroots voluntary effort. The Christmas Seal sale might fund the work of the travelling clinics of the Manitoba Sanatorium and all the preventive efforts of the Saskatchewan Anti-Tuberculosis League, for example, but with these bodies managing the funds, it would be easy to overlook the contribution from the local committees. And this contribution was impressive. In 1940 the total seal sale had reached about $226,000, and with this amount of money involved, it was probably no wonder that the CTA was pushing to organize it. [79] It was simply becoming too profitable to be run haphazardly.

As was the case with the conception of the disease itself, its diagnosis, and its treatment, the voluntary associations established to campaign against tuberculosis underwent profound changes and reorganization in the interwar period. Most of the significant developments reflected similar turmoil occurring in Canadian society as a whole, and they were, like the approach to TB itself, both an outgrowth of and response to social reform and wartime experience. The growth of foundation-style philanthropy mirrored the growth of the new big business, as we have seen. The increasingly important role of the specialized administrator was paralleled in the person of Robert Wodehouse, the executive secretary of the CTA, who was trusted as an equal partner and advisor by the life insurance executives because of his business acumen as much as his medical knowledge. (Wodehouse left in 1933 to become federal deputy minister of pensions and health. As such he would be instrumental in introducing the concept of health insurance in Canada a few years later.[80])

Like foundation-style philanthropies, the service clubs were also, as we have seen, a reflection of and reaction to the era: similarly emphasizing cooperation, organization, and service, with language infused by the social gospel, they represented members of the traditional middle class struggling to maintain their social and economic place while trying to adjust to the new business climate.

In the midst of such shifting circumstances, the CTA evolved as an intermediary – an advisor and administrative link between the sometimes contradictory impulses of the big business foundations like CLIOA, the government, and the resolutely independent and defiantly local service clubs. Such a position would increase its influence and authority immeasurably. And, after the close of another world war, as Canadians began to consider the risks and benefits of health insurance and federal grants, it would be to the CTA that the federal government would look for advice.

# 5 The Interwar Years: The Role of the State

In March and August of 1935, R.B. Bennett, the Canadian prime minister, received the following letters from two small towns in Alberta:

I am a farmer's wife and come to you with great confidence ... Our place is up for taxes there is $132 against it that means a family of 11 will be put on the road ... The Dr has ordered more beds in my home at present they are sleeping 4 in one bed we have no money to buy beds & covers we cannot get them on credit Dr said they will get TB if we leave it much longer, and before time would change it might be to late I do want to raise a healthy family ... all I ask to safeguard the children from TB.

I am an invalid. I have TB of the kidney and bladder. I was at the Marshall Hospital for 32 months and have been in bed at home now for 4 months. I am improving, but in 2 weeks I have to go back to hospital again to have another x-ray picture taken, and a course of treatment, and the picture and medicine are cash and we have know [sic] money for it ...
    We have not had a crop for 4 years and our crop this year is poor due to drought. I am a middle aged woman with three children are old timers of Alberta. I need help now more than ever before to fight my sickness, or else die.[1]

"We would never have eradicated smallpox," remarked David Stewart, superintendent of the Manitoba Sanitorium in 1935, who perhaps had tragedies similar to those of the letter-writers in mind, "if a man had had to mortgage his farm to pay for the treatment."[2] Because tuberculosis control in the interwar period was intended to benefit the community first with its attack on infection, it seemed logical that the community should pay. If the "closed-fistedness, selfishness, and short-sightedness of individuals and communities"[3] stood in the way, tuberculosis sufferers simply remained at home, further infecting their neighbours. The importance of free treatment was confirmed in Ontario when it was discovered that despite available facilities, only a disappointing 53 percent of the cases dying of tuberculosis in 1936 had received sanatorium care.[4]

As with the approach to the disease itself and the place of volunteers in the campaign, the role of the state, together with the responsibilities of different levels of government, was influenced by concurrent social, political, and economic changes in interwar Canada, and it was altered to accommodate them. The increasing importance of provincial governments in economic development, particularly with the resource industries, was paralleled in health care, while the close association between government and industry in new hydroelectric and mining industries was mirrored in public health by the association of government health departments with new, professionally administered voluntary associations such as the CTA. The postwar emphasis on scientific management and efficiency, promoted so consistently by the Rockefeller Foundation, would be developed in the public sector as well. If the Privy Council rulings encouraged provincial rights and restricted federal authority in the political sphere generally, the reluctance of the federal government to take on any more financial burdens in the depression led, by default, to further provincial authority.[5] By the time Canada mobilized for World War 2, the balance of power had been established. The municipalities, crushed by the depression, lacked the tax base and the resources to provide tuberculosis care, and the Dominion government abdicated responsibility by invoking the British North America Act. Responsibility for tuberculosis care – and therefore free treatment – settled on the provinces.

### State Duty

With the concept of "state duty" elevated to a right by the war and the cost and size of the tuberculosis program expanding, insistence grew for state involvement. "A citizen has his garbage removed and is given police and fire protection as part of a community service," the Montreal Health Survey Committee reasoned in 1928, "He is not asked to pay an extra charge, nor is he refused such a service even if he is unable to pay for it; he has paid for it in his taxes. Health services, including laboratory facilities, should be on the same basis."[6] If cars and gasoline were taxed for the upkeep of highways, why not taxes for health? "It is difficult to understand," penned a perplexed editor of the *Public Health Journal*, "why a country that has accepted free education as a state responsibility should evade the acceptance of the principle of the provision of medical and nursing care, when required in the public interest, as a state responsibility."7 And since treatment was not only for the benefit of the individual but to protect the community in general, it was only fair, as David Stewart pointed out, that "as the man is treated to make the state safe, the state should help with the burden of payment." If it could not afford to pay for everything, it should at least pay for maintenance; for, as those involved in the tuberculosis campaign frankly acknowledged, capital expenditures were easier to raise through voluntary contributions. Moreover, as the civilian sanatoria had already done their patriotic duty by caring for returned soldiers, "we have every right to expect that the federal authorities will show their gratitude by assisting us in our task for the civilian citizens of Canada."8

It was only a short step from this to a demand for government-financed free treatment for all patients – especially since most patients were already partially or completely subsidized during their sanatorium stay. In 1924 the CTA endorsed the principle of free sanatorium treatment for indigent patients at its annual meeting. By this point, Manitoba had demonstrated that when a municipal levy supported the poorer people completely and the rest partially, as many as five times the number of sufferers went to the sanatorium, thus protecting their communities.9 It did not seem fair to many people that veterans should be treated free, but not civilians, since the latter not only contributed to the nation's economy but had not caused their own infection – and so should not be personally bankrupted to pay for a cure.

More practically, it was impossible to forcibly segregate an infected father or mother unless it could be guaranteed not only that his or her treatment was paid for but also that the family would be supported if the breadwinner were removed. Solving both problems made long-term sense, for if a contagious parent were allowed to remain at home and infect the children, the government would have even greater costs to bear, especially if the province paid part of the treatment costs already, which was generally the case. "In one family," Peter Bryce stated in the Ontario Mothers' Allowance Commission Report, "seven children were infected because the tuberculous father was permitted to remain at home."10 Only state funding could ensure removal. In 1922, the five Western provinces were paying out $308,856 in mothers' allowances for tuberculosis. By 1924 the Ontario government alone spent $214,578, which was 13 percent of all payments for mothers' allowances made by that body. Added to the $315,290 that province paid out for institutional treatment for the tuberculous that year, it represented a substantial sum.11 As both provincial officials and tuberculosis workers noted with dismay, it would only increase unless infection was controlled.

## The Role of the Federal Government

It was federal government involvement for which public health workers pressured most – they demanded a federal department of health. The Canadian Medical Association had passed resolutions for such a department in 1902, 1903, 1904, and 1907, and it was supported by the *Public Health Journal*, CAPT, and the NCW among others.[12] Tuberculosis workers believed that the magnitude of the tuberculosis problem required a federal department as the central authority, with the responsibility of directing, controlling, and coordinating the campaign; educating; gathering statistics; and funding sanatoria, dispensaries, hospitals, model farms, and workshops.[13] A few even suggested a fixed tax to keep up a federal system of hospitals, nationalization of the medical profession, a universal, obligatory health and accident insurance scheme, and a special "tuberculosis tax" to care for victims of the disease.[14]

Not all wanted such extensive government involvement – the inspector of hospitals and public charities for Ontario believed that "The relation of the state to institutions for the care and treatment of tubercular patients should, we think, be supervisory, not proprietary."[15] But the majority of reformers would probably have agreed with the feminist prohibitionist Nellie McClung who argued that "More and more the idea is growing upon us that certain services are best rendered by the state, and not left to depend on the caprice, inclination or inability of the individual."[16]

The war changed their request for a federal department of health to a demand. Canada's citizens became "one of the most important natural resources,"[17] and because of wartime service, the state owed them proper health care – not as a dole, but as a debt. It was a profound change in attitude. "A federal bureau of health," resolved the Canadian Medical Association in 1917, "is a war measure of the first importance. Extra and unusual measures must be taken to make good to Canada the enormous loss of our young men in this war. Thousands of our boys have fallen in France and Flanders – a necessary and voluntary sacrifice in the cause of liberty and humanity, while thousands of those needed to take their place in civil life after the war are allowed to die needlessly, in the cause of nothing but ignorance and neglect."[18] The association found it particularly galling that despite an estimated loss to the nation of $50 million a year through human tuberculosis deaths, the government took better care of its animals. "In Alberta," commented one Edmonton doctor acidly, "the public health is administered through the Department of Agriculture, and takes second place to the killing of noxious weeds and gophers, to the health and happiness of our horses, our cattle ... and even of our hens ... Should any of these be sick, a paid provincial veterinarian will travel the length and breadth of the land to see them and cure their ills."[19]

It took the war to prove to the government the value of a healthy citizenry. "The time is fast approaching," Alan Brown, chairman of the pediatrics section of the Academy of Medicine, confidently predicted in 1919, "when the health of the community is going to be supervised by the state, in some such manner as education now is ... The state has begun to view the individual from an economic standpoint, and to realize that money spent in various ways to keep the individual well, improve his environment and promote his development, means a corresponding decrease later in the cost of providing for delinquents and defectives."[20]

The state may have begun to view the individual "from an economic standpoint," but in the early reconstruction period this usually meant that all levels of government were reluctant to admit financial responsibility – or liability. Despite the creation of a new federal department of health, support for tuberculous indigents was primarily municipal, and coverage varied widely.[21]

### The Role of the Municipalities

If a rising tuberculosis rate was directly attributable to "the indifference of the citizens who are not in office, and the criminal negligence of those who are," it was still the municipality's responsibility to carry out provincial legislation and to look after sufferers who were poor.[22] An exasperated Charles Hastings slammed errant municipalities in 1919 for evading their clear-cut responsibility: "Attend almost any church burial service today, and you will hear the officiating parson read from the service: 'The Lord giveth and the Lord taketh away, Blessed be the name of the Lord.' In the light of modern knowledge, can you conceive of anything more libellous on the Almighty? If the church is determined to retain this form, why not change it sufficiently to make it consistent, and have it read: The Lord giveth and the Municipality taketh away, Cursed be the name of the Municipality."[23]

Montreal exhibited patronage politics, municipal irresponsibility, and callous indifference at its worst. Tuberculosis workers unceasingly both pleaded for and demanded more enforced legislation, dispensaries, and accommodation for consumptives – to no avail. Ninety percent of the milk reaching the city in 1914, according to a bacteriological study published by the federal department of agriculture, was unfit for human consumption.[24] Tuberculosis death rates were constantly rising, from 187.1 per 100,000 in 1908 to 210 in 1913. As J.E. Dubé, the medical director of the Bruchesi Institute commented sarcastically: "When a city the size of Montreal has insufficient accommodation for her tuberculous persons, and refuses to provide more, excepting in the police stations and the common jails, those who are not fond of such luxury move to other towns and die there. These, at least, do not encumber our municipal statistics."[25]

If the "puerile timidity" and "backwardness" of the city moved the director of the Bruchesi Institute to angry frustration, it caused the director of the Royal Edward Institute to adopt an attitude of almost hopeless resignation. The Royal Edward Institute had been demanding reforms for several years longer than its French counterpart and had almost given up trying to inspire the civic leaders with any sense of municipal responsibility. "It seems futile to mention in our report each year," the director commented wistfully in 1914, "the institutions we ought to have and don't get, the things the city ought to do and does not do, the obligations of the province and government that they never fulfill. It seems that we must block out our own advances, forget our great handicap and do the best we can by using our inadequate artillery."[2] By 1919 J.A. Jarry, the medical director of the Bruchesi Institute, was still angrily demanding, "What is Montreal waiting for to decide her to take her part in this immense anti-tuberculosis work? Is she in need of examples?"[27]

Hardly – for Toronto had established such a model health department that the local anti-TB league gave up its charter in 1912, believing there was nothing left for it to do. As the nursing director, Eunice Dyke, put it, the city health department was becoming the "organizing centre in the tuberculosis campaign."[28] The city paid 70 cents a day for all patients sent to Muskoka, tried to enforce compulsory notification and disinfection, inspected buildings, distributed cuspidors and sanitary supplies, ran a laboratory that examined sputum samples, had medical inspection of the schools, and employed a staff of visiting nurses. In 1914, the mayor proudly informed the Canadian Club that the work of the tuberculosis nurses cost $23,921 that year, milk inspection cost $10,800, dental clinics $10,000, sanitary inspection (including housing) $19,540, and school nurses $75,000 to $100,000.[29]

By the postwar period it was becoming increasingly evident that Quebec was lagging behind most of the other provinces, and public health workers maintained that one did not have to seek far to find the reason for this sorry state of affairs: the problem was money. In Ontario, the tuberculosis death rate had fallen from 160 per 100,000 in 1900 to 89 in 1915; while in Quebec it went from 192 to only 155 in 1913. But the Ontario government granted $108,000 to its provincial board of health, while Quebec granted only $23,000; Ottawa and Toronto spent $1 and $.55 cents respectively per capita for sanitation, while Montreal spent $.39; Toronto (with a population of 376,240 according to the 1911 census) spent $158,496 annually on anti-TB work and had a mortality rate of 110 per 100,000 in 1916, whereas Montreal (with a population of 466,197) spent $17,432.50, and had a correspondingly higher rate: 189.6 per 100,000.[30] It was all too clear to the tuberculosis workers – without adequate government support they could not begin to hope to defeat the white plague.

Municipalities not only lacked the financial resources of the provinces but were frequently tight-fisted – especially the rural ones. Nothing demonstrated that more clearly than Nova Scotia, where, ironically enough, 75 percent of the patients in the provincially owned sanatorium had to pay their own way because the municipalities generally refused to take any responsibility for indigents. It was becoming evident, public health specialists believed, that everyone would have to be treated to run an effective campaign. There was a choice: either the municipalities had to be forced to care for their indigents (and the term had to be defined loosely – sufferers should not have to sell all their possessions to get support in a sanatorium, as was now occurring), or the province would have to shoulder the responsibility. The provinces were already paying for much, if not all, of the capital costs – especially in Nova Scotia, Alberta, Manitoba, British Columbia, and Saskatchewan, where the province or a provincially supported commission owned the sanatoria. In addition to sanatoria, all provinces were involved in other tuberculosis-related health work: travelling clinics, health units, and the establishment of formal tuberculosis divisions. To protect their investment, they would be forced to assume the burden of treatment. The depression would prove what the twenties suggested: even when willing, the municipalities had an inadequate financial base for a comprehensive anti-TB campaign.

### Provincial Responsibility

The federal government, by returning the DSCR facilities to the provinces and voluntary societies and instituting more costly programs and treatment procedures for veterans, had forced the provinces, whether they liked it or not, to take some responsibility for anti-TB work – the investment in sanatoria facilities and upkeep alone demanded it.[31] And once provinces became involved in paying, even if only partially, for patients' maintenance, it did not take officials long to realize that, paradoxically, to save money in the long term, the government would have to become more involved and spend even more money to isolate infectious cases and curb escalating costs. In the new postwar social climate of state responsibility, fueled by a pragmatic desire to avoid seeing their anti-TB programs, however limited, nullified by municipal inaction, the provinces reluctantly took action.

In keeping with the postwar philosophy of efficient scientific management, they began with a stock-taking, in the form of various provincial commissions, to determine the requirements of Canadian public health. A special subcommittee of the Quebec Superior Board of Health drafted a report in 1920 outlining an anti-TB campaign for that province, including the foundation of hospitals in Montreal and Quebec, and as a result the provincial government provided $100,000 per year for five years to undertake a general health campaign that included dispensaries, chest clinics, and education.[32] This step was followed by the establishment of county health units, partially funded by the Rockefeller Foundation, and the institution of the Grancher System, in which urban children considered at risk for tuberculosis were placed with rural foster families, so that by the end of the decade, the province was beginning to attempt to deal with rural health problems.

### The Pool System and Free Treatment in Saskatchewan

The most significant development occurred in Saskatchewan. That province had taken its comprehensive survey in 1921 that roused public opinion to such an extent that the government paid off the Saskatchewan Anti-Tuberculosis League's bank deficit, voted $520,000 for another sanatorium at Saskatoon, and raised the daily per capita grant from $.50 cents to $1 (about one-third of the cost of treatment).[33] This action, in and of itself, did not settle the issue of maintenance, however.

In 1919 and 1920, most patients in the Fort Qu'Appelle sanatorium had been soldiers; they outnumbered the civilians three to one, so that three-quarters of the cost of treatment was paid by the federal government. By 1924 the civilians outnumbered the soldiers by six to one so that almost five-sixths of the cost had to be paid by the individual, the province, or the municipality.[34] To deal with this altered situation, the "pool" system was devised at the request of the Rural and Urban Unions of Municipalities to provide for the cost of indigent patients in Saskatchewan and Manitoba – just as grain pools had been adopted to cope collectively with the agricultural situation. In Manitoba an annual levy on municipalities, based on an equalized assessment and not exceeding $120,000, was made by the government under a special agreement with the Union of Manitoba Municipalities (excluding the cities)[35] and paid through the department of the Municipal Commissioner to the provincial sanatorium at Ninette. In Saskatchewan, municipally funded urban and rural pools were established to maintain tuberculous patients in the sanatoria, so that by 1928 less than 2.5 percent of the treatment costs above the portion borne by the provincial government were paid by individual patients.[36] The pools caused the league some financial trouble, since accounts had to be financed into the following year, and many municipalities were behind in their payments; but they were still the first provincial schemes to extend government-funded sanatorium accommodation to the majority of the population and, as such, were a crucial factor in paving the way for the introduction of free treatment for all citizens.[37] The provision of free treatment was debated by the Association of Rural Municipalities starting in 1926; by 1928 both it and the Association of Urban Municipalities, two of the most influential and representative bodies in the province, had passed resolutions in favour and presented them to the Saskatchewan government. The province acted quickly. Effective 1 January 1929, the Sanatoria and Hospitals Act was amended to extend free treatment to all Saskatchewan residents.

In a sense, the government was recognizing an existing situation rather than instituting a new and radical reform. Again, as with the establishment of the federal department of health, the Saskatchewan Act Respecting Sanatoria and Hospitals for the Treatment of Tuberculosis of 1929 was important in what it symbolized: the right of all citizens to free treatment. A person needed only to be a resident of the province for six months and have a doctor's certificate to be entitled to receive care at the expense of the league.[38] Saskatchewan was the first province, therefore, to have free treatment for curative and isolation purposes and free diagnosis for prevention. The latter, like all the preventive work in the province, was supported by voluntarily raised funds, although it too was carried out by the league.

Initially, there was a marked increase in the total number of treatment days: from 178,723 in 1928 to 213,952 in 1929 (a 19.7 percent increase), with a noticeable increase in the number of early pulmonary and nonpulmonary cases. This increase was partly a result of the removal of financial barriers, but it was also due to a more active, voluntarily supported preventive program: two sanatorium doctors ran extension clinics to outlying areas, while the league began to pay family physicians in inaccessible areas $5.00 for every contact examined. With additional treatment days, costs had necessarily risen – and the provincial grant to the Anti-Tuberculosis League rose from $213,780 in 1928 to $281,380 in 1930. But total maintenance costs had been rising steadily throughout the decade as the province had built more accommodation – the provincial grant had been only $45,004.50 in 1923.[39] Moreover, although there was a 100 percent increase in the number of persons referred for diagnosis (which meant free diagnosis was effective – those unable to pay were referred), roughly the same percentage as before were found to have active disease. Under the pay-for-diagnosis policy operating in 1928, 19.2 percent of the referred suspects had tuberculosis, while under the free diagnosis policy of 1929, 20 percent did – this was statistical proof, not only for Saskatchewan residents but for the rest of the country anxiously watching the innovation, that the populace would not abuse the provision of free diagnosis or treatment should it be extended to them. And as R.G. Ferguson, medical director and general superintendent of the Saskatchewan Anti-Tuberculosis League enthused, "the effect of removing the financial barrier is earlier treatment, earlier isolation and an increase in the number of days treatment and the gross cost, but the end result will be more cures and a shorter period of disability, lessened spread of disease, a lower death rate, and eventually fewer cases."[40] Canadians would go into the thirties with a state-funded, truly preventive program pioneered, ironically enough, by a province that was probably the hardest hit by the depression. Not only would it be successful but, more importantly, it would allay fears that the public would abuse a free, comprehensive system of tuberculosis care.

### Manitoba

While Saskatchewan did its comprehensive stock-taking at the beginning of the twenties, Manitoba did its stock-taking at the end. In 1928 the Manitoba Department of Health and Public Welfare appointed a health and hospital survey committee to report to the Welfare Supervision Board on the care of the sick in that province, particularly the tuberculous. After a year of investigation, it brought down a report recommending, among other things, the provision of 250 extra beds (100 for children) and the concentration of all tuberculosis activities in the province under a central authority. As a result, the provincial government voted $250,000 to provide more tuberculosis facilities and reconstructed the old board of trustees of the Manitoba Sanatorium, creating a new sanatorium board with a more representative membership. With the conventional goals of efficiency and centralization, this board would unify anti-TB work in the province, supervising the activities of the Ninette Sanatorium and the newly established Central Tuberculosis Clinic in Winnipeg, and gathering data regarding tuberculous persons, contacts, and suspects, thereby ensuring that all who needed to be were examined and treated. Since the Sisters of St Boniface had offered to build a sanatorium, the board concentrated on establishing a central clinic that would act as a clearing house and diagnostic and teaching centre and would include a central case registry.[41] Plans were prepared, as well, for a small preventorium for children, but they were shelved with the onset of the depression. By 1930 Manitoba, too, had coordinated its anti-TB work – provincial, municipal, and institutional – into an organized attack against the disease.

### Ontario

In 1934 G.C. Brink, director of the tuberculosis prevention division of the Ontario Department of Health, reported that only 50 percent of the cases needing sanatorium treatment found by the department's travelling clinic in 1933 had received it a year later. In Ontario the chief reason was the municipalities' refusal to furnish necessary aid. "Of what use is a correct diagnosis of active tuberculosis," Brink demanded with impeccable logic, "if it is not associated with proper treatment and the prevention of infection to contacts?"[42] He might have demanded, as well, for what use was the province spending increasing amounts of money on diagnosis and extending its travelling clinics in an effort to find cases earlier and keep its tuberculosis costs in line when the municipalities would not or could not maintain their share of the burden? During the thirties it became obvious that to prevent the money it expended on diagnosis from being wasted, the province would either have to force the municipalities to provide for their residents or assume all the maintenance costs itself.

Providing enough beds was not the sole answer. The Ontario Department of Health, prompted by the discovery that only 60 percent of persons dying of pulmonary tuberculosis in 1936 had had sanatorium care and only 50 percent of the patients discovered by the travelling clinics and needing treatment had entered a sanatorium within a year of diagnosis, instigated an inquiry into the general tuberculosis situation that led it to the revamp the Sanatorium Act. This investigation found the number of beds to be inadequate, yet paradoxically many patients were being maintained in sanatoria unnecessarily because there was no organized program of postsanatorium care or pneumothorax refill facilities near their homes. The tuberculosis mortality rate varied widely throughout the province, and there were marked differences in both the cost of sanatorium treatment and the incidence of hospitalization among both rural and urban municipalities. The explanation for this situation simply highlighted what most tuberculosis workers had already discovered – the municipality was an inadequate financial base for an efficient, comprehensive anti-TB program.[43]

As public health came increasingly under provincial control, so public health nursing, an essential part of the anti-TB campaign, followed suit – especially in the rural areas, where nurses often operated through the growing number of health districts. In general, the depression encouraged development of public health nursing under provincial supervision and organization, for it was thought to be more efficient, comprehensive and, most importantly, economical. In Manitoba, the old system of the municipality paying half the nurse's salary and the province the other half was demonstrably unjust – especially to poorer municipalities and unorganized districts, which contributed to the provincial maintenance of nurses in districts able to afford their share of the burden, while they themselves could not. As a result, the service was altered so that the province payed the full cost – although, also as a result of the depression, the service was greatly reduced.[44] In 1933 a provincial survey of British Columbia health services, by Dr G.M. Weir, the provincial secretary had counted 1,521 nurses engaged in public health work in 1930 and suggested that this be doubled in the next decade, but the depression squelched that suggestion.[45] In the thirties, tuberculosis and other public health workers, dealing with tightening budget restrictions, could only struggle to maintain existing services.

*Organization and Coordination:*
*The Creation of Provincial TB Divisions*

With the tuberculosis campaign becoming a bigger and bigger "business," there was a pressing need to coordinate, organize, and supervise it on a provincial level, in a manner analogous to the organization occurring on the voluntary side. Saskatchewan with its anti-TB league and Manitoba with its sanatorium board had demonstrated already the value of unification and central direction, and those involved in anti-TB work began to promote the establishment of some sort of provincial divisions, connected to the departments of health, "to stimulate, unify and harmonize" all tuberculosis activity, both government and voluntary, in the other provinces.[46] Without a provincial division, the Vancouver survey committee noted, either some municipalities would have to shoulder an unjustifiably heavier load, or they would refuse to improve facilities for fear of an influx of cases. Hamilton was already dealing with this problem in its sanatorium. In the past there had always been cooperation; but as the British Columbia travelling medical health officer pointed out, "lacking a head, coordination was impossible."[47] And if they were to get the most value for any investment in the hard times of the thirties, anti-TB workers believed coordination was essential.

By 1938 tuberculosis divisions had been created in Nova Scotia, Ontario, Quebec, Alberta, and British Columbia. These were important not only in what they accomplished (provincial coordination, increased facilities, more efficient case-finding and treatment) but in what they symbolized: a final declaration of provincial responsibility for the control of tuberculosis. In British Columbia a treatment and diagnostic centre was built in Vancouver, existing services were overhauled, three travelling clinics were added, and case-finding intensified. Pooling of all institutional beds under one authority enabled the division to use all available accommodation immediately and to assign certain cases to specific institutions – the more advanced, more complicated surgical and problem cases, for instance, were sent to the Vancouver unit, which made for greater efficiency.[48]

Again, as in Saskatchewan, results were soon evident and encouraging. The number of known cases for each annual death rose from 7.02 in 1936 to 16 in 1939 (indicating intensive and successful case-finding), while the percentage of advanced cases entering the sanatoria fell from 75 in 1934 to 38 in 1937.[49] If the majority of cases were discovered at a minimal stage there would be a quicker turnover of beds, cheaper treatment, and less infection – and thus less expensive hospital and social welfare costs in the future.

In Ontario the creation of the tuberculosis division did not eliminate the still striking variations in tuberculosis mortality rates, in sanatorium maintenance costs, and in the incidence of hospitalization in different regions of the province. The underlying cause of that problem was money – more particularly, the inability of patients to pay for their own treatment and the refusal of the municipality to do it instead. With an amendment to the Sanatoria for Consumptives Act in 1938, the provincial government finally abolished this inequitable and unsatisfactory system of maintenance charges and assumed the cost of maintaining indigent patients in the sanatoria – and since only an estimated 5 percent could support themselves, for practical purposes this change meant free treatment.[50] Relieved of its sometimes overwhelming responsibility, the municipality was now required to provide post-sanatorium care, including artificial pneumothorax (for which it was reimbursed up to $3.00 for each refill by the province).[51] The government made sure the municipalities fulfilled this obligation by insisting that any municipality failing to arrange for former patients' care within thirty days of notification of their discharge was liable for the patients' maintenance charges in the sanatorium until they were provided for. Because sanatorium care was always more expensive than after-care, this stipulation ensured that the municipalities did not evade their assigned responsibility.

Results were immediate. A shorter time elapsed between diagnosis and admission to a sanatorium; and with after-care and pneumothorax refills provided, maximum-benefit cases could be quickly discharged, permitting more patients to be treated – a full 10 percent more in 1939 than in the last year of the old system. Moreover, the number of readmissions fell from 504 in 1937 to 386 in 1939, most likely the result of improved care for discharged patients.[52]

Since the province was now contributing over 98 percent of the operating revenue of the sanatoria (its share of maintenance charges had risen from $670,860 in 1937 to about $1.1 million in 1938 and $2.4 million in 1940), it began to exert its authority – for all sanatoria but one in Ontario were managed by voluntary associations, and before 1938 they had different systems for both financial accounting and medical statistics. The TB division inspected the institutions, reviewed the records, and by 1941 was attempting to initiate some uniform system to compare costs and statistics.[53] At the same time, the government was pumping more money into prevention: the travelling chest clinics had grown from two in 1934 to six in 1938, with an approximate increase in cost from $20,000 to $85,000, while the number of persons examined and new cases found had risen from 4,781 and 192, respectively, in 1935 to 13,591 and 707, respectively, in 1938. Tuberculin was distributed free of charge by the department in 1938. Even its expenditures on capital construction – once the preserve of the voluntary association – were growing steadily, with $750,000 spent in 1937 alone. As a result, the number of sanatorium beds rose from 2,990 in 1934 to 3,700 by 1938.[54] This assumption of treatment costs and partial funding of preventive work enabled the province, by the end of the decade, to exert firm supervision over the tuberculosis control program.

*The Results of Free Treatment*

Saskatchewan had extended free treatment to all residents in 1929; in 1936 Alberta followed suit, and Ontario, by taking over the responsibility from the municipalities in 1938, extended it in fact, if not actually in name. Manitoba continued to operate under the fixed levy system, which served the same purpose. And even those provinces still reluctant to assume the whole treatment burden were becoming more responsible – in 1936 Nova Scotia increased its grant to the sanatorium to reduce the cost of treatment to patients and municipalities to $1 per week and turned the responsibility of admitting patients to the sanatorium over to the department of public health.[55] New Brunswick increased its per diem grant so that municipalities were responsible for only 50 percent of the cost of hospitalizing patients, while British Columbia introduced a new system of fees graduated according to a patient's means. Even Prince Edward Island, in the throes of setting up a provincial department of health, increased the amount voted for the sanatorium from $18,000 in 1932 to $36,000 in 1937.[56]

With free treatment, tuberculosis specialists confidently predicted, patients would be admitted earlier and treatment would be shorter, so more beds would be available and facilities used more efficiently. More practically, the number able to pay even just a minimal percentage of their treatment costs was so small that, as the CTA secretary commented, "it would seem to be almost uneconomical to maintain collection departments to attempt to collect payment." With the additional problems of after-care and rehabilitation to worry about, forcing patients to bankrupt themselves before they qualified for support in a sanatorium seemed not only inhuman but uneconomical. "I cannot see the rationale," stated G.J. Wherrett flatly, "of extracting money from a tuberculous patient for treatment, and then paying it back for public assistance in after-care."[57]

With the financial barriers against treatment removed, results were soon evident. In 1938, 80 percent of the patients in Ontario, Saskatchewan, and Alberta were admitted within a month of diagnosis.[58] Since it was Saskatchewan that had first introduced the principle of free treatment to all residents, it was to Saskatchewan, struggling to deal with successive crop failures, that tuberculosis specialists turned to evaluate the visible results. They were impressive. The number of suspects referred by family doctors for diagnosis increased 100 percent from 1929 to 1931; patients were diagnosed and admitted earlier; under the system existing in 1928, only 14 percent of the discharged sanatorium patients had been admitted as early cases, while this rose to 24 percent in 1930.[59] By 1936 an encouraging 42.9 percent of the new cases were in the early stages of the disease. With voluntarily funded case-finding intensifying, there was still a decrease in the number of new cases discovered after 1930 – from 686 that year to 513 in 1936, which was a hopeful indication that the sources of infection were being systematically flushed out. Treatment was correspondingly more efficient: 83 percent of new tuberculosis cases treated after 1930 were still living four years later, a rate that the director of the anti-TB league reported was almost the same as that of pneumonia.[60] Saskatchewan's declining morbidity and mortality rates were proof positive, tuberculosis specialists believed, that the control program of adequate beds and intensive, organized case-finding and preventive work, with no financial barriers to treatment, worked.

It was ironic that the province that first set the example of government responsibility for its citizens' health should be the hardest hit by the depression. As successive crop failures struck, impoverished municipalities found it increasingly difficult, and ultimately impossible, to keep up their share of the maintenance costs. Provincial per capita income had fallen from the 1928–29 average of $478 to $135 in 1933, and by the winter of 1937–38, two-thirds of the rural population was destitute and almost half the total population was on relief. Rural tax collections broke down almost completely, with rural municipalities collecting a mere 8.5 percent of the total arrears and current tax levies outstanding in 1937.[61] By that point they owed the league approximately $769,000 in back payments, while that organization's borrowings to keep going had risen from approximately $467,000 in 1936 to $584,000 the following year. On 30 June 1938 the league owed the provincial government $125,000. Without this aid it was doubtful, the board of directors reported, if the league could have continued to operate. Over and over again, the league directors pleaded with the municipalities for their contributions – but it was only with the harvest of 1939 that the municipalities began to pay their levies again.[62]

The very fact that the league did *not* collapse, however, that the municipalities paid the amount they owed as soon as their economic situation improved, and that the province staved off bankruptcy with a series of loans demonstrated just how deeply the belief that free treatment was a government responsibility had become ingrained in the Saskatchewan public's mind. Now, even in the hardest times – and perhaps because of them – treatment was a right, not a privilege. And it was only a short step from demanding health care for tuberculous citizens to demanding health care for all.[63]

### Case-Finding and Treatment: More Beds

Even in the financially hard-pressed thirties, anti-TB work was considered important. The success of the campaign could be estimated in several ways: the traditional number of deaths per 100,000 population, the number of known cases per death, the number of available beds per death, and the number of beds per 100,000 population. The first provided the mortality rate; the second was used to evaluate the extent of reporting and the success of case-finding procedures, while the last two were used to determine how competently a province or municipality treated its active or infectious cases.[64] There appeared to be a close connection between the mortality rate and the amount of accommodation available, which tended to fuel arguments in favour of more beds. As the death rate was falling and aggressive case-finding techniques were turning up more and more tuberculous sufferers who were treated and survived, the old standard of one bed per death became outdated. By 1935 the CTA estimated that roughly 2.5 beds per death were required (depending on the facilities for home treatment and ambulant pneumothorax) and had upped this estimate to three by 1941.[65] Saskatchewan, the model province, had 2.3 beds per death by 1935 – and if aboriginals (who generally did not use the sanatoria) were omitted from the calculation, over 3. With close to 10,000 beds in Canada by 1939, the country had almost two beds per death – although the situation in the Eastern provinces compared very unfavourably to Ontario and the West. Quebec alone desperately needed another 2,000 beds.[66]

While the Western provinces had grappled reasonably successfully with the related issues of indigents and municipal responsibility by the end of the decade, the Eastern provinces had not. All lacked sufficient accommodation (especially Quebec) to cope with their high death rates, and this problem was compounded by relying on municipalities for maintenance charges, a treatment system that tuberculosis workers had complained about throughout the twenties. Both Nova Scotia and New Brunswick desperately needed some form of uniform cost system to spread the maintenance burden over the whole province (although Nova Scotia saw an increase in the number of cases admitted to institutions once a law was enacted vesting admission to a sanatorium in the department of public health). Nevertheless, the increase in the number of indigents accommodated was too slow. And the situation was equally discouraging in New Brunswick, where the travelling diagnosticians were continually frustrated in their efforts to reduce morbidity by the reluctance or refusal of county authorities, who were pleading financial difficulties, to provide hospitalization. By 1940 the chief medical officer was still demanding more beds and a solution to the financing problem.

Quebec, in particular, lacked an adequate control program, adequate facilities, and beds. As usual, the Montreal region was particularly bad. Despite the studies and surveys carried out by various groups over the previous decades, Montreal had the worst tuberculosis death rate, after Quebec and Halifax, of all Canadian cities, and its rate of 84.9 deaths per 100,000 population in 1937 compared particularly unfavourably to a rate of 35.6 in Toronto, 26.1 in London, and even 11.9 in Saskatoon.[67] For the tuberculosis workers witnessing consistent improvements in other cities and constantly and unsuccessfully trying to inspire the local authorities with a sense of responsibility for disease prevention, it was both frustrating and depressing. As the medical superintendent of the Royal Edward Institute observed bitterly in 1939, "The lack of beds and the lack of financial resources have crippled our work all through the year ... Weekly staff conferences have become almost a farce, since it is useless to recommend something that does not exist, and we might just as well tell our patients to go south for the winter."[68]

By the end of the decade, civic awareness and responsibility, if not good, were improving. The city established a tuberculosis section in the contagious diseases division of the department of health in 1938 and began to organize the city into health districts, modelled on those of New York and Toronto in 1939. By 1940 it had even established a municipal x-ray clinic to examine poor contacts referred by their family doctor.[69] However, the problems of funding treatment facilities and, what was most critical, providing beds were still unresolved.

### The Role of the Federal Government: Noninvolvement

There were probably three influential government actions around 1920: the 1921 Saskatchewan Commission, the institution of free treatment in that province, and the creation of the federal department of health (1919). The Saskatchewan Commission was not only a stock-taking but also a symbol of government readiness to accept responsibility in the field of public health; with the institution of free treatment the government shouldered that responsibility in the case of tuberculosis. The creation of the federal department of health, however, was important in what it symbolized, rather than in what it actually did: the state's responsibility, generally, in maintaining the nation's health. The new department did very little, especially in terms of tuberculosis: it provided the CTA with funds for educational work (which the federal government had done previously) and, after 1928, supported the veterans through the DSCR. The dominion government's main anti-TB work was funding research through an associate committee of the National Research Council – again, a form of education – and initiating the campaign to eradicate bovine tuberculosis carried out by the department of agriculture. Both actions were largely a result of cattlemen's agitation.

This behaviour is consistent with the federal government's role in public health generally in the interwar period: despite initial optimism, it failed to expand in any meaningful way beyond its traditional realm of health promotion and quarantine.[70] By the mid-thirties, when the depression had demonstrated all too clearly that the provinces and municipalities were overextended and overwhelmed, there would be a new impetus for federal involvement – but in the two decades prior to that, the dominion would invoke the putative limitations of the BNA Act to avoid any long-term responsibility.

The new Act Respecting the Department of Health ratified in a striking way the federal government's consistent attitude of noninvolvement. Health, to the dominion, was a "one shot deal." It was willing to finance wartime sanatorium construction and equipment and aid in improving treatment methods, but as soon as the war ended, it hastily handed back all facilities to the respective organizations involved, making it clear that although it could not avoid supporting the veterans, it had absolutely no intention of getting caught up in any maintenance program for civilians.

The veterans were a significant investment. By 1925 the total capital expenditure of the federal government for tuberculosis buildings and fixtures was roughly $3.5 million, while the value of hospital equipment furnished by the department in such institutions was $506,000. In addition, the estimated cost of treating tuberculous former servicemen to 31 March 1925 was $9.5 million, the estimated cost of vocational training $900,000 ($250,000 for the actual training and $650,000 for the pay and allowances), with $21 million already paid to tuberculous pensioners, not including the dependents of those who died. The total *annual* liability for these men and their dependents was estimated at $3.6 million.[71]

It was understandable, then, that the federal government was leery of further permanent financial commitments; but while a policy of lump-sum funding of provincial activities – leaving the organization, control, and long-term maintenance in the hands of the provinces – permitted more mobility in the short term, it stimulated provincial responsibility and caused the dominion to lose any real authority it might have had over provincial health programs. The dominion was willing, sporadically, to invest by erecting sanatorium accommodation or voting $200,000 for venereal disease control but, by refusing to make long-term commitments, it was unable to exert much control. A case in point was the Dalton Sanatorium in Prince Edward Island. The DSCR had expanded it, then handed it back to the province, which claimed it could not maintain it – so the sanatorium remained closed. It seemed to some disappointed activists that the government took great pains in its new act to ratify its lack of responsibility, since it included the proviso that "Nothing in this Act or any regulation thereunder shall authorize the minister or any officer of the department to exercise any jurisdiction or control over any provincial or municipal board of health or other health authority operating under the laws of any province."[72]

To many, such as the president of the CTA in 1924, the government was involved in "an evasion of the issue through the invocation of the BNA Act"[73] – and a department had been created that, as one member of the House acidly observed, was "all dressed up and [had] no place to go."[74] It seemed that in the name of "provincial rights" the federal government could avoid instituting any costly health care scheme and confine its attention to education and occasional grants. The exceptions – the venereal disease program and the veterans' maintenance – were results of the war, and the former ended in the thirties as Canadians' concern lagged.

"Provincial rights" was for some a specious argument, as W.S. Fielding pointed out incisively, if somewhat cynically, in the House: "in many things which are distinctly within the control of the provincial legislatures, we are yet dabbling a good deal. The Road question is distinctly a provincial one, and yet we are delving into it ... I find that while we are all sensitive in this matter of provincial rights, when any proposal made to encroach upon provincial rights is accompanied with a generous grant, there is not generally very much objection."[75]

If roads were a national matter, why not infectious diseases? Especially one so extensive, chronic, and costly as tuberculosis. Even the chief medical officer of Ontario, J.W.S. McCullough, asserted as late as 1930 that the health of the people was within the jurisdiction of the federal government.[76] But the government had already, with its 1919 act, made the definitive statement concerning its role: the new department would maintain previously established federal institutions, such as quarantine hospitals, involve itself in education, and only occasionally fund a larger project. It generally abdicated responsibility for instituting, maintaining or directing health care programs – even the ones it funded. It was left to the provinces, by default, to organize and systematically support health care for their residents.

In fact, the federal government, despite provincial willingness in the depression to share the financial burdens of public health, not only refused to institute any additional federal health grants but also refused to fund the development or continuation of any health units. Since only provinces with medical schools were eligible for Rockefeller Foundation support to establish such units, both Prince Edward Island and New Brunswick were disqualified.[77] By 1936, when the provinces were still asking for support in this effort, Wodehouse, as federal deputy minister of Pensions and National Health, stated frankly that not only would the federal government not take over any costs from the Rockefeller Foundation, but that "We, as a Dominion department, could bury our pride sufficiently to accept money, if we could get it from him."[78] By the end of the decade the federal division of epidemiology was successful in obtaining Rockefeller funding to study the extent of sylvatic plague and Rocky Mountain spotted fever in the Canadian West.[79]

As a consequence of the federal position, there would be no central supervision or standardization in Canadian health programs, including the tuberculosis campaign. The plea of provincial rights, which seemed to be promoted by a desire to avoid any more financial outlay, ironically enough served only to strengthen those very provincial rights so that, in another postwar period, when the federal government was finally prepared to seriously enter the health field, it had no choice but to do so by funding provincial organizations. By then, the authority so lightly and consistently denied in the twenties could not be assumed.

### Native Peoples: A Reservoir of Infection

In the twenties, tuberculosis specialists noticed the pitiful state of rural areas when they contrasted them to the increasingly health-conscious urban centres. It was inevitable that once they had seen improvement in the countryside, another group would stand out sharply as a "reservoir of infection" – native Canadians. [80] In the twenties, tuberculosis specialists concentrated on setting up travelling clinics and attempting to convince rural municipalities to clean up their milk and water supplies and hire full-time medical health officers and sanitary engineers, thus standardizing public health. They soon realized it was hopeless to try to eradicate tuberculosis from some communities if their next-door aboriginal neighbours were a continual source of infection. This was especially true in the Western provinces, where tuberculosis-ravaged native Canadians were considered most dangerous – ironically enough, as we have seen, the successful prevention campaign had left unexposed children and young adults least able to deal with a potentially massive infection. It was possibly, as D.A. Stewart observed, "nothing but poetic justice that the Indians should now be unwittingly bringing back to us this infection their fathers as unwittingly got from ours," but that statement had little bearing on the problem at hand. [81] In Manitoba in 1934, native Canadians formed 2.2 percent of the population but accounted for 31 percent of tuberculosis deaths; in Saskatchewan the figures were 1.6 percent and 27 percent, respectively; in Alberta 2.1 percent and 34 percent; and in British Columbia, 3.7 percent and 35 percent. As David Stewart demanded of the representatives of the Union of Manitoba Municipalities in 1934, "Suppose you had done your best to clean the smut spores off all the wheat in your granary, what would you think if a granary adjoining yours, with a door opening into yours, had wheat in it far more smut-infected than yours had ever been? Would that not upset all your fine plans for clean seed?"[82] G.J. Wherrett, executive secretary of the CTA, spoke for most tuberculosis specialists when he observed in the 1936 annual report that "our programme cannot be successful in the White population until the programme has also been adopted for the Indian."[83]

Unfortunately, it was not that simple. Tuberculosis case-finding and treatment programs were supervised and at least partially funded by provincial governments – and native Canadians were outside their jurisdiction. Not only was it not their responsibility to look after the native people's health, but the provinces had no authority over the living conditions and general sanitation levels on the reserves. With a goal of tuberculosis-free communities, tuberculosis specialists found this situation increasingly frustrating. "Indian reservations and settlements within provinces have been likened to slum areas in cities," wrote the superintendent of the Manitoba Sanatorium in exasperation to John Bracken, the premier of the province in 1934, "but that is not an adequate comparison. They are like slum areas would be if the cities they are in had no control over them, could make no regulations and set no standards for them, could not deal with any of their delinquencies; if they had no connection with any city systems or facilities, and if the only control exercised over their ways of living centred one to three thousand miles away."[84]

Self-interest thus demanded that the tuberculosis problem among native Canadians be dealt with – and by the federal government, which, with a fine impartiality, had thus far not demonstrated an overwhelming urge to aid any tuberculous Canadian citizen, irrespective of his race or colour. But tuberculosis specialists – both voluntary and official – began demanding aid. It seemed unfair for the provinces and volunteers to fund preventive work if the federal government took no responsibility for a large source of infection over which it alone had control. All felt that it was the dominion government's duty to provide native Canadians with proper diagnostic and treatment facilities. And when the government did act, its efforts were considered insufficient. The CTA recommended in a brief to the Rowell-Sirois Commission on Dominion Provincial Relations that to carry out an adequate tuberculosis program among native Canadians, an additional expenditure of $500,000 a year was required.[85]

## The Role of Immigrants

Anti-TB advocates also fretted about immigrants – especially those coming from countries with much higher death rates than Canada. A

Saskatchewan study over a five-year period showed the tuberculosis death rate among those in Canada less than five years to be one and a half times that of the remaining white population, which was a forewarning of what might occur once immigration increased. In Manitoba, 51.5 percent of tuberculous deaths were among immigrants, who made up only 35 percent of the population.[86] Often overworked, able to afford only cheap food and clothing, and too often coming from a highly tuberculous area, an immigrant was an easy prey to the disease. Having few resources, immigrants were almost invariably a burden on the community. Nevertheless, when they fell ill, they had to be cared for, for reasons beyond mere humanitarian considerations: as one sanatorium specialist observed practically, "tuberculosis treated and isolated – at whatever cost – is cheaper than tuberculosis neglected and allowed to spread."[87] Nonetheless, with the municipalities and provinces burdened with treatment costs and relief rolls, it seemed only just to demand federal support for aliens who were ill, particularly those recently repatriated after a long residence in the United States.

## The Limited Federal Role: Research and Cattle

With World War 1 demonstrating the practical implications and applications of scientific research, Canadian cattlemen demanding government action on bovine tuberculosis, and a newly announced BCG vaccine, it was not surprising that the federal government became involved in a form of education for the TB specialist: research. As has been mentioned, it appointed an associate committee on tuberculosis research at the National Research Council that represented all interested groups (including departments of health and agriculture, the CTA, cattlemen, universities, and sanatoria) and financed, with up to $30,000 annually, research on the human and bovine forms of the disease and on tuberculin and the BCG vaccine.[88] This, together with the printing of two pamphlets and the CTA's quarterly *Bulletin*, and, after 1923, a $15,000 grant to the national association, was the main federal initiative against tuberculosis. And this initiative, in turn, increased the importance of the CTA: it evolved into both a referral and advisory centre for the country, including provincial health departments.

By the end of the thirties, the federal government was continuing in much the same fashion as it had begun in the twenties: it combated tuberculosis in livestock, extended to the CTA its grant for educational purposes, and continued tuberculosis research under the aegis of the National Research Council.[89] Also, the Dominion Bureau of Statistics aided the CTA in devising some standard cards for keeping records.[90] But these activities were not enough. In its submission to the Rowell-Sirois Commission, the CTA suggested that the federal government improve its care of native Canadians and extend grants-in-aid to the provinces. The cost of the tuberculosis campaign, all agreed, was now simply too immense for provinces to handle alone. Half the total expenditure of provincial health departments in 1937, according to the *Canadian Public Health Journal*, was required only for sanatorium maintenance and the tuberculosis control program.[91] R.J. Collins, CTA president in 1939, pointed out that in both England and the Scandinavian countries the national government contributed 50 percent of maintenance and capital costs, and he saw no reason why that system should not be adopted in Canada – especially since the 12,000 beds needed in the campaign would cost $9 million a year to maintain.[92]

Taking a pragmatic approach, few tuberculosis specialists now worried about the intentions of the Fathers of Confederation – instead, tackling the situation as it now existed, they turned to the dominion government and demanded, first, that it look after its clearly assigned responsibilities (native peoples) and second, that it grant the provinces financial aid to run their *own* tuberculosis programs. Now specialists wanted federal funds to plug provincial gaps in tuberculosis programs and rural health care and to ease regional disparities, but they relied on provincial departments of health to provide the supervision and maintenance and on voluntary associations for education and support of preventive work.

"Tuberculosis is today," the *Canadian Public Health Journal* had written in a 1931 editorial, "our greatest public health problem." It was still the biggest killer of people between the ages of fifteen and forty-nine – when they were most valuable economically to the state.[93] The following year, David Stewart estimated that Canada's loss was twenty-two lives and one-third of a million dollars a day.[94] Public health activists had believed that the depression could only worsen the situation. Poverty, with its associated malnutrition and poor housing, not only lowered resistance but, by forcing whole families to crowd into a few small, cramped rooms, immeasurably increased contact with the disease. The inevitable results, the *Canadian Public Health Journal* gloomily predicted, would be "an increase not only in the tuberculosis death rate, but also in tuberculous infections – and these will add to the toll of tuberculosis and to its cost for years to come."[95]

Despite this ominous prediction and the national dislocation and misery, the tuberculosis death rate continued to fall. During the thirties, anti-TB workers attempted to treat more cases, examine more contacts, and educate more people – but where that was impossible, they usually managed (sometimes with salary cuts) to maintain most existing services. Moreover, the depression would lead many Canadians to question their health care system and conclusively demonstrate to doubting provincial governments that the costs of tuberculosis in particular were far beyond the means of the average individual – or even municipality – to pay. By the end of the decade, free treatment would be extended in fact, if not in name, to residents of Ontario, Manitoba, Saskatchewan, Alberta, and British Columbia. With the rate of infection among school children and young adults falling and collapse treatment increasingly successful, the future seemed promising, despite hardship.

Perhaps equally important, a division of responsibility had been firmly established among various levels of government that would affect not only the anti-TB campaign but the evolution of state responsibility in Canadian health care generally in the years after World War 2. Finally, encouraged by Rockefeller Foundation funding, an underlying philosophy of efficient, organized, centralized, and specialized scientific management not only influenced the manner in which both voluntary and government departments were established but promoted the development of new public health professionals who were administrators as much as physicians. Employed by both voluntary associations and governments, it was this new group who became the entrenched leaders of the anti-TB campaign in the interwar period. It was their policies and their direction that would guide and control the campaign against the disease for the next two decades.

"Our first slogan," reminisced R.G. Ferguson, medical superintendent of the Saskatchewan Anti-Tuberculosis League, the province probably hardest hit by the depression, in a 1936 address to the CTA, "was 'Tuberculosis is curable'; it is now 'Tuberculosis can be prevented'; and for the future, 'Tuberculosis can be eliminated.'"[96]

# 6 Childhood Tuberculosis

I once saw a strong healthy woman wheeling a consumptive daughter along, and on turning around to look at them, a genteleman said, "That woman is wheeling to the grave the last of a family of five. She has buried within three months her husband and four sons.

Extract from a letter received by the secretary of
the Toronto Free Hospital for Consumptives

Tuberculosis, Canadians soon realized, presented unique problems in childhood. With the advent of the tuberculin test, the amount of infection in a given community could be measured – and it became evident how widespread tuberculosis was among children. Anti-TB workers had been slow to recognize it because the childhood disease frequently affected the glands, bones, and joints, rather than the lungs; but the international conference on tuberculosis held in Washington in 1908 brought the problem to everyone's attention. Encouraged by wartime experience, the theory began to take root that tuberculosis began in childhood and blossomed only when the individual became an adult. Consequently, to deal properly with the disease, workers had to focus on the child. No longer were children merely "a resource for family welfare."[1] With the new century, they were worthy in their own right.

## Childhood Tuberculosis:
## A Different Presentation of the Disease?

As recognized today, childhood pulmonary tuberculosis frequently differs from the adult form and presents in a myriad of ways. *Neonatal* TB is now considered an acute, disseminated variant of the disease, likely secondary to infected amniotic fluid or hematogenous spread from the mother. *Miliary* TB presents as multiple small pulmonary lesions, while unilateral or bilateral hilar adenopathy (increased lymph nodes in the hilar area of the lungs) with an associated infiltrate (local lung disease) is the most common form. Chronic TB (secondary reinfection, or adult type) can occur in the pediatric population, with the associated typical features of the adult form: common involvement of the apex of the lung, cavitary formation, less prominent lymph nodes.[2]

Although fully alive to the danger of human tuberculosis, turn-ofthe-century anti-TB workers were in a quandary about the bovine form. Koch had stated flatly in 1900 that this form of the disease could not be communicated to humans – hence, there was no need to worry about diseased meat or infected milk. Many experts disagreed. The British government appointed a Royal Commission to investigate the thorny question in 1901, and, after exhaustive study and several interim reports, it pronounced in its final report of 1911 that the disease was communicable between humans and animals, noted that a large percentage of childhood tuberculosis was caused by infected meat and milk, and urged effective regulations to minimize the danger. Meanwhile, the American Veterinary Medical Association appointed an international commission on bovine tuberculosis in 1909 with members from both the United States and Canada. Its report of 1911 confirmed the British report, and a pamphlet was published offering advice on how to deal with the problem of diseased cattle.[3]

By World War 1 it was becoming generally accepted that although the chief cause of tuberculosis, particularly the pulmonary form, was the human bacillus entering through the respiratory tract, bovine tuberculosis infected a significant percentage of children, usually through the food they consumed.[4] The implications were far-reaching. A constant, pure supply of milk and meat was now necessary, and this requirement involved the profits of an influential, vocal segment of society – farmers, dairymen, stockbreeders, meat producers, and meat packers. As with tuberculosis in general, reformers would adopt the traditional two-pronged approach to the problem of diseased food, especially milk: prevention and cure.

*The Childhood Public Health Movement and the Fight against Childhood TB*

Influenced by the same concerns molding the adult campaign – the postwar emphasis on infectivity and bacteriology, centralization, efficiency, and professional expert leadership – the fight against childhood TB can also be seen in the context of a larger reform movement to improve the lives of Canadian children in general. Initiated largely by school boards in urban centres (since public health departments were initially unenthusiastic or unable to take responsibility), the childhood public health movement focused first on improving sanitation in school buildings and then, bolstered by new knowledge in infectious disease and bacteriology, expanded its focus to quarantines, school inspection, and, finally infant welfare. As with adult public health, advances in urban centres were extended to rural areas in the twenties. In an attempt to be more comprehensive and efficient, infant and child health services eventually merged under public health department supervision. With new importance placed on the the child in the reconstruction period following World War 1, the emphasis changed from controlling disease to ensuring good health. In the rural areas, this strategy required provincial involvement, because, mirroring the experience with adult TB, municipalities lacked an adequate tax base and population to manage by themselves. Provinces had to provide the appropriate supportive legislation, financial aid, professional health staff, and administrative structures. As with the adult campaign, this development would encourage provincial autonomy.[5]

Anti-TB work itself was only one part of the campaign to purify the milk supply. In the early years of the twentieth century roughly one out of every five to seven Canadian infants died in the first two years of life, and many deaths were linked to infected or adulterated milk.[6] New York statistics had proven that infant mortality in the hot summer months was related to the kind of milk consumed and that infantile diarrhea could be reduced by breast feeding. The Canadian movement for "pure milk" began in 1908 with the Canadian Medical Association Milk Commission, which publicized that milk carried typhoid, scarlet fever, diphtheria, infantile diarrhea and TB and which recommended hygiene standards for milk production, storage, and delivery.[7]

Initially the goal of pure milk was conceived in terms of infectious disease: prevention and cure. To lower infant mortality and reduce the number of children suffering from bone and joint TB, the milk supply could be "certified," (that is, produced from a clean, regularly inspected dairy and thus prevented from becoming infected), or it could be treated after the fact but prior to sale (that is, pasteurized). Many public health activists, disgusted by the milk peddled to consumers, believed they could achieve more in the short run by militantly demanding that all milk be pasteurized. As late as 1914, 90 percent of the milk reaching Montreal was unfit for human consumption, and only one-quarter of the city's milk supply was pasteurized (and only by dairies in the English-speaking West End).[8] Dr J.E. Dubé informed the *Montreal Star* in 1901 that the milk supply of Quebec City was the worst in the world.[9]

## Case-Finding and the Medical Inspection of Schools

To treat tuberculous or predisposed children, anti-TB crusaders first had to identify them. As part of the more general public health movement, reformers began pressuring for proper medical inspection in the schools, since a teacher could not be expected to spot symptoms early enough to prevent a child from infecting others. Moreover, school inspection had other reputed advantages: the doctor could diagnose such physical defects as undernourishment, bad teeth, diseased tonsils, and diseases like measles, all of which "predisposed" a child to tuberculosis. The doctor could also check the physical environment to ensure that the school room was adequately lit and ventilated: as early as 1883, the Ontario board of health's committee on school hygiene had set a minimum standard of 500 cubic feet of air space for each pupil to help prevent TB.

Therefore medical inspection was, the Canadian Association for the Prevention of Tuberculosis insisted, a state duty: not only should children have compulsory medical examination on entering school, but both students and teachers should be instructed in the basics of personal hygiene to avoid habits which spread the disease.[10] Montreal began the first regular system of medical inspection of Canadian school pupils in 1906. By 1910, inspection had been extended to Sydney, Nova Scotia, Vancouver, Hamilton, Halifax, Lachine, Toronto, Brantford, Winnipeg, Edmonton, and Nelson, British Columbia, while that same year British Columbia passed an act calling for an annual medical inspection of all school children, teachers and janitors in the province. Local tuberculosis leagues in British Columbia, Montreal, and Ottawa distributed pamphlets on the subject. How useful this strategy was in reducing the spread of infection is questionable, however, since at least 70 percent of school age children were believed to have tuberculosis in a latent or active form in 1910.[11]

It was Toronto, in 1910, that began to establish the model of school inspection for the country. By 1915 the board of education had a chief medical officer, twenty medical inspectors (who worked mornings), including a tuberculosis specialist, one chief dental officer and thirteen part-time dental surgeons, one superintendent of nurses and thirty-five full-time nurses. The city was divided into districts with one medical inspector and two nurses in charge of each.[12] A school medical inspector usually referred an exposed or suspected tubercular child to the special examiner for diagnosis, but a child could also be examined by the family doctor or a chest clinic at one of the local hospitals. Results and recommendations were reported to the municipal board of health and the visiting nurses operating under the board of health and board of education.

The school nurse undertook the basic organizational work. She arranged for the examination (which required the parents' written consent) and administered the tuberculin test. Doubtful cases were continually reexamined until they were deemed either positive or negative. Sometimes clearing up related problems was treatment enough. Tuberculous children, the chief medical officer reported, often had sore eyes, defective teeth, discharging ears, enlarged glands, or diseased bones, joints, or skin, which, it was believed, wore down their resistance and made them particularly susceptible to disease.

Health workers constantly pointed out the relationship between poor dental hygiene and disease in general, but especially tuberculosis. A dental inspector checked the children's teeth in Toronto schools. The Royal Edward Institute sent its open-air students to the Montreal General Hospital dental clinic. In Hamilton the Mountain Sanatorium arranged for free treatment of its child patients from that city's dentists, since fully 90 percent of the children they treated for tuberculosis had decayed teeth.[13] Such statistical evidence was unsurprising – a child who was in poor health generally due to poor nutrition and living conditions would be particularly prone to tuberculosis; and such a child's family would have little money for luxuries such as dentists.

With an increasingly bacteriological focus, Toronto school nurses educated the children about personal hygiene, running nose-blowing and tooth-brush drills and issuing comprehensive instructions on everything from cleaning fingernails and carrying a handkerchief to taking a bath (not always easy for a slum child). As a result, the school nurse gradually assumed a central position in the prevention of childhood tuberculosis in the prewar period.

Toronto's organization soon extended out from prevention to treatment, for it was evident that inspection and diagnosis alone were of little value unless some solutions to the identified problems could be found. Dental conditions were corrected at school or at a municipal clinic, while ear, nose, and throat disease was referred to the family doctor or a hospital. When advice went unheeded, school nurses in Toronto and elsewhere were not above using the juvenile courts to coerce parents to carry out school medical officers' orders for operations on adenoids and enlarged tonsils.[14]

### The Role of Departments of Health

It was Toronto again that set the pace in organizing institutional treatment for tuberculous children through its departments of health. Most cities, like Hamilton, diagnosed children through a dispensary, then had a visiting nurse treat them at home, or they placed them in the children's section of the local sanatorium. In Montreal, the Royal

Edward Institute established a preventorium for tuberculous children. But Toronto, through its department of health and various hospitals and voluntary organizations had a well-organized, detailed, and specialized system. By 1912 there was, theoretically, compulsory reporting of tuberculosis in Ontario, and municipal nurses visited the homes of reported adult cases. If children were in the house, the authorities tried to remove the source of infection by sending the adult to a sanatorium or hospital, and then the health officer disinfected the home and examined the child. An advanced case was sent to the children's department at Weston; older children with slight, open tuberculosis went to the Muskoka sanatorium; children with nonpulmonary tuberculosis went to the Heather Club pavilion for a number of months; those requiring surgery went to the Toronto Hospital for Sick Children, and closed patients who needed only to be removed from the dangerous environment of their homewent to the IODE preventorium. Health department visiting nurses supervised those remaining at home; they attended open-air or "forest" schools (discussed in a moment) to build up their resistance. The last group also had to report to a clinic at suitable intervals for periodic examinations.[15] For the first time in Canada a government had accepted more than minimal responsibility for the health of its citizens and had established a systematic and comprehensive – although, it might be argued, rather coercive – system to supervise and deal with the situation.

By 1915 Toronto's system of integrated health care for school children was considered, as mentioned, a North American model. Although statistics were sketchy and scientific analysis nonexistent, public health workers were pleased with the results. In 1917 the chief medical officer reported that while 85 to 95 percent of children had had dental defects in 1915, the rate had fallen to an encouraging 51 percent in eighty-six Toronto area schools. This result, combined with the fact that 3,000 children had been operated on for diseased tonsils or adenoids in 1916, obviously was, they believed, an important step in preventing and treating childhood tuberculosis.[16] And without childhood tuberculosis there could be no adult breakdown.

*Special Education:*
*The Forest School and the Preventorium*

By World War 1, reformers had noted that some children were not robust enough to cope with the often unsanitary, ill-lit, and ill-ventilated environment of regular schools, and they therefore promoted open-air and forest schools as a solution. Based on the principle of fresh air and good food, these schools were run by both voluntary

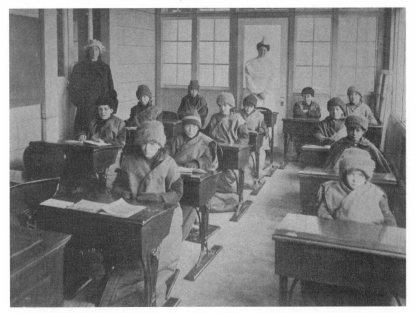

Open-air school. Free class for consumptive children, ages 5 to 15, opened on the verandahs of the Royal Edward Institute, December 1912. Reproduced from Royal Edward Institute, *Annual Report* (Montreal 1912)

associations and departments of education and aimed at building up the strength of delicate children to enable them to return to the normal education system. In 1912 the Toronto Board of Education established two forest schools in Victoria Park and High Park to run from May to October for children who "bear the earmarks of incipient disease and whose poverty precludes any hope of summer vacation away from the dirt and degradation of their homes."[17] Although public health workers consistently extrolled their virtues, forest schools were not a generally available, alternative means of education but a form of special education for the physically weak.

For children at higher risk – more sickly, or frankly tuberculous – the preventorium was established. The term was sometimes vague and encompassed institutions that were little more than summer camps, on the one hand, and specialized children's buildings attached to a local sanatorium, on the other. The preventorium was premised on the observation that children often suffered from a different form of tuberculosis – of the bone and joint – and required different care and discipline from that required by adults. Moreover, as the recommended length of stay increased from months to years, they required formal schooling.

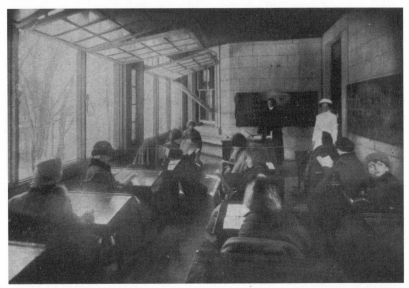

The open-air school, a February morning. Reproduced from Royal Edward Institute, *Annual Report* (Montreal 1912)

In 1909 the alumnae of the Toronto Hospital for Sick Children formed the Heather Club (taken over by the IODE in 1913) to aid tuberculous children in their homes, instruct their parents, and protect the other children. The club distributed clothing and food, employed a visiting nurse, and erected a summer shack for the young patients to sleep outside on the grounds of the Lakeside Hospital on Toronto Island. It was the first preventorium in Canada where a delicate or undernourished child, predisposed to tuberculosis, was cared for and fed nutritious food to strengthen natural resistance. Hamilton established an open-air classroom in 1910 at a preventorium attached to the sanatorium and supported by the school board, and the Royal Edward Institute opened a class for the actively diseased (twenty students were in the class).[18]

Whether they were attached to a sanatorium or were independent structures, both open-air schools and preventoria followed roughly the same routine. Children studied their lessons in unheated rooms with all the windows open, regardless of the weather. Like adults taking the cure, preventoria residents bundled up in mittens, scarves, and coats to sit behind their desks in the Canadian winter. Adhering to the tenets of fresh air, good food, and rest, children were fed nourishing meals indoors at school and required to take an afternoon nap. Limited government support of these schools (by the Toronto school board, for example) demonstrated a dawning awareness of the economic advantage of childhood prevention over cure – especially since the state already paid for the child's compulsory regular education. Initially infant mortality had been a problem distinct from that of the health of school children, but the two problems began to merge as tuberculosis workers extended their activities into the younger group. Because the child was viewed more and more as the primary source of adult infection, it seemed logical that if ill health and exposure as a child left an adult prone to relapsing with tuberculosis, ill health as an infant was far more likely to result in weak, unhealthy, and susceptible children, as well as increased infant mortality. In addition to the milk depots (in Montreal, *gouttes de lait*) established to distribute pure, fresh milk to needy infants, educate their mothers, and, ideally, lower the infant mortality rate, special babies' wards were opened at the IODE preventoriums in Toronto and in the Saskatchewan sanatorium; child welfare exhibitions were held and "little mothers'" classes organized.[19]

## Anti-TB education in Childhood

Such specialized accommodation as the preventorium was designed to cope with the unique *clinical* manifestation of childhood TB, with its more common nonpulmonary presentation. Treatment incorporated sunlight, or heliotherapy, and dealt with the *social problems* of caring for and disciplining younger patients. However, another social reform tenet, the need for education, also fostered a focus on the child, as anti-TB crusaders tried to overcome public ignorance and apathy, which they were finding unendurably frustrating. Osler had optimistically observed that "The public is awake, sitting on the edge of the bed, not yet dressed, but still it is an improvement even to get the public awake."[20]

But most social reformers were too impatient to take this prosaic approach. "I have myself," an exasperated C.J. Fagan, secretary of the British Columbia Anti-Tuberculosis Society and the secretary of the provincial board of health, asserted in 1910, "distributed some 40,000 circulars explaining this whole subject in the simplest way, and in popular language, and sent them to every church and school in British Columbia. And yet every man or woman whoever came in contact with me afterwards didn't have the simplest rudimentary idea of what it was. Anything official coming to the public ear does not enter the brain. We have decided, therefore, to give up the old people and get after the next generation."[21] By educating the child, who was more malleable, reformers could, as another commentator observed with typical social reform optimism, convince parents, and thus government, to pass legislation. The inevitable result, he concluded, would be "the rapid eradication of tuberculosis, not only in Canada, but in the world at large."[22] Concentrating on the child, therefore, would battle the disease on two fronts: preventing childhood infection would not only reduce the number of adults breaking down with the disease in later life but would also indirectly stimulate public education, awareness, and action.

The child took on added importance after the war. "Our children are our greatest national asset," asserted the president of the Canadian Association for the Prevention of Tuberculosis in 1919.[23] With the "fittest and finest" killed in the war, Canada could not afford to waste potentially good citizens. "Every child's start to a healthy, normal family life," R.W. Bruce Smith, the Ontario inspector of hospitals and public charities stated firmly, "must be regarded as a legitimate claim by the province or state."[24]

### A Comprehensive Approach

Viewing children as a precious commodity in the postwar reconstruction period, anti-TB workers had to deal with them in a comprehensive fashion. Their approach mirrored the themes in the adult campaign: standardization, organization, and efficiency. Before the war, campaigns for school inspection and a lower rate of infant mortality had been separate and distinct – now they were merged into the child welfare movement, which included the care of the pregnant woman, as well as the infant and the child. Just as visiting nurses had discovered in the course of their work that it was more efficient to combine all aspects of public health nursing in one person rather than maintaining separate tuberculosis and infant welfare nurses, so public health workers realized that it made more sense to coordinate and concentrate their efforts on the whole child. This was especially true in rural areas, where the great distances and scattered population made an uncoordinated system sketchy and inefficient. The limited municipal tax base virtually mandated provincial support and organization – and this, in turn, promoted centralization.

Anti-TB and public health specialists began to view individuals as *whole entities* developing through states of infancy, childhood, and adulthood, and they treated them as such. District health units were premised on this concept, as the provincial health officer of British Columbia outlined in 1929. Ideally, the vital statistics branch of the provincial government forwarded the medical officer of health a list of births each week. The public health nurse immediately took charge of the infants for the first two years; then preschool children were supervised by "well baby" clinics, their physical defects were diagnosed and corrected, and mothers attended talks to teach them health care and preventive medicine. Upon entering school, children were supervised by the medical officer of health and routinely examined by the nurses. However, such comprehensive district care was costly and available only in select spots across the country.[25]

Industrial hygiene was, incidentally, an outgrowth of this focus on the whole individual. Tuberculosis specialists began to realize that child care was meaningless if adults were allowed to overwork in a poor environment, break down with the disease, and become a burden to the state at the very time they should be paying back the state's investment in their health. The tuberculosis examiner of the Massachusetts-Halifax Health Commission noted in 1922, for example, that three-quarters of the children in the area left school to work at the age of sixteen: they were at high risk for tuberculosis and yet were no longer getting medical examinations.[26]

## The Source of Infection: Bovine or Human?

Various surveys had forced Canadians to confront the extent of childhood infection. The solution, activists asserted, lay in prevention; and with pasteurization of milk employed more frequently in the twenties, an increasing emphasis was placed on *contact* as the primary source of the disease, rather than food or milk; tuberculin was used to determine infection. No doubt this shift in focus was at least partly due to the increase in available accommodation since the war. With more beds to isolate the infectious parent from the child, tuberculosis specialists could afford to promote this approach. And since they also agreed, in the main, that the war had proven adult tuberculosis to be a reactivation of childhood infection, it seemed even more important to isolate the open case. Although institutional treatment began to be extended to rural children for the first time, traditional methods were relatively unchanged. Open-air schools, preventoria, and children's wings of sanatoria continued to flourish; summer camps were established, often by a service club, for the undernourished or sickly. Light treatment was popular, and ear, eye, nose, throat and dental clinics continued to discover other defects.

In 1910 the infant mortality rate had been 197 per 1,000 births in Toronto. By 1914, with a milk bylaw rigidly enforced, a public health system established, and a water filtration plant built, infant mortality had fallen to 60 deaths for every 1,000 births. The death rate for tuberculosis alone for children under two in that city fell from 6.3 per 100,000 in 1918 to 3 per 100,000 in 1927.[27]

As Neil Sutherland has demonstrated, however, it is difficult, if not impossible, to determine how much of any decline in infant mortality is attributable to the public health work discussed here. Although improved milk supplies undoubtedly lowered the total number of gastrointestinal diseases, sanitary reforms and an improved standard of living also affected survival. Moreover, mortality statistics are a tenuous basis for evaluating a city's progress, since their collection varied extensively from place to place. Under-registration of births had artificially increased the infant mortality rate; as registration improved, the situation reversed itself. Early infant deaths were unlikely to be recorded as comprehensively as the births of the survivors, so that infant mortality rates would decline for this reason alone. In general, however, the decrease in the proportion of infant deaths attributable to infantile diarrhea and the decline in the proportion of younger age groups in the total death rate suggests that such public health work probably had some beneficial effect.[28]

### Pasteurization

While wartime expansion of sanatoria facilities and the increasing emphasis on bacteriology focused attention on the role of contacts in childhood TB, the philosophical emphasis on state responsibility and the importance of the child continued to fuel demands for a pure milk supply in the interwar period – ironically, particularly in the previously neglected rural communities. A committee appointed by the Canadian Public Health Association reported in 1926 that milk caused more disease than any other single food and asserted that it was the duty of the local authority to safeguard the milk supply as much as the water supply.[29] Although it was argued that with 35 to 50 percent of cattle reputedly infected, a milk famine would result if all diseased cattle were destroyed, anti-TB activists also pointed out that it cost roughly $75 per month to treat a tuberculous child in a sanatorium and that for that price a first-class dairy cow could be replaced. Of course, later infection of the milk by tuberculosis and other diseases could still occur through improper handling.[30]

The answer increasingly lay in pasteurization. As the twenties progressed, public health specialists began to agree that certification of cattle was impractical, more expensive, and even unsafe, since tuberculosis did develop in certified herds. The Canadian Public Health Association committee went so far as to state that with pasteurization, tuberculin testing was "no longer an essential from the public health viewpoint."[31]

By 1922, most major Canadian cities pasteurized much of the milk sold.[32] Not all Canadians – particularly dairy farmers – were convinced of the benefits. Dr W.F. Roberts, the first minister of health in New Brunswick, who introduced pasteurization of milk in St John in 1923, was defeated in the 1925 election at least partly because of this action. Such public ignorance and intransigence infuriated health specialists like J.W.S. McCullough, the chief health officer of Ontario, who, agreeing with those who complained that the pasteurized product tasted "different," acidly observed that "there is less cow manure in milk subject to rigid inspection and to the other safeguards, including pasteurization."[33]

A Toronto study of 500 tuberculous children begun in 1926 added credence to the advocates of pasteurization, since every one of the bovine-infected children (9.6 percent) had come from areas outside the city, where pasteurization was not enforced.[34] "Compulsory pasteurization," insisted the *Canadian Public Health Journal* dogmatically, "is the only method by which municipal milk supplies may be rendered safe."[35] Public health specialists hotly refuted the old charges that compulsory pasteurization would squeeze out the smaller producer or lower the nutritional value of the milk and pointed triumphantly to the Certified Milk Producers of America, who agreed in 1935 to have their "certified milk" *pasteurized,* as irrefutable proof of its outstanding advantages.[36]

In 1938, Ontario became the first province to pass a compulsory pasteurization law. The Milk Control Act of 1934 had chiefly regulated price, while a 1938 amendment, although it set standards for raw-milk dairies and pasteurizing plants, vested administrative control in the milk control board, a branch of the department of agriculture, rather than the department of health. With compulsory pasteurization in 1938, the latter took over, and each plant was required to obtain a yearly certificate of approval.[37] Although over 85 percent of the milk in the province was pasteurized by 1937 and although Ontario milk distributors and public health officials had advocated compulsory pasteurization for two decades, successive provincial governments had failed to require it because of the opposition of small dairy farmers.

It was Mitch Hepburn, the exuberant, fast-talking, politically shrewd, larger-than-life premier of the province from 1934 to 1942 who finally pushed the measure through. Suffering from chronic bronchitis and particularly prone to respiratory infections himself, his health problems may have given him a personal interest in the issue. Dr Alan Brown, chief pediatrician at Toronto's Hospital for Sick Children, provided Hepburn with a National Research Council report that proved that over 10 percent of the 490 tuberculous children at the hospital suffered from bovine tuberculosis acquired from raw milk. Despite the statistics, Brown apparently told the premier bluntly that because of the farm lobby – part of Hepburn's support – he doubted the politicians had the "guts" to pass compulsory legislation.

Touring a TB ward with the pediatrician, just before the legislative session opened, Hepburn is said to have confronted two long rows of cots filled with bovine TB patients. None of the children would have been there, Brown informed him, if Queen's Park had been courageous enough to pass compulsory pasteurization. "Your government has the power – if it wishes to use it – to empty hospital wards like these." "Done," Hepburn is said to have replied.

The subsequent protest threatened to divide Hepburn's cabinet and alienate his key rural support. An Ontario Agricultural Council delegation, including some of Hepburn's own neighbours from Elgin, met Hepburn at Queen's Park in February 1938 to present their opposing arguments: the necessary machinery was expensive; there was no evidence that untreated milk caused the disease.

According to one biographer, Hepburn is said to have recognized one of the men in the delegation:

"How many children do you have?"

"I have five," replied the surprised farmer.

"Didn't you have seven?"

"Yes, two died."

"They died of bovine tuberculosis, didn't they? They drank milk from your own cows and died?" Hepburn persisted angrily.

"You came here today to protest against the pasteurization of milk. You have already lost two children to bovine tuberculosis, but that doesn't prevent you from coming here to ask this Government to withdraw its bill and leave your children and other children open to the threat of death. What kind of man are you?"[38]

Opposition didn't cease with the passage of the bill in 1938. "I thought we had a real leader," a St Thomas farmer wrote, "but I find we have a damn stool pigeon." Others were equally abusive. Hepburn did not back down, and he was proud of his decision. "I had to take the hard way, not the popular way," he told his own supporters at a farmers' meeting in Aylmer, "and I am going to live to see the day when the children of Ontario will be safe from the dangers of bovine tuberculosis."[39]

Such a dramatic confrontation and defense may have been apocryphal. Compulsory pasteurization applied only to urban municipalities and towns in 1938 but was soon extended to rural areas, so that by

1941 over 98 percent of the milk sold in Ontario in fluid form was pasteurized. Local centres no longer had to make a controversial choice of whether or not to pasteurize, and, more importantly, pasteurizing plants now had to conform to uniform standards set by and under the supervision of the department of health. Results were quickly evident: by 1939, cases of undulant fever had been reduced 45 percent and of typhoid fever by approximately 50 percent.[40] The protection Toronto and other urban centres had received for so many years was now finally extended to the residents of rural townships and smaller centres. To the public health specialists, it was a landmark decision in terms of provincial responsibility for public health – especially for rural areas. The *Canadian Public Health Journal* even maintained it would stimulate tourism![41]

## BCG and the Grancher System

It was in the prevention rather than treatment of childhood tuberculosis that the greatest innovations were made in the 1920s. "It is easier," David Stewart observed in an essay on tuberculosis, "to correct criminal tendencies than to cure crime," and most public health workers agreed. One medical health officer from Nova Scotia confidently proclaimed in 1922, "Prevent contacts in children and infection will largely disappear."[42]

The most obvious means was with BCG, the attenuated live TB vaccine that was described in chapter 3. As has been mentioned, Dr J.A. Baudoin began a series of clinical trials in Montreal in 1925, in cooperation with the Bruchesi and Royal Edward Institutes and several hospitals, vaccinating new-born infants exposed to the disease. This research would continue for over twenty years.[43]

Quebec was the most obvious place to begin – in 1926 the death rate for the non-native population was 82.5 per 100,000 in Canada, but 118.6 in Quebec; sanatoria were few, and the anti-TB campaign was localized and disorganized. The extent of the disease in that province was still unknown, for doctors did not always report new cases, and they avoided mentioning TB on death certificates. Cases were frequently diagnosed too late – 50 percent of the tuberculous patients in the province died within five years of the initial diagnosis of their disease.[44] Mass vaccination – if safe and effective – would have been a solution for Quebec. But in the twenties both these factors still had to be determined.

Quebec also pioneered the Grancher system in Canada in 1929, another preventive measure, theoretically, first developed in France (in 1903). Children exposed to an open case of tuberculosis were removed from their infected city homes and placed in the family of a farmer who either had no children of his own or whose children had grown up. Selected children, with the Royal Edward and Bruchesi Institutes, were three to twelve years old and otherwise in good health. The system in Quebec was directed by the provincial bureau of health, which paid $10 a month for board and lodging for each child, with the bureau usually supplying clothing and paying school fees. The local public health nurses, the curé, and the local physician supervised the children. According to Emile Nadeau, director of the Quebec Bureau of Health, Grancher had calculated that 60 percent of exposed children, if left with their parents, became tuberculous, with 40 percent dying from the disease; while under his system, he maintained, less than 1 percent even became infected.[45] Not only that but, as Nadeau observed enthusiastically in 1929, under the Grancher System "the child is raised as a peasant, acquires a taste for rural life, goes to the local school and later, as observed in France, there is considerable probability that he will remain on the land, a farmer like his foster family, healthy, robust and forever freed from the danger to which he would have been exposed had he remained in the city."[46] To be exact, Grancher had found that a full 33 percent of the children chose to remain on the land on turning thirteen.[47] Statistical support for the success of the system in Quebec was not available, however. It was in fact, it might be argued, not merely a public health measure or even a residue of the prewar "healthy life on the farm" attitude but also a thinly veiled resettlement scheme to control a growing urban proletariat.

A "religion of right living," with an organized, bacteriological approach, had become more important than social reform in improving adults' health.[48] It was therefore not surprising if the same philosophy extended to children. As the Montreal Anti-Tuberculosis and General Health League expressed so clearly in 1925, "To those who ascribe our high infant death rate to large families and low wages, we would point out that neither of these explains away the deaths from Diarrhoea and Enteritis, which are due to ignorant mothers and impure milk in the vast majority of cases."[49] When one veteran social reformer at the 1920 annual meeting demanded that the association interest itself in economic conditions, George Porter, the executive secretary, agreed that "We should have decent living wages," but stressed "education as well."[50] His remarks set the tone for the interwar period.

### The Junior Red Cross and the Children's Health Crusade

Medical inspection of schools had emphasized the health of children but, in the process, their physical health had become separate and

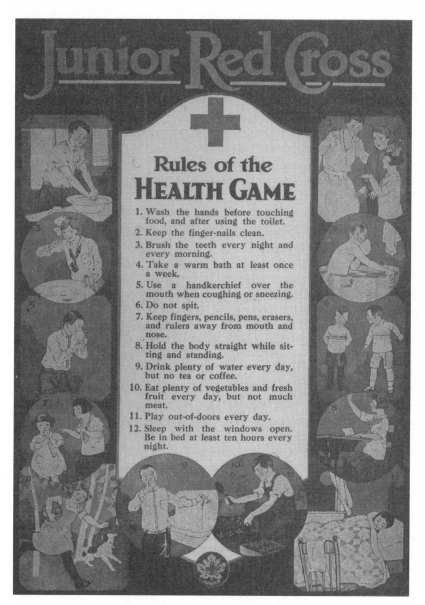

The Junior Red Cross Rules of health. Reproduced from the frontispiece of a textbook used in Canadian schools, Ritchie and Caldwell, *Primer of Hygiene*

distinct from their mental and moral education. Those interested in "health education" proposed to merge these three again under the direction and supervision of the class teacher. Health, they argued, should not simply be a half-hour class taught by the school nurse, since it affected everything a child did. "Home-nursing" and "care-of-the-baby" demonstrations were organized. Health talks given one day formed the subject of a writing lesson the following day. In Halifax a "health crusade" was begun in which 3,000 pupils in grades three through five appointed one pupil for each class to ensure health rules were obeyed, awarding the obedient students a crusade pin. To carry this policy out teachers would have to be properly informed, and thus there was a growing emphasis on hygiene in normal school curricula.[51]

Mirroring the growth of large, professional voluntary associations in the adult anti-TB movement, the children's health crusade was most effectively organized through the Junior Red Cross. Begun in the World War 1 as a means of having children "do their bit" for the men at the front, the organization evolved into an instrument of public health in the twenties. If medical inspection and treatment were, as the director of this new movement commented, only repair work, then the Junior Red Cross taught children to remain healthy in a comprehensive, systematic fashion. Its stated goal was to enrol every child in the country, and its medium was the schools. Children in previous decades had been told what to do – now, with the emphasis on education through demonstration and example, children were *shown* what to do and were encouraged literally to practise it in the classroom. By 1925 there were 100,000 members (Juniors) in Canada who followed the "Twelve rules of the health game": by 1929 membership had burgeoned to 200,000 under 7,000 teachers, with roughly 20,000 joining each year.[52]

Organized for "health, service and good citizenship," the Junior Red Cross was also a very effective means of inculcating middle class standards and values in all school children. It promoted the maintenance of a healthy environment, proper nutrition, and personal hygiene, but Juniors were also encouraged to aid in community health programs and service work. They were being trained to be healthy, responsible citizens and, possibly more importantly, future members of service clubs and voluntary associations. Public health workers had long recognized that children were most receptive to new thought and instruction – now, through a national organization, not only personal hygiene, but the doctrine of voluntarism, with its underlying middle class belief in the modification – but not the wholesale overthrow – of the social system, was systematically propounded in the schools.

By the end of the twenties, results seemed encouraging. As milk became pasteurized and as more cases were treated, more contacts examined, and more cases discovered early on, children were inspected and instructed, and prevented from falling prey to tuberculosis. Public health for children was becoming more organized, and, as it expanded into previously neglected areas, it was receiving more provincial support. The tuberculosis rate began to fall in many places, and treatment facilities had to adjust accordingly: the St John County Hospital closed one children's ward, while the IODE preventorium in Toronto began admitting hearing conditions and choreas, along with bone and chest cases.[53]

By the thirties, tuberculosis specialists were reevaluating their campaign against childhood disease. Because of the rapidly falling rate of infection in areas with proper case-finding machinery, along with the federal government's program to eradicate bovine tuberculosis and the fact that most milk was now pasteurized, it appeared that tuberculosis, as a childhood disease at any rate, was fading fast.[54] Although most established methods, including medical inspection of schools, forest and open-air schools, summer camps, and especially the Junior Red Cross, continued to flourish, specialists began to question whether the money that had been pumped so enthusiastically into the campaign to protect the child could now be better spent elsewhere – perhaps on preventing the disease in young adults.

The role of the preventoria came under the closest scrutiny – despite intensive searching, even at the height of the depression, tuberculosis workers were finding them impossible to fill. The Mountain Sanatorium reported in 1936 that its child population was only one-quarter of what it had been previously. The East Windsor Sanatorium actually closed its preventorium, while the preventorium at the St John Tuberculosis Hospital slowly evolved into an institution for the care of childhood orthopedic cases. From 1935 to 1937 a comprehensive survey was made of the IODE preventorium in Toronto, and although no conclusions could legitimately be drawn from the statistics collected,[55] it was indicative of the changing attitude that such a task had been attempted – twenty years earlier, the value of the preventorium would never have been questioned.

By 1942, the Ontario health department's survey of the Toronto health department (the survey was done by the Phair Committee) had pointedly condemned the forest schools for serving only 500 pupils and not enhancing the children's health.[56] Specialists had come to believe that it was more sensible and less expensive to improve the home situation than to institutionalize the child. "It is cheaper," the

Vancouver Survey Committee remarked succinctly, "to remove the tuberculosis from the home than it is to remove the children from the tuberculosis" – especially when there was more than one child.[57] The interwar expansion of beds encouraged this shift in emphasis – just as it had with adults. If beds were in short supply or if the home situation was irremediable, foster homes were the favoured alternative (particularly in Quebec, which, lacking adequate sanatorium accommodation for infectious adults, had established the limited Grancher system).[58] With years of tuberculin tests and school surveys giving a clearer idea of the prevalence of the disease, specialists noted that even if the number of children infected rose rapidly from the ages of two to fourteen, the number of active cases did not. Yet it was these children, who had recovered from a primary infection, who were frequently found in the preventorium. If the source of infection was removed, they were unlikely to develop further disease until they were past preventorium age. In terms of tuberculosis control, preventoria had all but outlived their day.

As the depression deepened, specialists concentrated their efforts on adolescents and young adults. With the rate of infection falling rapidly among school children, it was plainly evident that, provided a child was not born into a tuberculous environment, the first serious exposure to the disease would probably not occur until after the age of fourteen – when many left school and began associating frequently with infectious adults. Experience with student nurses, who too frequently became infected with tuberculosis upon entering training, bolstered this theory. In addition, many adolescents were of course suffering from the physical, mental, and emotional strains of puberty; they were perhaps working for the first time or studying intensively under poor conditions; they had new responsibilities and were possibly bearing children while burning the candle at both ends. It was no wonder that the death rate of adolescents and those in their twenties continued to be high.[59] TB specialists consequently pleaded for health education to prepare students for the grinding rigours of modern life and for a more serious concentration by experts on the general health of Canadian youth. Those under thirty were "working hard and playing far too hard" and now, if exposed to disease, had no resistance against it.[60] Again, the elimination of infection became crucial.

At the same time, tuberculosis workers were seeing the success of the campaign against the disease in children repeated with cattle. Largely through the continuing efforts of the federal department of agriculture, bovine tuberculosis was slowly being eliminated. Livestock owners found few markets for untested cattle and their products and so were willing to take advantage of any plan for which they qualified, even those that paid no compensation.[61] Results were apparent: the percentage of cattle slaughtered for food with tuberculous lesions had fallen from 4.71 in 1924–25 to 1.81 by 1932–33. By the end of 1940, 46 percent of Canadian cattle had been tested under the federal department's plans, with a total of about $13 million paid out since compensation policies had been initiated. Perhaps more importantly, not more than 2 percent of the cattle in the country were tuberculous by the end of the decade.[62] Bovine tuberculosis was gradually becoming extinct – in 1938 the CTA, revealingly, placed its eradication eleventh in a series of policies designed to deal with tuberculosis in humans.[63]

By the World War 2, childhood tuberculosis, if not yet a concern solely of the past, was fast becoming an inconsequential part of the tuberculosis campaign, especially in Ontario and the West. Both pasteurization of milk and aggressive case-finding were promoted as the causes of the accelerating fall in the rate of infection – in Saskatchewan the percentage of primary school children (ten to eleven years old) reacting to tuberculin fell from 51 in 1921 to 6 in 1947, while the percentage for normal school pupils (eighteen to twenty years old) fell from 75.6 in 1921 to 9.4 in 1948.[64] Yearly patch tests were still advisable, if only to ensure that all was well and to provide an index of infection. Even in Quebec, where tuberculosis had yet to be systematically controlled, the president of the newly created tuberculosis commission, J.A. Vidal, reflecting on the methods of treating childhood tuberculosis, summarized them as part of the *past*: open-air schools and summer camps he now considered "an admirable social institution" but not specifically anti-tubercular. He recommended that the leagues entrust their administration to a separate organization – as they did in Montreal, where the Bruchesi Health Camps, though still in existence, were handled by the Federated Charities.[65]

Perhaps the most obvious sign of the times was the change in 1940, by order-in-council, of the old Toronto IODE preventorium for children from tuberculous families to the IODE Hospital for Convalescent Children, associated with the Toronto Hospital for Sick Children. A survey of the institution at the end of the previous decade had revealed a great amount of money had been spent on "predisposed" children; and specialists now argued that if the same amount had been spent to improve home conditions, perhaps more could have been accomplished. Nevertheless, as George Wherrett, the CTA secretary, summed up unemotionally in 1944, "The Preventorium probably served a useful purpose when it was first operated. It aroused a good deal of interest in the community, focused attention on the care of children from tuberculous families and no doubt influenced public opinion so that there was a demand for adequate sanatorium accommodation to treat the original source of the infection."[66] But now its time was past.

The campaign against childhood tuberculosis evolved as part of both a general movement to improve the well-being of children generally in Canadian society and as a branch of the larger campaign against tuberculosis in Canada. Such specialization was justified both socially and clinically. Children were seen as patients distinct from adults, with specialized needs: formal education and appropriate age-related discipline and control. The importance of bovine tuberculosis and infected milk reinforced this specialization, which emphasized a treatment – heliotherapy – for the bone and joint form of the disease, which was more common in childhood. Heliotherapy was unsuccessful with the adult, pulmonary form of the disease.

In other ways, however, the campaign against the childhood form of the disease closely paralleled the adult campaign. There was a shift into rural areas in the twenties, with a concomitant increase in provincial involvement and responsibility. Organization, efficiency, specialization, and scientific management became the watchwords here, too, as public health specialists gradually assumed responsibility for children's health from the school boards and public health nursing evolved into a recognized specialty. Large, professional voluntary organizations were represented in the role of the Junior Red Cross. And the professional managers – the public health officials – were clearly in charge.

# 7 Tuberculosis and World War 2

It is an appalling reality that, during the first five years of World War II, 36,000 Canadians died from TB, while 38,000 Canadians were killed by enemy action.                    *Saturday Night,* 1945

"The older men will remember," warned the president of the CTA, R.J. Collins, in a 1939 address, "the difficulties that arose because of our lack of knowledge regarding tuberculosis in the last war."[1] And those difficulties had been costly. For every hundred Canadians killed in action, six had died of tuberculosis, while for every hundred pensioned for wounds, twenty-five had been pensioned for tuberculosis.[2] The cost of the disease alone as a direct result of World War 1 was estimated to be $150 million for Canada[3] – and it was a cost that neither the government, which was responsible for treatment and pensions of soldiers and veterans, nor the tuberculosis specialists, who were trying to control infection, wanted repeated.

Canada on the eve of World War 2 was very different from the nation in 1914. Farming, fishing, and lumbering now employed only one-third of the labour force, while the service industries – transportation, communications, trade, finance, and the professions – accounted for 39 percent of wage earners and salaried employees. Although the depression had halted economic growth, over 54 percent of the population lived in cities or towns by 1941.[4] And by 1939 the combined federal and provincial expenditures for health amounted to $32 million.[5] The depression had ended an era of western settlement and expansion – World War 2 signalled a new beginning when the country would change not only its direction but its character.[6]

The anti-TB campaign had also changed in the interwar period. The death rate had been cut to one-third of that existing in 1914; sanatorium beds had increased from two thousand (primarily in Ontario) to over ten thousand across the country; a network of clinics and travelling diagnosticians had been established; and, most important of all from the point of view of the Canadian government, x-rays had come into general use.[7] There was now a reliable, simple, and inexpensive method of eliminating diseased and tuberculosis-prone recruits that would save enormous postwar pension costs. It took little time for the federal government to see the wisdom of the CTA's immediate recommendation that every recruit be routinely x-rayed. *Maclean's Magazine* publicly endorsed it in an editorial in November 1939.[8]

### TB and the Military

Soon after the outbreak of war, the Department of Defence x-rayed the entire army and instituted chest x-ray examinations for everyone on admittance to and discharge from the armed forces.[9] Roughly .9 percent were rejected, with about one-third of those requiring treatment or observation – usually they were minimal cases who were reported to their provincial health departments. This practice sometimes caused problems in areas where treatment facilities were already overtaxed. In 1940 one army expert estimated a saving to the Canadian government of $25 million for the first 100,000 troops examined, at an estimated cost of $200,000 for the x-ray service. It was, exulted the executive secretary of the CTA, "the greatest case-finding project ever attempted in our history."[10]

As a result, tuberculosis in the armed forces presented a very different picture in World War 2 than in World War 1: simply put, it was controlled. The incidence of pulmonary tuberculosis was only one-quarter of that in civilian life, and tuberculous pleurisy was about the same. The rate rose in the army overseas where tuberculin-negative troops, unresistant products of intensive control programs in Ontario and the West, fell prey to pulmonary tuberculosis on contact with the tuberculous environment. Their rates of infection rose to be three to four times higher than corresponding civilian rates and double those in the army at home. It was a situation specialists had encountered before with student nurses, and it brought home once again the critical problem of uninfected, and thus theoretically unprotected, individuals exposed to the disease.[11]

### Wartime Industrial Experience

Soldiers were only part of the war machine. Equally important were war workers – especially since an estimated one-half of all Canadians employed in manufacturing were engaged in the production of wartime needs. In the first two years of the war the number of unemployed

Canadians fell from half a million to less than 200,000. Iron and steel production doubled, and the gross national product rose by 47 percent. Supplying arms and equipment to the country's allies started Canada on a period of prosperity that would last another three decades.[12]

In modern industrial warfare, healthy workers were essential if assembly lines were to be kept running at top speed – "without them," Grant Fleming, professor of public health at McGill, observed bluntly, "money is of no avail in speeding production."[13] Manpower shortages enhanced the value of workers. As they had been during World War 1, Canadians were shocked to discover how unhealthy their fellow citizens were: 43 percent of young men called up for military training by November 1941 had been rejected on the grounds of poor health. "It should not be necessary to have a war," noted the *Canadian Public Health Journal* sensibly, if idealistically, "to make the people realize that the health and physical fitness of children and of young people are of paramount importance to the country."[14]

Paradoxically, and much to the specialists' dismay, tuberculosis, which had decreased during the hard times of the depression-ridden thirties, increased with the greater prosperity and low unemployment of the war. Several factors were believed to account for this blow: rapid shifts in population, especially into urban centres to work in war industries, a housing shortage and resulting overcrowding, longer working hours causing lowered resistance, food shortages, and the more nebulous wartime anxieties and stress.[15] "Our unemployed," observed the chief of the tuberculosis section of the Montreal department of health, "undernourished for several years, were obliged, within a few days of the outbreak of the war, to work for long hours, sometimes in daytime, sometimes at night, in temporary quarters, erected hastily and not often very healthful."[16] The strain of war was even affecting the nation's hens, noted the veterinary-general; they were threatened with an outbreak of poultry tuberculosis, due to overcrowding in the chicken-houses.[17]

Capitalizing on wartime zeal and rhetoric, the CTA pointed out that the anti-TB campaign itself was nothing less than a patriotic duty, while money raised from selling Christmas Seals was "a war fund that will provide the means to keep our workers free from tuberculosis, keep our factories in full operation and bring nearer the day of the five freedoms": freedom from want and from fear, freedom of speech and of thought, and a new freedom, freedom from disease.[18] With mass x-ray surveys demonstrably so successful in weeding out sources of tuberculosis in the armed forces, it was only logical to apply them in turn to war industries, beginning in the Kitchener-Waterloo area, with a postwar objective of examining the whole nation.[19]

*Sanatoria and Wartime Shortages*

Two pressing problems occupied tuberculosis specialists during the war: a shortage of staff and an acute shortage of beds. In vain did the CTA tell the federal government that the disorganization of the sanatoria in World War 1 must be avoided if sanatoria were considered an essential war service; in the first four years of war, although the number of beds in use increased 10.7 percent, staff decreased 5.1 percent.[20] As J.H. Holbrook, superintendent of Hamilton's Mountain Sanatorium, noted in frustration in 1942, all the best orderlies, nurses, doctors, laboratory workers, and other employees had left early in the war, leaving old men and women and less qualified individuals to replace them, including "a group of floaters who are untrained and irresponsible and are liable to sign up for work today and to disappear after their next pay day."[21]

The problem was aggravated by the burden of war work, especially the examination of recruits and the interpretation of their x-rays. By the end of 1942, five of the original health districts in New Brunswick (with 55 percent of the province's population) lacked medical health officers. Both Nova Scotia and Manitoba were forced to close beds because a nurses' shortage caused a reduction in the follow-up program for former sanatorium patients and in supervised home treatment. In Ontario, due to lack of qualified personnel, surgical procedures fell from 3,350 in 1940 to 2,678 in 1942.[22]

Something obviously had to be done. In British Columbia, to deal with the shortage of specialists, travelling clinics were altered: a public health nurse ran the x-ray surveys, while rural doctors had x-rays taken of suspicious patients at the expense of the health division and forwarded the films to it for interpretation. A similar arrangement operated in Ontario, where individuals ineligible for war services were given intensive training as x-ray technicians to conduct clinics unaccompanied by doctors, while the central office in Toronto read the films. But these were only temporizing measures. The continual turnover of staff decreased sanatoria efficiency and increased costs. There was also the nagging worry that well-trained personnel would not return after the war ended unless their salaries were increased – especially if promised health insurance was introduced, for physicians would fare better in private practice.[23]

The war also affected available treatment facilities and equipment – especially beds. Wartime restrictions made it difficult to obtain x-ray or pasteurization equipment, or even to construct new buildings, while the increasing number of military cases aggravated pressure on existing accommodation.[24] By 1942, with more rigorous case-finding encompassing surveys of the armed forces and industry, sanatorium accommodation throughout the country was inadequate even for civilian needs. The Department of Veterans Affairs was forced to set up 1,200 temporary beds in clinics until military patients could be treated in provincial sanatoria, and by 1945 it had to operate tuberculosis hospitals in Nova Scotia, New Brunswick, Quebec, and Ontario, while treating tuberculosis patients in Veterans Affairs' hospitals in Alberta and British Columbia. Despite a 10.7 percent increase in sanatorium beds by 1944, demand had far outstripped supply: there were still twice as many deaths from tuberculosis outside the sanatoria as in them, with 3,500 to 4,000 people dying yearly at home.[25] A story blazoned across the front page of the *Vancouver Sun* that same year threw the problem into sharp relief, denouncing the unforeseen cruelties inflicted on helpless citizens in the widely praised tuberculosis-detection drive and giving voice to public worry by pointing out that "the same government which tells them they are forbidden to work until cured [also] tells them that it can't find beds for them in institutions and consigns them to a lingering disintegration on relief."[26] Lack of beds threatened to impair more comprehensive case-finding. It was an old problem with a wartime immediacy: why find cases early if they could not be treated?

Although sanatorium accommodation was a problem in all provinces, it was worse in areas that had begun the war lagging behind – particularly in Quebec. Half the beds required for Canada were lacking in that province alone. As the provincial committee observed in 1944, although all provinces suffered from staff and accommodation shortages, "the trouble has been that facilities in Quebec are less adequate and less able to deal with these difficulties ... the mortality rate from tuberculosis in Quebec is two and a half times that of Ontario, but that Ontario still has more treatment beds than Quebec." In Montreal 1,500 sufferers could not find a bed, while the committee demanded that the government provide another 4,000 beds for the province, since Quebec was 50 percent short of a minimum requirement of three beds per death.[27]

Inevitably, institutional costs were rising, due to climbing building costs, commodity prices, and wages. The cuts taken by various staff members during the depression now had to be adjusted. In the space of a year (from 1941 to 1942), the daily sanatorium cost in Saskatchewan rose from $2.45 to $2.67 per patient – a total increase of about $57,000. On the other hand, with new wartime prosperity, the Saskatchewan Anti-Tuberculosis League was finally relieved of its debt load – by 1944 the municipalities were paying their current levy accounts promptly and had taken care of all but $6,324 in arrears, which permitted the league to expand its survey program.[28]

## State Planning, Management, and Responsibility

World War 2 would alter the anti-TB campaign as profoundly as World War 1 had. With the rapid growth of the armed services and the war industry, the federal government acquired new prominence and authority. The wartime Prices and Trade Board, established in September 1939, restricted the supply and distribution of commodities and established a ceiling on prices to prevent the runaway inflation and profiteering that had caused so much bitterness and resentment in World War 1.[29] If such "equality" could be imposed on the whole country during the war, it seemed reasonable to expect that the state – in particular, the federal government – would provide similar social services in the postwar period. Sir William Beveridge's *Social Insurance and Allied Services* suggested that such a welfare state was possible in Britain, and Leonard Marsh, one of the founding fathers of the Cooperative Commonwealth Federation (CCF), adapted it to Canada.[30]

The war had made state planning and management legitimate. Federal officials had feared a recurrence of the depression that had followed World War 1, leaving another generation of Canadians uncared for – which was unthinkable in the socially responsible postwar state. At the Dominion-Provincial Conference on Reconstruction in the fall of 1945 the federal government proposed that its wartime monopoly of personal and corporate income taxes be extended indefinitely, and in exchange it would assume most responsibility for welfare benefits, pensions, and unemployment insurance and pay 60 percent of the cost of provincially administered health insurance plans, provided they met national standards.[31] Conditional grants would also be made for tuberculosis, venereal disease, mental health, crippled children, the blind, and public health in general.

A new generation of civil servants had arisen during the war, convinced that they could "promote, direct and control" the economy, and that "positive and forceful action was the first duty of government and that full employment and social welfare were its highest aims." This conviction ran into a wall of jealously guarded provincial independence after the war, and although new tax agreements would be negotiated and federal grants established, the comprehensive, federally controlled postwar plan outlined at the Dominion-Provincial Conference on Reconstruction had to be abandoned.[32] Nonetheless, a new managerial bureaucracy, disciples of Keynes and Beveridge and of efficient scientific management, had grown not only in numbers and experience but also in confidence during the war, and it would be firmly in control in the reconstruction period.[33]

Perhaps a more significant effect of wartime experience on the anti-TB campaign than the use of mass x-ray surveys and more sophisticated rehabilitation was a reinforcement of the concept of state responsibility. The provinces had accepted responsibility for their residents' health after World War 1; now, with memories of the depression still painfully clear – including its revelations of the inadequacy of much of Canada's health care – and with the example of massive federal funding of the war machine, there was no reason why, public health advocates maintained, the dominion could not fund the nation's health in the same way. Provincial inequities, most tuberculosis specialists believed, made this necessity obvious. By this point, each province had developed its own individual program; but even if a global federal plan and national health insurance scheme failed, there was no reason why federal grants-in-aid, suggested at the close of the previous decade, should not be established – especially for tuberculosis. "Surely the time is approaching," reflected J.H. Holbrook in his 1942 presidential address to the CTA, "when this phase of the problem must be considered from the federal standpoint. In this the tuberculosis problem of our soldiers points the way, for it is administered as a federal problem."[34]

Members of the federal government agreed. "Our enemy today," announced Brooke Claxton, federal minister of health and welfare in 1945, "instead of being Germany or Japan, is disease and unhealthy conditions."[35] With the coming of federal grants, it would be a new beginning in Canadian health care too.

# 8 The Triumph of Technology, Bacteriology, and Scientific Management

And today, not so good. "How's my x-ray, Doc?"

"No change."

"The other tests?"

"Not so good," Up to G4? No, not so good. I wonder – am I getting any better? Or is it going to be just: "Died in a Vancouver hospital, after a long illness ..." Wonder what the family is doing? Wonder if I'll ever get home ...

When you get to that stage, brother, you turn the radio off and ring for the nurse. "Nurse, a phenobarbital, sleeping pill or a 292." Something quick and powerful. Otherwise your thoughts will begin to squirrel-cage.

L. Postill, "Bed's Eye View," *Maclean's Magazine*, 1946

Instead of the bleak depression feared by many Canadians, the end of World War 2 ushered in a new era of unparalleled prosperity. From 1941 to 1956 there was a 40 percent increase in population, fueled by both new urban immigrants and a "baby boom," so that almost a third of the population was younger than fourteen by the mid-fifties. Encouraged by the unbroken rule of the Liberal Party in federal politics and a sense of state duty inspired by the war and justified by postwar prosperity, an ethos of scientific management and state planning moved triumphantly into the foreground of Canadian society, organized and led by an ever-enlarging class of bureaucrats, administrators, and managers typified in many respects by the great administrator, C.D. Howe.[1]

Public health in general and the anti-TB campaign in particular, not surprisingly, reflected and reinforced such trends – most obviously with the establishment of federal health grants. But if the postwar era saw the ascendancy of scientific management and the expert administrators, it also witnessed the triumph of bacteriology and technology in TB diagnosis and treatment: new miniature x-rays allowed mass surveys of the whole population, while breakthroughs in chemotherapy

– first streptomycin and then isoniazid – made TB, for the first time, a curable disease.

## Mass Surveys

Although surveys of select groups were carried out in the interwar period, tuberculosis specialists in areas with low infection rates had begun to question their value – especially surveys of school children, which, experts in both British Columbia and Manitoba complained, were simply not justified economically as a case-finding measure, although they had some educational value. In fact, British Columbia continued them only as a research tool to establish the incidence of infection.[2]

With the advent of the war, however, surveys were extended into industries and factories on a mass scale. By 1941 the mining industry was extensively x-raying employees in an effort to reduce compensation costs.[3] With an x-ray machine set up in a section of a plant, it only took ten minutes to x-ray a worker's lungs. By 1948 many firms, especially those in urban centres, required an x-ray before offering a candidate a job. As the Montreal league had bluntly observed in a 1943 fund-raising letter, "Industrial management is in the best position to understand the connection between good health and a high rate of production."[4]

The development of miniature x-ray films had given a new impetus to this somewhat outdated case-finding method, making it both physically and financially possible to x-ray not only a whole industry, or even community, but a whole province – and by 1943 R.G. Ferguson was suggesting that a worthwhile objective might be x-raying the *whole population* of the country within the next decade. At a cost of fifteen to twenty cents per person (including the salaries of doctors and technical staff) the new x-rays cost about one-tenth the price of the standard plate, and with the ever-increasing Christmas Seal funds, "there is no city or municipality, small or large," Ferguson asserted dogmatically, "that cannot raise voluntarily the cost of such a survey."[5]

Not only were the films cheaper and easier to store, but tuberculosis specialists soon discovered that although 10 percent of the abnormalities discovered on a full-size chest x-ray were missed on the miniature films, more than two and a half times the percentage of minimal active cases would be found by mass surveys than by ordinary clinic methods.[6] To the optimistic, it appeared that there was finally an affordable means of examining "well" people and hunting out the unknown pockets of disease. The mass surveys were, as the CTA executive secretary enthusiastically commented, "a genuine first-aid project which

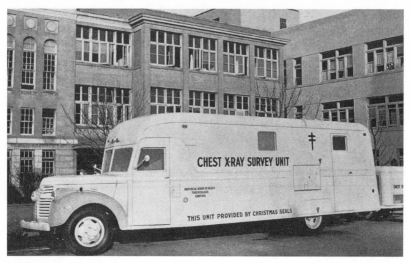

British Columbia division of tuberculosis control mobile unit used to conduct surveys taking miniature x-ray films. Reproduced from Hatfield, *Handbook on Tuberculosis*, 118

if carried through will finally make tuberculosis as rare in Canada as smallpox."[7]

As a plan to eliminate tuberculosis, the mass surveys presented some difficulties. An estimated four million individuals had to be x-rayed yearly, requiring highly trained technicians and doctors who were liable to miss the very people who should be examined, because they would not attend: "the improvident and careless."[8] A conference of provincial tuberculosis secretaries held in 1948 wryly noted three additional groups that cut down survey attendance: men over sixty who felt it was a good idea for other people to be x-rayed, but not busy individuals like themselves; former servicemen who had had so many plates taken in the service that they considered themselves safe for the next twenty-five years; and former patients.[9] Although not a simple cure-all, mass surveys indicated the level of infection in a community and discovered active cases earlier (in Ontario 50 percent of the cases discovered were in the minimal stage, compared to 20 to 25 percent discovered by the usual chest clinic methods), and as an added bonus, they uncovered other conditions, especially lung cancer and heart disease. In British Columbia, mass x-ray surveys found four times as much heart disease as tuberculosis, leaving the department of health with the thorny problem of how much responsibility it should assume for the discovery of previously unknown heart disease in the province.[10]

Perhaps the greatest advantage of mass surveys was, in the end, the most difficult to evaluate: education. Nothing else made a community so tuberculosis conscious, especially since they were usually carried out with the aid of service clubs and local volunteer associations, accompanied by as much fanfare as possible. They fostered an interest in a more prompt use of x-rays in general diagnosis and, paradoxically, increased attendance at regular clinics, encouraging the public to seek medical advice about chest problems at an earlier date. As well, the CTA reported with satisfaction in 1945, they sparked a demand for educational material.[11]

Results even of selective surveys were promising. In 1941, Ontario, which was still x-raying only selective groups, reported 2 percent more individuals in sanatoria between twenty and twenty-nine years of age, but the percentage with far-advanced disease fell from 35.6 to 27.6. Saskatchewan initiated the policy of x-raying whole communities in 1941, and as soon as equipment was available at the end of the war, other provinces followed suit. By 1945 the Ontario department of health, representing an attitude prevalent in most provinces, had abandoned its policy of selective surveys in favour of surveying whole communities using mobile x-ray units, with at least 75 percent of the cost borne by Christmas Seals. By 1947 Saskatchewan had completed a survey of its whole population, with Manitoba quickly following in 1948; and by 1950 Saskatchewan had even finished a second overall survey and started a third. These mass surveys clearly demonstrated a fall in the incidence of infection, and they were an encouraging sign that tuberculosis was being eradicated, albeit slowly: in the first province-wide mass survey, the Saskatchewan league had discovered one new case in every 1,300 individuals examined; in the second, one in every 2,300.[12]

In contrast, the situation, although fast improving, was still gloomy in Quebec: by 1949 less than one-third of the population had had an x-ray examination. The provincial committee for the prevention of tuberculosis reported that work had centred mainly on industrial, commercial, and educational establishments, with little attention as yet paid to women in the home or the rural population.[13] Ironically, the war had been a partial cause of this state of affairs – in 1944 some parishes had absolutely refused to be examined because, according to the medical director of the St Georges Sanatorium, "a rumour had spread that this was a 'subterfuge from Ottawa to enlist all the young men for military service.'"[14] In Canada as a whole, however, the number of individuals examined in this fashion alone rose from 439,610 in 1944 to about 1.9 million in 1950, topping the two-million mark in 1951.

Mass surveys, experts believed, were only one part of a well-balanced tuberculosis control program, and in those provinces where the death rate was falling at an escalating rate, they were becoming uneconomical as a case-finding method as early as 1950. That year, the pioneering Saskatchewan Anti-Tuberculosis League again changed its emphasis, now carrying out an intensive drive to eradicate the disease by tuberculin testing and x-raying only in highly infected areas, with special emphasis on hospital admissions as a suspect group and on follow-up of treated cases. Meanwhile British Columbia began to eliminate the tuberculosis division's mass x-ray survey, replacing it with x-ray equipment installed in general hospitals and local health units, so that x-ray facilities would be available on a day-to-day basis and case-finding would be a responsibility of local health services. Manitoba, too, concentrated on both the sparsely settled areas with a higher incidence of disease and on special suspect groups.[15] In a decade, the emphasis in case-finding had nearly, but not quite, gone full circle: from an examination of select groups in the thirties, to comprehensive mass surveys in the forties, to a shift in emphasis again to specific suspect groups and districts beginning in the fifties.

## Immigrants and Hospital Admissions

Together with a focus on specific suspect groups (contacts, native Canadians, nurses, and hospital employees), postwar efforts began to focus on two other groups: immigrants and general hospital admissions. "We are still suffering and paying for the tuberculosis that was brought to us by the mid-European immigrants early in this century," announced J.D. Adamson, president of the CTA in 1946, "and it is our duty to prevent a repetition."[16] With the example of unresistant soldiers succumbing to the disease in highly tubercularized areas of Europe at hand, as early as 1940 the Canadian Public Health Journal was militantly demanding compulsory x-raying of all postwar immigrants, and tuberculosis specialists were warned of the impending catastrophe should unrestricted immigration take place.[17] Adamson ominously pointed out that, presumably, many immigrants would settle in sparsely populated parts of Canada (in other words, in the Prairies) where tuberculosis death rates were among the lowest in the world and the younger generation had no previous infection to offer even slight protection. The resettlement of 2,876 Polish soldiers sent to Canada in 1946 without x-rays demonstrated this possibility all too clearly: 86 had tuberculosis, for an astounding (in Canadian terms) rate of 3,094 per 100,000. The consequences if this continued, Adamson warned, would be "devastating."[18]

There was a monetary consideration as well. Dr Charles F. Bennett of the Fort Qu'Appelle Sanatorium argued in 1940 that, had x-rays been taken of the 55,976 immigrants settling in Saskatchewan from 1926 to 1930, the province would have saved $98,118 in treatment costs alone.[19] Although T.A. Crerar, the federal minister of mines and resources, had not thought a chest x-ray of all postwar immigrants to be practical in 1943, by 1947 the federal immigration authorities had come around and were adopting a policy whereby all prospective immigrants would be x-rayed before leaving for Canada and all those with active or doubtful lesions rejected.[20]

Closer to home, tuberculosis campaigners demanded that general hospitals routinely x-ray all admissions. The high rate of infection noted among nurses in the previous decade made it obvious that unsuspected TB sufferers, admitted for other conditions, were infecting hospital personnel, while routine x-rays of patients proved it. Because they uncovered a higher percentage of tuberculosis sufferers than the mass surveys (three per thousand, instead of one) routine x-rays of hospital admissions were a more valuable means of flushing out pockets of infection. They were also, theoretically, another way of making the medical profession and hospital staff tuberculosis-conscious.[21]

Routine x-rays were expensive, however, and although most specialists agreed that they were desirable, if not essential, lack of funds was, as ever, the perennial problem. Most provincial tuberculosis associations and local hospitals were incapable of assuming the burden. Only in Alberta was the x-raying of general hospital patients completely the responsibility of a voluntary provincial association. Saskatchewan introduced the practice in 1947 as part of the newly established free hospital services, but others needed the assistance of federal health grants for equipment and operating costs to give the movement any impetus. By 1950 the practice had begun in all provinces, though it was less comprehensive in Quebec and the Maritimes.[22] In that year 306,347 Canadians were examined, increasing to 560,359 by 1953.[23]

*Tuberculin Testing*

With the rate of infection falling, tuberculin became more valuable as a diagnostic tool. It was now used extensively by clinics, private doctors, and public health nurses, both to check for infection and to determine who among high-risk subjects (nurses and contacts) was to receive BCG. In the initial enthusiasm for mass x-ray surveys, some specialists rejected tuberculin testing as nothing more than a very rudimentary case-finding technique, and a few even queried whether, considering the low cost and potentially universal use of x-rays, tuberculin testing was becoming unnecessary.[24]

More to the point, what tuberculin testing indicated was now also, to a limited degree, open to speculation. In the past, a negative reactor had always meant an escape from infection; now, with Canadians exposed less frequently to open cases, loss of allergy was becoming more common, and it was impossible to differentiate between loss of allergy and an escape from infection. Both reactors were negative. Thus, a negative reaction now indicated a lack of *recent* exposure. A positive reaction was more significant, for, especially in the case of a child, it signified current, intimate exposure and generally led to an open case. One assumption seemed obvious: with tuberculin tests increasingly negative, Canada was, as one expert warned, "on an immunological hotspot from which we dare not retreat for fear of disaster ... since we are bringing up the younger generation with negative tuberculin reaction, we must provide an uninfected environment."[25] It was another argument fuelling demand for compulsory x-ray examinations of immigrants.

### BCG

With a falling infection rate, some specialists looked to BCG, the only available vaccine, as an aid in warding off disease among those unavoidably exposed, especially nurses in training and contacts. The CTA had even recommended its use in the armed forces for this reason.[26] As in the past, it was used most extensively in Quebec: 264,570 persons had been vaccinated from 1926 to 1949 in that province, compared to the nearest runner-up, Saskatchewan, with a mere 6,055. By 1948, 20 percent of the newborn babies in Quebec received it, and by 1950, with the aid of federal grants, it was dispensed through the health units to children, adolescents, and even adults.[27]

The precise value of the vaccine was still in dispute, however, as were the ethical and clinical implications. "Are we," demanded W.H. Hatfield, director of the British Columbia division of tuberculosis control, "to adhere to the principle of elimination of infection? If so, why give infection? We usually state that a patient with primary tuberculosis does well and that it is the secondary infection that causes our trouble. Should we then give primary infection even in a measured dose to anyone? Giving infection to study immunity is probably an unorthodox experiment. What knowledge have we of immunological factors in tuberculosis?"[28] Aside from this conundrum, the effect of BCG was difficult to assess. In 1946 the chairman of the National Research Council tuberculosis panel commented that the panel regarded R.G.

Ferguson's work with native Canadian children in Saskatchewan "as the only complete scientific experiment with BCG yet carried out."[29] The executive secretary of the CTA agreed. Although BCG had been used in Quebec for approximately two decades, the statistics compiled in Montreal were not analyzed independently until 1939, when the panel excluded many of the vaccinated and control subjects. In addition, infants were taken at birth and hospitalized until the test was positive – for four to eight months. With no "controls" other than babies born under similar circumstances and without the benefit of four- to six-months care under medical and nursing supervision, the immunity BCG guaranteed was impossible to estimate. "When you consider the large number of infants that are born in Montreal," observed G.J. Wherrett practically, "to give them all four to eight months hospital treatment seems to be entirely out of the question."[30] Without proper controls, data from the Montreal vaccinations were meaningless. Still, by 1946 Ferguson had demonstrated that BCG could reduce tuberculosis in nurses to one-quarter of its former incidence, so that it had merit.[31] It was no cure-all – it was only, like the mass surveys, one more adjunct to the campaign.

*Clinics*

Paradoxically, mass surveys helped increase the importance of the established preventive method: stationary and travelling clinics. Surveys made both the public and the medical profession more tuberculosis-conscious, so that general practitioners referred more patients. Moreover, clinics did the follow-up work, not only of former sanatorium patients but of those found by mass surveys. The more new cases the surveys uncovered, the heavier grew the workload of the clinics. Since these clinics were primarily for known cases, contacts, and suspects (although, as in the past, clinic staff might examine specific groups as a whole, such as normal school students or industrial groups), they usually continued to use regulation-size x-rays. Sometimes they were, like the surveys, supported by Christmas Seals – in Ontario, for example, 131 out of a total of 183 were funded in this fashion.[32]

Health units, too, continued to be formed under provincial supervision to deal with rural health problems. Quebec had sixty units operating by 1947. Instead of a travelling diagnostician, they used stationary clinics, which were held monthly in major centres for referred patients from the surrounding area.[33] In 1945 the Manitoba legislature provided for the establishment of full-time health units and hospital facilities, and in the following year the British Columbia government took over the administration of health units from local authorities and had nine units of a proposed eighteen in operation by 1950.[34]

## Changing Concepts of the Disease

With the war, the advent of mass surveys, and, finally, chemotherapy, it was inevitable that the standards used to evaluate the effect of the tuberculosis control program would be in a constant state of flux. In 1939 it was generally accepted that the required number of beds per death was two, and although the president of the CTA reported in 1942 that not all provinces had lowered their mortality rate to a point where it was economically feasible to increase the bed ratio to three per death, only a year later this ratio had become the generally accepted goal.[35] By 1947 Canada had a national average of three beds per death – but a declining death rate and a growing number of cases (a result of the surveys and improved case-finding) caused more minimal cases to be treated, with more recoveries and fewer deaths; so the value of any established ratio seemed questionable. "Obviously," G.C. Brink, director of the Ontario division of tuberculosis prevention, observed impatiently in 1946, "the number of sanatorium beds should depend upon the extent and the result of diagnostic activities, not upon the false index 'beds per death.' If there are patients with tuberculosis awaiting admission to sanatoria, it is self-evident that there are insufficient beds, irrespective of the ratio of beds to deaths. Waiting lists indicate shortage of beds."[36]

Not only was the number of beds open to question – the very nature of the disease itself seemed to be changing. More frequently cases were discovered in older age groups (in Alberta in 1944 more tuberculosis was found in individuals over forty years of age than under), with some apparently developing tuberculosis for the first time.[37] It was debatable whether this pattern was due to a lack of exposure and thus a lack of opportunity to acquire limited immunity in childhood (the problem of the nurses) or, conversely, to residual disease from an earlier period with a higher incidence of infection when individuals had been subjected to more intense exposure, leaving them more susceptible to a later breakdown. In fact, with first infection now often postponed until adulthood, there was constant debate over the process of the disease.[38] Everything, it seemed, was open to question – "What shall we do with a young man or a hundred young men," a perplexed D.A. Carmichael asked CTA members at their annual meeting in 1943,

in perfect health if judged by any standard which he and his family can comprehend, fully occupied with his daily pursuits and plans for the future, who is found to have an area of disease in his lung? Shall we provide expensive sanatorium beds, place him in one under observation and treatment, withdraw him from industry, disrupt his future? Who knows which of our hundred will ever become ill or really need such treatment? Certainly, many will not. And what shall be the status of tuberculosis as a communicable disease? Shall it be notifiable whether infectious or not – suspect or definitely diagnosed, perhaps over-diagnosed? Must it be rigidly isolated and by what clinical or laboratory test shall it be certified for release? Or shall we depend on protection from massive infection, training and education of the carrier and the community, improved living standards and continuously higher dilution of the infecting agent?[39]

Which individuals will need such treatment, indeed? With a bed shortage, the most sensible approach from a community standpoint seemed to be to isolate at least all infectious individuals – and then others, if possible. "No sputum, no tuberculosis," stated Grant Fleming in 1941,[40] and this concern for the community over the individual, developed in the interwar period, was carried to the point that both Alberta and British Columbia refused free sanatorium treatment to those whose disease was not dangerous to others.[41] The aim of the campaign was tuberculosis control – and the treatment of the individual was important insofar as it furthered this aim in the *community*.

### Bed Shortages and Standards of Care

The postwar period brought no relief from the chronic wartime staff and bed shortage. Increased construction costs and difficulties in obtaining building materials precluded an immediate solution to the accommodation problem; moreover, there was such a shortage of doctors and nurses that some existing beds had to be closed – seventy in Alberta alone in 1946. Doctors preferred more lucrative private practice. British Columbia was particularly hard hit; as late as 1949 the tuberculosis division reported that consulting work could only be meagrely carried out in rural areas, and it called for a revision of salaries as a solution.[42] The nursing situation was equally acute, although by the end of the decade higher salaries, expanded training programs, and grants led to improvement. Nonetheless, Ontario reported two hundred sanatorium beds vacant in 1949, while roughly the same number of patients awaited admission.[43]

Even after building restrictions eased, the bed situation was both encouraging and discouraging: encouraging because, despite rising costs, accommodation was steadily increasing, from 13,594 available beds in 1946 to 17,302 in 1950, and yet discouraging because, as always, this increase did not seem to be enough. It was, as the CTA

president observed dispiritedly in 1946, "a catalogue of blasted hopes
– all showing to what extent our accomplishments have fallen short
of our aspirations."44 Demand for facilities outstripped supply with
monotonous regularity. And yet, specialists insisted with an obsessive
passion, an adequate supply of beds was crucial to the campaign –
Hugh Burke of Montreal's Royal Edward Institute pointed out in 1950,
that Ontario, which had the highest percentage decline of the tuberculosis death rate in the past twenty years and now had the lowest rate
in Canada, had long had adequate or nearly adequate treatment
facilities. In 1948 it had a respectable ratio of 5.5 sanatorium beds per
tuberculosis death. Quebec, on the other hand, had had only an
intermediate percentage decline in its death rate for tuberculosis in
the past two decades; it still had the highest rate in Canada; and it
had never possessed adequate treatment facilities – in 1949 it had a
miserable ratio of 1.8 beds per death. The lesson could hardly be
clearer.45

Mounting costs made sanatoria (particularly those in Ontario, managed as they generally were by local voluntary associations) leery of
starting building programs without government aid. By 1948 new
construction cost as much as $12,000 *per bed*, while the costs of tuber-
culosis treatment (in constant 1949 dollars) in Canada rose from
about $14.9 million in 1945 to $21.8 million in 1950. The cost per
patient-day rose from $2.85 in 1944 to $5.24 in 1950.46 In fact, the
Ontario government estimated that the cost of simply *discovering* active
cases through clinics and surveys was $166 for each case in 1945.47
Quite obviously, only the government could bear this kind of burden.
And it became another reason for federal involvement.

Although more and more disease was diagnosed at an early age,
there was still a need for convalescent care for chronic, active cases
who required isolation but no extensive treatment. Instead of setting
up another specialized institution to deal with chronic "maximum
benefit" cases, the tuberculosis specialists, especially the national office
of the cta, concentrated on bringing already existing institutions up
to par. Even at this late date standardization was, they agreed, lamen-
tably lacking. "We have little agreement," observed W.H. Hatfield, "on
how to build sanatoria or tuberculosis hospitals. Our systems of
records are far from uniform. In treatment some believe in long
hospitalization, others in short. We don't even seem to agree on who
should be hospitalized. In the various provinces our ratio of beds
differs vastly and opinion on actual need for beds also differs. Various
methods of therapy have their enthusiasts and there are those who
temper these enthusiasts."48

Money – or the lack of it – was again considered to be the major
issue. Reflecting yet again an emphasis on scientific management,

organization, and efficiency, as early as 1943 the CTA was looking to the promised federal health insurance, with its attached health grants, to bring standards of tuberculosis service up to a minimum level.[49] "I can see no reason," G.J. Wherrett complained in 1941, "why pneumothorax should be given to only 25 percent of the patients in one institution and to 60 percent in another institution; or why thoracoplasty should be used in less than 1 percent of discharged patients in one institution and in 10 percent of discharged patients in another." It sometimes depended, as one expert noted, "upon the enthusiasm of those administering the treatment."[50]

### Antibiotics: Finally a Cure

If mass surveys had caught the public imagination as a preventive method, it was chemotherapy that revolutionized treatment. Ever since Koch had discovered the bacillus, researchers had been vainly attempting to discover a specific cure for the disease. In 1943 an American researcher, Selman Waksman, isolated streptomycin, the first antibiotic found to inhibit the growth of tuberculosis bacilli. After years of disappointment, specialists found it difficult to believe an effective drug had truly been found. However, it was introduced in Canada in 1947, and aid from federal health grants began in 1948; it was quickly distributed throughout the country. Although not a miracle cure, it did increase the number of cases eligible for surgery, and it saved or prolonged the lives of many patients previously considered hopeless. In combination with para-amino-salicylic acid (PAS) and isonicotinic hydrazide (INH) discovered soon after, it was responsible for a spectacular fall in the death rate.

Ironically, with such dramatic results from a long-sought "cure," it was easy to overlook the important role of the accelerated case-finding programs in controlling the disease. More pragmatically, the introduction of chemotherapy paradoxically increased the strain on available accommodation, for now formerly fatal cases were recovering – but only after months of treatment. Adequate bed facilities had seemingly never been more essential.

### Surgery

The use of surgery had grown steadily since World War 1, so that by the late thirties pneumothorax was even attempted on early, sputum-negative cases in order to ensure that the disease was arrested. By 1942, 37.2 percent of the patients in Canadian sanatoria had some form of collapse therapy.[51] Perhaps surprisingly, the use of drugs signalled a new era in the *surgical* treatment of TB – not only could the more traditional methods be carried out more safely and more extensively, but now surgical excision or resection of diseased tissue was possible.[52] Patients were treated with drugs for several months, after which any significant residual focus was resected. Older procedures, such as pneumothorax, pneumoperitoneum, phrenic crush, and even thoracoplasty (techniques discussed in chapter 3) were fast falling into disfavour as this new, combined approach was making a true cure seem possible.[53] "Our whole concept in the approach to treatment has changed," enthusiastically proclaimed the director of the British Columbia division of tuberculosis control; "we now attempt to achieve a cure, whereas formerly we had to be satisfied to bring the disease under control ... and through careful control of the patient to hope that the disease would remain arrested."[54] Antibiotics were very definitely a supplement, not a substitute, for sanatorium treatment. They were still too new; their ultimate effectiveness was unknown; and the threat of a drug-resistant strain of disease developing was very real. By the early fifties specialists were worrying that the public, lulled into security by the falling death rate, would neglect prevention. "Useful though the drugs are," Wherrett warned sternly, "we must not use them as an excuse to slacken our efforts to prevent tuberculosis or decrease our facilities for fighting it."[55]

*Follow-up and Rehabilitation*

With the postwar developments in the treatment and preventive aspects of the campaign, it was not surprising to see corresponding activity in follow-up, aftercare, and rehabilitation work. Since sanatorium costs were rising and roughly 25 percent of the patients were readmissions,[56] the motive for demanding adequate aftercare was not solely humanitarian – proper care, support, and supervision would permit patients to be discharged earlier, utilize beds more efficiently, prevent individuals from breaking down and becoming foci of infection, and – most important of all to economy-conscious government officials – save money. In essence, proper aftercare of patients and their families was not a charity but "an investment or insurance by the state or municipality against future and large expenditures which will undoubtedly follow," warned Ontario's G.C. Brink, "if a niggardly policy is followed. Penny-wise policies will only add to the burden of the future taxpayer."[57]

British Columbia was the only province to heed this advice. In Ontario, although legislation in 1938 had placed the responsibility for aftercare squarely on the shoulders of the municipalities, its effect too often depended, as Brink sadly admitted, on "the enlightenment and attitude" of local officials – hardly a reliable source of support.[58] Patients in the past had received aid under mothers' allowances, but British Columbia was the first, in 1944, to introduce a special tuberculosis allowance. Under its terms, patients no longer had to be destitute to receive assistance – instead, they could apply on the basis of cessation of income. The allowance therefore provided a form of disability insurance. Individuals could now retain some assets for their rehabilitation, while the allowance benefitted the province by allowing patients who otherwise would have been hospitalized to remain at home, and it shortened the institutional stay of others. By 1943 the Metropolitan Health Committee and Family Welfare Bureau of Vancouver had jointly begun an experimental homemaker service to help out tuberculous families.[59]

Since a growing number of professional social workers were available to deal with the now-specialized problem of a patient's social and economic situation, the social condition of the individual tuberculosis sufferer received more attention now than it had since the age of social reform. This change was yet another example of the increasing emphasis on specialization and expert management in Canadian society. Both inside and outside the sanatorium, Osler's dictum, "What a patient with tuberculosis has in his head is more important than what he has in his chest," was unearthed and quoted with renewed fervour.[60] With the example of the veterans in mind, it became abundantly clear to TB professionals that aftercare, however desirable, was not sufficient – "the next and already overdue step," insisted one professional in 1940, "is to arrange, particularly in the larger centres, for a rehabilitation scheme."[61] W.H. Hatfield, director of the British Columbia tuberculosis division was even blunter. "We have left our job half finished," he stated flatly. "How have we equipped our patient to face the rigors of economic life? Are we not asking for breakdowns, for upset homes, for a new nidus of infection in the community? Can we continue to close our eyes to this problem? Our present course is not only inhuman but illogical and uneconomic."[62] Tuberculosis specialists had been demanding rehabilitation for victims of the disease since World War 1. By 1940 occupational therapy had become solidly entrenched as part of sanatorium care, but rehabilitation had been little more than discussed.

Manitoba led the way officially by establishing a rehabilitation division under the Sanatorium Board in 1942, but it was the war that, once again, brought the question to the forefront. The casualty rehabilitation section of the federal Department of Veterans Affairs studied rehabilitation as it affected service personnel, and a conference was held in Ottawa in 1946. The CTA believed that the success of the rehabilitation of veterans in provincial sanatoria hinged on whether a rehabilitation program was already in place for veterans and civilians alike – a definite incentive to organize postwar programs. As a result, with the aid of federal government grants in some cases and Christmas Seal funds in others, all provinces had some sort of rehabilitation service by 1949, and all but Quebec and Saskatchewan had full-time rehabilitation directors.[63]

Although the veterans created a demand for a serious attempt at rehabilitation and the federal grants gave added impetus to the movement, these were not the only factors promoting it. Improved case-finding and treatment methods had led to patients being discovered earlier and treated more effectively, permitting a greater number to return to the labour force. More generally, modern technological advances meant machines were doing more of the heavy manual work and placing a premium on skill – an incalculable benefit to the tuberculosis victim.[64] There was still talk of sheltered workshops for those too delicate to cope with a regular job, but there were now few jobs from which former patients were barred because of their physical strength. Thus, the successful rehabilitation of tuberculous patients and their return to productive roles in society was, if not easy, at least possible. Those who did not receive any vocational training and returned to unsuitable jobs were increasingly prominent among the relapsed patients, thus adding a strong economic argument for a proper rehabilitation program. Overwork alone, R.G. Ferguson asserted dogmatically, was to blame for 30 percent of the relapses.[65]

A more nebulous incentive to rehabilitate patients had been in existence since Koch had isolated the germ: public prejudice and ignorance. Although the hysterical "phthisiophobia" of the turn of the century had dissipated, lingering doubts remained. As late as 1949 the CTA passed a resolution encouraging industry and the civil service to hire rehabilitated patients, while the Manitoba Sanatorium Board reported the following year that in one or two cases employees were not accepted back into their old jobs because of their tuberculosis history – although apparently employers as a whole were becoming more "enlightened." Despite close to half a century of public education, the average person, *Maclean's Magazine* reported dramatically, "conjures up a false vision of a sanatorium as peopled by an emaciated throng condemned to a living death in some place akin to a leper colony. The result is that the cured TB patient, returning to normal life, faces a barrier which places him in a position comparable to the Untouchables of India."[66] Given the long lists of people waiting to gain admittance to the sanatoria, the situation could not have been quite so bleak. Nevertheless, it was one more reason to give vocational training to tuberculosis victims: they needed to have a saleable skill that would be in sufficient demand to compensate for employer prejudice.

What did rehabilitation involve? The old concept of sheltered workshops and industrial colonies had changed. No longer did the specialists concentrate on modifying the environment to suit the needs of the patient; instead, they attempted to train patients to take a normal place in the business and social world. Postwar rehabilitation, specialists insisted, ideally began the minute patients were diagnosed and ended only when they were reestablished in suitable jobs. Thus, every patient was a potential rehabilitation problem, and yet another specialized, expertly administered organization, a – "rehabilitation division" – was expected to include vocational counselling, vocational training, placement guidance, and supervision of aftercare and relief. Under a director, it coordinated the work of other specialists – medical staff, public health nurses, and social service departments – and it used occupational therapy and employment services where they existed. Ostensibly, it focused primarily on patients as individuals, and was geared to their personal welfare, but it reflected the underlying, all-pervasive emphasis on the community: for former patients were to be trained to fit into society as it existed. Unless there was no other alternative, the environment was not to be modified to suit *their* needs.

Reflecting the pervasive postwar emphasis on professional administrators, rehabilitation by the end of the decade was no longer the prerogative of isolated voluntary associations, as it had been ten years earlier, but instead it was considered essential in most comprehensive tuberculosis control programs. The first national conference on the rehabilitation of the physically handicapped, sponsored by the federal departments of Health and Welfare, Veterans Affairs, and Labour in 1951, demonstrated this new focus – although for some, like George Wherrett, the focus was not changing fast enough.[67] "We have reached the point," he succinctly summed up to the members of the CTA in 1950,

where everyone is saying it's a good thing. They are in favour of it. They look suitably impressed when we tell them that 25 percent of the patients in sanatoria are there for the second or third time and we think maybe 50 percent could have been saved the return trip if they had been able to go to suitable work, but they have not yet been impressed to the point where they are willing to expend money that is necessary to provide these services. There is a sort of willingness but we are a good way short of the place where those in charge of the expenditure of funds will figure out what it costs to get the facilities for giving needed training – the personnel, the courses, the staff to scout out job possibilities and establish good relations with public and employers, and then give consent for that amount of money to be spent.[68]

The establishment of a rehabilitation program simultaneously highlighted a fundamental failure and a success of the tuberculosis control program thus far. Rehabilitation was necessary only once an individual had succumbed to the disease – it therefore reflected a failure of adequate prevention. On the other hand, rehabilitation could concern tuberculosis specialists only once their treatment facilities were approaching an acceptable level, for beds were still a first priority.

Nothing illustrates this double-edged situation more effectively than Saskatchewan and Quebec, the only two provinces that did not have a rehabilitation director or division by the end of the decade – but they do so for contradictory reasons. Quebec was still concentrating its energy and funds in attempting to improve its pitiful accommodation and reduce active disease with the wholesale use of BCG. It had no resources to start a provincial rehabilitation program, and consequently relied on limited in-sanatorium programs and on what the voluntary association, the Cross of Lorraine, could do. Conversely, Saskatchewan, with its consistently low rate of mortality and infection, had no need of a rehabilitation division. Sanatorium medical superintendents informally supervised whatever education and vocational training was required. Specialists acknowledged the fact that most Saskatchewan patients returning to their former occupations in the predominantly agricultural province might have had some influence, but the key factor in reducing the need for rehabilitation there was seen to be the emphasis the league placed on prevention. With the number of cases falling and those that were discovered being treated at an early stage, rehabilitation was simply not an issue.

*Provincial Responsibility*

By the postwar era, most of the responsibility for and maintenance of the tuberculosis control program had fallen on the provinces. By 1950 Wherrett was instructing tuberculosis workers not to use Christmas Seal funds for treatment, relief, or major construction projects, since the provinces were required to assume these services by law. In keeping with the emphasis on centralized management, divisions continued to be established to supervise and administer the programs in Prince Edward Island (1948), New Brunswick (1947), and Quebec (1947), where the division was termed a "commission."[69]

Free treatment continued to be extended. As of November 1943, Winnipeg acknowledged an existing situation by officially instituting free treatment for its residents – only $3,665 had been paid out of the $165,319 cost of treating tuberculous patients in Winnipeg hospitals in 1941. New Brunswick established free treatment in 1945, and Nova Scotia followed suit in 1946. By 1949, not more than 5 percent of tuberculosis sufferers in any province paid anything towards their maintenance costs. Experience proved that free treatment caused patients to be hospitalized earlier and to stay longer, for better results: while 40.4 percent had left the sanatoria against advice in 1938, the figure had fallen to 18.4 percent by 1946. In addition, the Ontario government began to pay for all patients' (not just indigents') pneumothorax refills in 1949, while free treatment was extended with the aid of federal grants to nonpulmonary cases in Alberta.[70]

The depression had demonstrated the need for some form of social security, while the staff shortages in the war had focused attention on health personnel. In an effort to attract prewar health personnel back to their old jobs and as an incentive to others to stay, provincial governments began making tuberculosis a compensable disease. Beginning with British Columbia in 1943, employees of hospitals and sanatoria who did not have the disease at the time of employment were covered by workmen's compensation. Ontario followed suit in 1950, hoping to encourage more young women to become nurses and alleviate the nursing shortage. The CTA and the National Sanatarium Association adopted pension plans in 1947 and 1944, respectively, both to reward faithful employees and, more practically, to stop the rapid labour turnover.[71]

"Horizons have broadened in the entire concept of public health," announced the president of the Alberta Tuberculosis Association, without a trace of irony, at the end of the decade. "Now we know that adequate tuberculosis control requires the whole gamut of psychological, social and economic, as well as medical services."[72] British Columbia had set an example with its tuberculosis allowance, and it employed social workers in all division institutions, but in the other provinces allowances varied considerably, sometimes from city to city or municipality to municipality – and the rising cost of living, reported the CTA in 1947, aggravated the problem. Some form of social security was, in the wake of the depression and the war, considered to be a government responsibility. Once again, the CTA demanded financial aid – from the provinces as well as the federal government.

By continuing to assume the burden of ventures pioneered and proven by the voluntary associations and by extending free treatment, provincial governments were adding to their responsibilities: the government of Prince Edward Island took over the public health nurse who was working with the tuberculous in 1944, freeing funds for the league to purchase a mobile x-ray unit; the tuberculosis division took over the occupational therapy department from the Alberta Tuberculosis Association in 1949; dominion grants helped the British Columbia government take over the responsibility of maintaining the Tuberculosis Institute and of performing rehabilitation work from the Tuberculosis Society that same year; and the New Brunswick department of health assumed part of the burden of mass surveys.[73]

There was also growing cooperation among the provinces themselves. A considerable movement of the population during the war had created problems in establishing residency so that "Some citizens," British Columbia's Hatfield observed dryly, "legally have no residence, yet they still appear to themselves to be living in Canada."[74] Proof of residence was an essential requirement for free treatment. Following a resolution passed by the Dominion Council of Health in 1942, the CTA executive secretary investigated the problem. He discovered that during the previous nine years New Brunswick, Ontario, and Manitoba had more nonresidents dying in their provinces than each had residents dying in other provinces. British Columbia reported that fully one-fifth of the division's new cases in 1944 had come to the province since 1942.[75] The solution seemed straightforward: uniform residency requirements (instead of six months in one place and a year in another) and reciprocal arrangements between the provinces. J.H. Holbrook, superintendent of Ontario's Mountain Sanatorium, even suggested that the federal government pay for patients until their residency was established and then continue to pay if they were not sent to the province in which they officially resided.[76]

By 1946, reciprocal arrangements were agreed upon between Ontario and Quebec, Ontario and Saskatchewan, and Ontario, Manitoba, and Alberta. Although this partially eliminated the messy problem of returning patients to their "native" provinces and consequently disrupting their family lives, it did not deal with the problem of capital expenditure – if, for example, a large number of patients preferred the facilities in one province over another, a mass movement to that province would unfairly overburden its facilities, while the less attractive province would have empty beds. It was another argument in favour of national standards.[77]

### Changes in Quebec

Probably the most spectacular activity in the provincial arena during this decade took place in Quebec. After decades of indifference, the province finally began to grant adequate funds to establish a serious tuberculosis control program. Although the provincial committee had been exhorting and educating public and government officials since its establishment, it was only after the war that the legislative assembly finally took action, passing Bill 31, An Act to Combat Tuberculosis, in 1946. This bill authorized an expenditure of $10 million by 1950 for case-finding, enlarging, equipping, and building sanatoria, hospitalizing needy patients, and training tuberculosis specialists – but not for rehabilitation. A director general of tuberculosis and a provincial tuberculosis commission was appointed to organize and supervise the campaign. By 1948 the province had spent approximately $16 million toward the construction and expansion of sanatoria, while the cost of other services (for example, treatment and clinic maintenance) brought the budget for tuberculosis up to $5 million annually, for a total outlay of an impressive $26 million in just two years.[78]

Results were encouraging. By 1950, hospitalization was free for 98 percent of the cases and, while there was still a bed shortage (especially in the Montreal area), large-scale construction and a falling mortality rate had caused the number of beds per death to rise from 1.4 in 1941 to 3.2 in 1950.[79] From 1938 to 1947 – before chemotherapy was introduced – the mortality rate in the province decreased 32 percent, while the number of x-ray examinations increased eight times, from 51,000 to 400,000, partly due to the establishment of a municipal chest x-ray clinic in 1940 and the activities of the newly created Montreal Anti-Tuberculosis League.[80]

But if the figures showed, at last, the provincial government taking steps to deal with the disease, they also showed Quebec still lagging behind the other provinces. The non native Canadian mortality rate averaged below 40 per 100,000 in 1946, and Quebec's rate of 70.4 contrasted even more starkly with a rate of 17.5 in Saskatchewan.[81] Although it was encouraging to see Montreal's rate fall from 74.8 in 1941 to 56.4 in 1947 and 42.5 in 1949, it was somewhat discouraging to realize that Toronto's rate was only 25.2 (1948) while Winnipeg reached a new level of 9 per 100,000 (1949).[82] G.J. Wherrett neatly summed up the situation existing at the end of the decade in a letter to the chairman of the CLIOA health committee. "I am reasonably satisfied," he wrote in 1948, "with the [tuberculosis] programme in all the provinces, with the exception of Quebec. While great progress has been made, the problem still sticks out like a sore thumb, as compared to other provinces. The deaths now are 45% of the total, while the population is 29%. The organization in the province lacks the force that other provinces have. There is not the unity of purpose found in the other provinces, resulting in wide gaps and even overlapping. The provincial organization is spread too thin. What is needed is some means of better co-ordination and organization."[83]

*The Role of the Federal Government*

Of all levels of government, it was the role of the federal body that changed most radically in the postwar period. Traditional federal responsibilities – gathering statistics on tuberculosis institutions and clinics under the Dominion Bureau of Statistics, funding research through the National Research Council's associated committee of medical research (for example, research on BCG in Montreal and Saskatchewan), controlling bovine tuberculosis, and conducting the campaign among native Canadians – continued, but fueled now by a wartime-inspired ethos of state duty that was encouraged by an increasingly influential class of bureaucrats and administrators, the government struck out in a new direction. Fairly strong anti-TB programs had been developed individually by each province, but few could afford, as the *Canadian Public Health Journal* pointed out in 1941 and again 1942, to finance *all* aspects of a comprehensive public health program. Tuberculosis consumed a sizable fraction of provincial health department budgets – over half in 1937. And while $20 million was spent annually to maintain patients in general hospitals, sanatoria, and mental hospitals, a mere $2 million was spent on preventive medicine. The solution was simple according to the *Canadian Public Health Journal* and like-minded citizens: provide federal grants to fill in the gaps and standardize Canadian health services.[84]

From the start of the decade, the topic of health insurance had been hotly debated among politicians, health professionals, and the public press.[85] The CTA was intimately involved, since the proposed federal Health Insurance Bill included a scheme of federal grants to develop tuberculosis services in all provinces, particularly those with a higher rate of tuberculosis than the Canadian average. The national association had already recommended such grants to the Royal Commission on Dominion-Provincial Relations as a means of augmenting, improving, and standardizing tuberculosis services across the country. Moreover, the federal deputy minister of health actively involved in the negotiations, Robert E. Wodehouse, had been the executive secretary of the CTA before his appointment to the government.

By 1941, public health workers had noted that the provision of federal funds under the American Social Security Act of 1937 had not only improved health services in every state but had, more significantly, caused both state and municipal governments to appropriate greater amounts of money for public health. "If this arrangement is necessary in the United States in order to provide adequate health programs," asserted the Nova Scotia deputy minister of health, "it is equally essential in Canada."[86] Just as it had supported tuberculosis demonstrations in the past, CLIOA threw its weight behind the principle of health grants, although, predictably enough, it was strenuously opposed to such aid being associated with health insurance. As far as grants alone went, it had seen the advantage of improving public health since 1926, when it had begun to aid the provinces on its own.[87]

It was hardly surprising when the CTA, presenting a memorandum to the Select Committee of the House of Commons on Social Security in 1943, endorsed such grants once again.[88] In a letter to Ian Mackenzie, the minister of pensions and national health, Wherrett also strongly recommended that a national committee similar to the Invalided Soldiers' Commission, established at the close of World War 1, be appointed to study the situation and lay down minimum standards that the provinces had to meet before grants were disbursed.[89] To ensure that the minimum standards were high enough, the CTA itself drew up a list of conditions to be met by the provinces (Wherrett revised the list in 1945 at the request of J.J. Heagerty, the director of public health services),[90] including provisions for free treatment, clinics, mass surveys, adequate sanatoria with surgical facilities, aftercare, rehabilitation, an educational program, and the compilation of statistical data – everything, in fact, that made for a comprehensive tuberculosis control program.[91] There was even talk, while the issue of health insurance was still being heatedly discussed, of establishing a federal division of tuberculosis control, supervised by a director, within the Department of National Health. The CTA proposed a list of duties and qualifications for this director and volunteered to find a well-qualified candidate.[92] When this plan fell through in 1946 (grants had not yet materialized, and the salary range quoted was too small), Wherrett suggested to Dr G.D.W. Cameron, the deputy minister of the department of health, that the CTA, whose executive secretary had already acted in an advisory capacity to numerous federal departments and bodies, expand its functions slightly and fulfil the role of the proposed division.[93] By that point, the CTA was not only supplying most of the educational material on tuberculosis used by the country but seemed to have placed itself in the position of preeminent theorist and organizer in the anti-TB campaign. In a sense, Wherrett's suggestion was a public assertion of the influence of the postwar administrators in public health. When the grants were finally approved in 1948, Wherrett did serve as an advisor to the government concerning their use.

An annual grant of $3 million (to be raised to $4 million) was available to the provinces through the federal Tuberculosis Control Grant. Twenty-five thousand dollars was to be given outright to each province, and the balance divided 50 percent on the basis of population and 50 percent on the basis of the average number of deaths in each province over the five-year period from 1942 to 1946, in an attempt to extend more aid to those provinces with the biggest problem. As a result, Quebec alone was entitled to more than one-third of the available funds: more than $1 million.[94] Another $1,500 per bed was provided under the Hospital Construction Grant to stimulate provinces to increase accommodation, so that in 1950 alone, approximately $3.7 million was spent under the Tuberculosis Grant and another $3.8 million under the Hospital Construction Grant.[95]

Grants were used to extend all facets of tuberculosis control programs: additional staff and equipment for sanatoria, regular and travelling clinics, mass surveys and hospital admission x-ray programs, and rehabilitation. Significantly, the grants financed the free distribution of the costly new drugs, especially streptomycin and PAS, and so made it possible for them to be used as quickly and extensively as medically indicated. Physicians, nurses, and technicians were trained, the use of BCG extended, and research funded. As a result, programs such as rehabilitation and x-raying general hospital patients were given a much-needed boost out of the planning stage, while case-finding and sanatorium facilities, if not completely standardized, began to approach minimum standards.

The federal contribution, although impressive, still paled in comparison to provincial support. By 1953, an estimated $45 million was spent for tuberculosis services *annually* in the country, with the hospitalization of tuberculosis cases (a provincial responsibility) alone accounting for $40 million of this. For a six-year period (1948 to 1953) the *total* federal expenditures under the Tuberculosis Control Grant were less than half this annual amount: about $20.8 million.[96] The major part of the burden was, quite obviously, still a provincial responsibility.

Perhaps as significantly, the situation was analogous to the federal role in World War 1, when the national government had extended accommodation, donated equipment, and pioneered new programs (for example, occupational therapy), only to withdraw and leave the maintenance of those programs and the facilities to the provinces. Once again, the dominion government funded new ventures (rehabilitation, x-rays for general hospital admissions) and encouraged the extension of existing facilities and procedures (travelling clinics, beds, surgical and x-ray equipment, additional and specialized staff). Although the grants paid for capital costs and even maintenance costs in limited cases, they added to the long-term provincial financial burden. For example, Alberta used part of the grant to extend free treatment to nonpulmonary cases, but the province assumed all costs in 1954. When Quebec added 1,800 new beds, the cost of each was

$10,000. The federal government contributed $1,500, but the province provided the rest. With additional funds available, provinces were encouraged to take over programs pioneered by voluntary groups, such as rehabilitation and x-rays for general hospital admissions, saddling themselves with additional responsibility.[97]

The grants also fostered increased provincial *authority* as well as responsibility in the health field. As B.D.B. Layton, the chief of the venereal disease control division of the Department of National Health and Welfare, bluntly stated to the members attending the annual meeting of the Canadian Public Health Association, "a point which is of fundamental importance is that the funds are made available *to the provinces.* Thus, in order to obtain financial support under any of the grants, all dealings must be made with your own provincial health department. There is no direct channel to the federal source of supply."[98]

It was under provincial authority that funds were allocated, administered, and expended. Since the provinces had assumed control of the health field during the interwar period, this arrangement in itself was not a striking departure. Federal grants functioned in a fashion almost identical to the CLIOA and Red Cross grants after World War 1: they extended services and demonstrated and pioneered new ones to encourage the provinces to reach minimum standards and assume increasing responsibility – but the federal government was leery of funding maintenance costs. In fact the federal purpose of *stimulating,* but not assuming, provincial responsibility – a job that had been almost the sole prerogative of CLIOA and the voluntary associations in the past – was so similar to CLIOA's purpose that it rendered traditional CLIOA aid unnecessary. By 1949 George Wherrett had informed J.K. Macdonald, chairman of the CLIOA public health committee, that further grants were "unjustified."[99] It was the end of an era.

### The Role of Volunteers

With such government involvement increasing, what was the role of the volunteers? Paradoxically, in no period since the end of World War 1 had they been so important – for local associations were now responsible not only for the success of the Christmas Seal sale, which paid for much of the preventive work, but also for organizing the mass surveys. By 1950 there were three hundred committees across the country, raising over $1.5 million per year.[100] Most of it was in small donations, with over three quarters of a million Canadians contributing roughly $1.80 each, which, the tuberculosis specialists believed, not only indictated grassroots support of the campaign but was a tremendous force for health education. More practically, the Christmas Seals also paid for travelling and stationary clinics, mobile x-ray units, public health nurses (in New Brunswick, Prince Edward Island, and Alberta), education, occupational therapy, rehabilitation, relief (occasionally), tuberculin, BCG, and x-rays of general hospital admissions. In Ontario alone, 75 percent of the cost of mass surveys in 1948 was borne by Christmas Seals, which also supported 123 of the 182 chest clinics in the province.[101]

On a local level, the Christmas Seal committees and service clubs (often the same organization) continued to organize the sale and distribute funds. It was a measure of just how entrenched service clubs were in the campaign that the president of the Alberta Tuberculosis Association could comment quite seriously in 1947 that "this 'citizen's war' on tuberculosis was not always the responsibility of the service clubs."[102] It was the mass surveys, however, that appealed to the public's imagination. The CTA reported with satisfaction in 1946 that most new committees were formed with this objective in mind, believing, perhaps naively, that the mass survey demonstrated a desire on the part of the Canadians to help wholeheartedly in eradicating the disease.[103]

### Mass Surveys

The mass survey's grassroots appeal was understandable, for although the health department supplied medical and technical personnel to take and interpret the x-rays and sometimes advised on the organization of the survey, it played a minor role overall. The real success of a survey hinged not on technical knowledge but on fostering public awareness, support, and involvement, a job for which the service clubs, women's organizations, and local associations were ideally suited. The professionals themselves recognized this. "Consider the number who won't get out to vote," wailed one expert. "Why, if they are too careless to use their franchise, should it be expected that they would turn out without compulsion to be x-rayed?" Massive publicity and personal contact with all residents of the community, convincing them it was in their own best interests, were the reasons for the turnout. And this task was too immense for public health officials alone, no matter how well equipped. "If you want your survey to be a success," proclaimed another observer, "place the responsibility on women's groups."[104]

Ongoing educational work carried out in a province, together with publicity from previous surveys in smaller centres, familiarized Canadians generally with the idea of a mass survey. When it was ready to canvas a city, the league or health department staff obtained the consent and support of the city council and enlisted the aid of women's groups, service clubs, the chamber of commerce – any and all volunteers. Sometimes local clubs expressed interest first. In Regina, for example, the Women's Voluntary Services got 1,300 women out to help: 800 canvassed the city, house by house, while another 500 manned the office, did the clerical work, and assisted as hostesses to the three units.

The canvassers, organized by districts or streets and armed with answers to possible questions and reasons favouring an x-ray examination, whether one had tuberculosis or not, filled out a "request card" or "survey card" for every household agreeing to participate. To ensure an even flow of people through the clinics, these cards were sorted at the central office, which sent out a notice telling people the location of the nearest clinic and an approximate time to attend. To avoid bottlenecks, the examinations of fairly large groups, such as school children, were specially arranged. In Regina, roughly 2,600 to 2,900 were examined daily in a clinic.

Canvassers listed individuals who refused, and they were later visited by a member of the city health department. Clinic records were checked each night against the request cards from residents notified to attend that day, and reminders were sent to those who had not appeared, with alternate times suggested. The volunteer office staff arranged transportation for disabled people, sent out cards for individuals who were to be rechecked (they were examined by the city health department), and answered the telephone, fielding often mundane questions, reassuring fellow citizens, and encouraging a high turnout: "No madam," a *Bulletin* writer in the Regina survey overheard someone saying, "your cold won't make you look as if you had tuberculosis. If your cold is slight enough to permit you to go out, then it is all right to come to the clinic."[105] With the full support of local press and radio, a mass survey was considered to be not only a successful case-finding technique but a major force in community education. Regina, Lethbridge, Medicine Hat, and Trail all reported a turnout of over 90 percent. In Edmonton the turnout was over 80 percent.[106]

In Quebec the mass surveys were handled differently. Instead of relying on service clubs, women's groups, and other local volunteer associations to get the people out, health officials relied on the clergy. While the health department turned to the local Lions or Kiwanis Club in Northern Ontario, in Quebec the travelling diagnostician sent a letter to the curé of each parish, advising him of the visit of the mobile x-ray unit, explaining the usefulness of the survey, and asking him to announce it from the pulpit. Local doctors and the medical officer of the health unit and his staff were informed, as well, but "social clubs" were almost an afterthought – "where there are such organizations," commented one observer, Dr Herman Gauthier, revealingly.[107]

The comprehensive grassroots organization and the responsibility of the lay volunteers that predominated in the rest of the country was lacking in Quebec. There the surveys were imposed from the top – by the medical profession, public health officials, and the clergy. In English Canada, with its structure of service clubs, women's institutes, the IODE, and other local associations, at least a good part of the middle class was actively involved, if not the whole community.[108] The difference was apparent in results: Trail, Regina, Lethbridge, and Medicine Hat all reported turnouts of over 90 percent; 70 percent of some of New Brunswick communities and 60 to 70 percent of the adults in Nova Scotia were surveyed, while Quebec diagnosticians did not hope to reach more than 30 percent of the population. "Where the local people organize the survey and arouse interest," Wherrett wrote to K.L. Dawson of the Nova Scotia Tuberculosis Commission, "participation goes up to about 90% or more."[109]

Independently of their medical value, the mass surveys served two functions. First, they increased public awareness of the antituberculosis campaign and consequently aided the Christmas Seal sale – for the community was always more prone to donate when it could literally see and participate in the results. Second, the surveys put a heavier demand on the growing Christmas Seal funds. "We have found," Wherrett reported, "that the surveys arouse interest in the Seal Sale and the Seal Sale in turn arouses interest in the surveys."[110] As a result, the specialists felt, local communities in charge of the Christmas Seal sale could no longer be left to meander along happily in whatever fashion they chose. Organization and direction was mandatory, the CTA believed, so that the Christmas Seal campaign could be run more efficiently on a comprehensive, uniform basis in order to generate more profit and so that the money raised could be spent on the "right" things: prevention, rehabilitation, education, and research, not, Wherrett reiterated, on treatment and major construction projects. And who was better fitted to direct, the national association believed, than itself?

It was easier said than done. Toward the end of the previous decade the CTA had encouraged the establishment of provincial associations with full-time secretaries to inject some order and efficiency into what it saw as local chaos, and it continued to push this approach into the forties. But the very fact that local associations were volunteers made the situation volatile – provincial secretaries, although hired to organize the surveys and promote the Christmas Seal sale, were still paid with funds raised by volunteers and still employed by a provincial association composed of representatives from their groups: they therefore had to avoid being dictatorial. C.R. Dickey, the newly appointed secretary of the Alberta Tuberculosis Association, typified their plight. "Would you give me some information on how the local committees function," he begged in bewilderment to George Wherrett in 1943. "Do they operate under any sort of license or supervision from you, or are they accountable only to themselves? My relations with those I have met are most friendly, but I have discovered that some of them regard Seal Sale funds as their own private possession, and they feel it unnecessary to account to anyone. In some cases seal receipts have been used to buy turkeys, Christmas hampers and other things that seem a bit beyond a strict interpretation of 'preventive' or even 'rehabilitation.'"[111]

Anne Grant, the CTA Christmas Seal director, touring the country in 1944 in an attempt to bring some semblance of order and coordination into the seal campaign, ran up against the same problem of local autonomy. The reasons why a committee did or did not bother with cards, posters, letters, or any other part of the campaign paraphernalia as set out by the central office had little to do with efficiency or even principle; the reasons were as many and varied as the committees themselves. Sometimes it was simply the result of the prejudice of a strong-minded individual member. In Windsor, Grant reported, the reason the committee neglected to use follow-up cards lay with the treasurer: "She doesn't like them. Mrs. Stuart said comfortably that Miss Bartlett had never had to worry about money in her life and didn't understand that people who were busy making a living had to be jogged about things like that."[112] While on the East Coast the Yarmouth sale was "an outstanding example of a seal sale run with no troublesome routine ... [t]he word 'campaign' or 'drive,'" Grant acidly observed, "would not be fittingly applied to it. Dr Morton is a happy warrior who spends the money happily on the wrong things."[113]

It was the Newcastle committee that typified the easy-going, disorganized, and unbusinesslike approach to the seal sale that the small local committees sometimes demonstrated, and she is worth quoting in full for that reason. In a letter to Wherrett, Grant observed whimsically that "Cousin Waldo" (the man in charge)

has the situation loosely but I think competently, in his grasp. He said amiably that he didn't think anyone had ordered supplies – but then as far as he knows nobody had ordered them last year, but they had arrived. I said I thought it was customary to order them. Said Cousin Waldo, "Well just send along the usual amount – maybe a little more."

"Oh yes," he added, "and send some cards." I thought he meant cards for names but it turned out he meant follow-ups.

So will Betty send them supplies as usual, plus enough for a couple of hundred extra names – though they may not add that many. Still they may. They told me they were surprised at how well the new names did, and how well the follow-ups did.[114]

With the surveys making efficient fund-raising more crucial, and the seal sale ever increasing, such a lackadaisical approach could not be tolerated for long by the professionals. At the instigation of the CTA and with CLIOA aid, provincial voluntary associations were established as a coordinating link between the national office and the local committees. They stimulated the setting up of more local associations in uncovered areas, did educational work, fostered rehabilitation, and, most important of all, aided in organizing mass surveys and increasing seal sale returns.[115] By the middle of the decade the basis of the campaign had changed from local units responsible to a national office to a provincial association with local units cooperating in a provincial campaign. Another layer of professional administrators had been added.

This businesslike approach brought quick financial results. In Alberta (where a contract was drawn up between the provincial association and its "agents" regarding seal sale funds) the returns increased from $23,000 in 1942 to $81,000 in 1945.[116] By 1949 the Alberta Tuberculosis Association had eleven full-time and six part-time employees, including a general secretary, a rehabilitation director, and a directory of surveys. In Quebec, the receipts rose from $16,000 in 1941 to $130,000 in 1947. Within a year of the formation of the Ontario Tuberculosis Association, the number of Christmas Seal committees climbed from eighteen to eighty-five, and revenue increased 162 percent.[117]

The volunteers were not completely malleable. The Alberta association, despite stated CTA disapproval, was still spending $12,000 a year by the end of the decade on supplementary relief allowances, including milk and cod liver oil.[118] Meanwhile Wherrett, reporting on the situation in Ontario, was still advising more uniformity in the names and organization of local committees, in an effort to "make them feel more a part of the provincial association and wean them away from the present, perhaps exaggerated, idea of local autonomy and instil in them more responsibility in regard to the future unified provincial organization."[119] Beginning in 1950 the women's groups and service clubs forming the local committees in that bastion of "local autonomy" were being organized into county and district associations.[120]

## Volunteers and the Christmas Seal Sale

With so many local associations jealously guarding their own turf, provincial associations establishing authority with an expanding, specialized staff, and the national association trying to direct the campaign and ensure the increasingly lucrative seal sale profits were funnelled into approved channels, there was plenty of opportunity for friction. And friction did occur.

First there was the question of a fair distribution of costs for the seals. Since 1927 the national office had received 10 percent of the gross returns of all committees except those of Montreal and Toronto, and, calculated on a per capita basis, the Western provinces and Prince Edward Island were paying more than their share.[121] This revenue was important to the national office, since its sole support was the federal government grant, membership fees and donations. By 1948, at the suggestion of the Ontario Association, local committees began instead to purchase their seals and educational supplies at 130 percent of the cost. Although the net return to the CTA was about the same as before, the scheme protected it against increased prices and was considered equitable.[122]

The problem in Montreal was not so easily solved. The stubborn insistence on "local autonomy" by the Kiwanis-run seal committee had been a constant irritant to the national office. That committee had added to CTA costs by demanding a special index card and different sized envelopes from the rest of the committees – and then it did not use any personal solicitation or follow-up of the letters that were mailed. Just instituting these two features alone, Wherrett predicted in exasperation in 1940, would increase the amount of money received by more than 50 percent. "Saskatchewan," he pointedly informed Henry Fyon, the seal committee chairman of the Kiwanis Club, that year "with a population approximately the same as Montreal and with much less per capita wealth, has a mailing list of approximately the same size. They use personal solicitation and follow-up and will reach a total this year of at least $24,000." Montreal had a net collection of about $15,669.[123]

The situation worsened when the CTA, together with the Quebec Provincial Committee for the Prevention of Tuberculosis, set up the Montreal Anti-Tuberculosis League in 1942. From the very beginning, the local association refused to take any direction from either of the parent bodies. "Since they are so self-sufficient," Wherrett penned angrily to J.A. Couillard of the Quebec Committee, "and in a short space of six months have learned more about the seal sale than other people have been able to learn in twenty years, I feel inclined to let them go ahead and take the consequences. They will probably do as well as last year and by that time the other people working with them will probably be so fed up that they will be ready to take some action as to straightening things out."[124]

Relations became even more acrimonious when the league, adopting the method of personal solicitation once suggested by Wherrett to the Kiwanis, absolutely refused to be "taxed" by either the provincial committee or the CTA on any money not raised strictly through selling seals.[125] This refusal was particularly galling since the CTA, to set the budding association on its feet, had picked up the full costs of its first campaign in 1942: about $8,800.[126] The league was quite prepared to pay the CTA for the materials used, the president, C.O. Monat, explained. But the money collected in Montreal, however it was collected, "should be spent for the benefit of the citizens of this city and … the latter should not be always called upon to pay for the rest of the Province" – especially when the provincial committee "limited their activities to publicity," which was "often more detrimental than helpful," and was willing only "to preach and to do nothing to prevent the contagion and spread of tuberculosis."[127]

The members of the Quebec committee were furious. "I esteem that last year we did not hurt the anti-tuberculosis effort in Montreal by inviting His Eminence Cardinal Villeneuve to speak on the CBC," Dr Georges Grégoire, the secretary, responded sarcastically.[128] The provincial committee was particularly frightened that the refusal of the Montreal league to turn over 15 percent of its gross receipts would result in the other twenty-eight local associations refusing on the same grounds[129] – and because at least twenty-three appealed by personal solicitation as well as by mail and four did personal solicitation alone, it would likely mean the collapse of the provincial committee and the end of its educational work.[130] "They will refuse to walk if Montreal is out of the movement," a desperate Jean-Marie Turgeon, the publicist, penned anxiously to Wherrett. "From the other side, we can't give to Montreal a treatment of favour and oblige the other committees to pay the 15 percent on the postal sale and the solicitation. We can't even exempt them from the 15 percent of the solicitation, because they will neglect the postal sale and practically all the work now in way."[131]

His fears were not realized. The other associations continued to cooperate, but Montreal remained intransigent, isolated, and fiercely independent. Over ten years later, a bitter George Wherrett summarized the situation as he saw it:

The League has developed only the mass survey programme. For this purpose it has set up a large organization which [has] made survey costs the highest in Canada. In order to expand the programme, it has withdrawn support from the Bruchesi and Royal Edward Laurentian Hospital dispensaries. It has branched out in twenty-two counties adjacent to Montreal, employs its own nurses and organizers, rather than developing community services or using those already in existence.

... The main source of revenue seems to be from Federal and Provincial grants, plus a direct charge to industries for work done. In addition there is a subscription campaign which capitalizes on the publicity of the National Christmas Seal Campaign.

... On the credit side of the ledger, the League has developed a fairly large volume of work accomplished by the mass survey, although costs are high and there is overlapping in the follow-up. No other phases of the campaign are covered by the League.

"Since the Montreal Anti-Tuberculosis League is not affiliated with either the provincial group or the Canadian Tuberculosis Association," he concluded, "we have no reports as to revenue received and expended on the work done, other than what appears in the press."[132] For the CTA, working to establish comprehensive, provincially organized campaigns across the country under its aegis, it was a frustrating defeat.

The Associated Canadian Travellers (ACT), an organization of salesmen on the road, presented a different problem. They had become involved in the campaign in 1934 to create greater interest and cohesion among their members, and they were primarily interested in some charitable enterprise they could eventually support across the country. They had members throughout the West, but only the locals in Saskatchewan and, to a lesser extent, Manitoba, became actively involved in the anti-tuberculosis campaign.

By 1946 they were becoming more ambitious. The Saskatchewan locals wanted the anti-TB campaign to be the national work of all the clubs in Canada, which would mean expanding into Ontario, Alberta, and British Columbia. They wrote to Wherrett, demanding that the CTA pay the expenses of sending a Saskatchewan ACT member to Ontario to set it up. The prospect was enough to make the executive secretary quail – not only would it be a possible distraction undermining the Christmas Seal sale, but there would also be "conflict and misunderstanding," he pointed out with admirable understatement to R.G. Ferguson, should ACT move in on already established campaigns. "It is very difficult to get the provinces to take a consistent stand in these matters," he complained in turn to E.L. Ross, medical director of the Sanatorium Board of Manitoba, whose province also profited from ACT fund-raising.

I remember that, about ten years ago, the Association of Kinsmen Clubs were anxious to get into tuberculosis work and were prepared to raise a considerable sum on a national basis. At that time Saskatchewan was very much opposed to it on the reasonable grounds that it was introducing two tuberculosis appeals by two different organizations in the same year. Then, however, they got mixed up with the Travellers and although Dr Ferguson admits that fundamentally that is wrong, they have to play along. I think the same applies to the situation in Manitoba and at present my considered opinion is that their participation on a Dominion-wide scale would not be advisable, and in fact, I think we would have a great deal of difficulty persuading the other provincial organizations to adopt it.[133]

## The Role of the CTA

The CTA executive office was becoming a troubleshooter, advisor, and coordinator, as it attempted to set up provincial organizations, bring sometimes stubborn and independent local associations into line with uniform standards, and prevent other organizations, such as ACT, from interfering with other people's business. The CTA also acted as a national spokesperson and advisor: the executive secretary presented a brief to the select committee of the House of Commons and prepared a memorandum on minimum standards for provincial eligibility for federal grants-in-aid (1943), surveyed and reported on health services in the arctic region (1944), helped the research advisory committee of the Department of National Health and Welfare by reviewing applications for support under the National Health Program, and generally advised federal departments.[134] The CTA represented Canada at international conferences; it was a representative on the committee meetings of the National Tuberculosis Association (United States) and the American Trudeau Society (the medical division of that association); and it arranged a scholarship exchange program with the British association, which the latter had suggested as payment for the seals the CTA had supplied that association from 1941 to 1950.[135]

The most important functions of the CTA were the organization and management of the seal sale and health education. Mass surveys had increased the importance of each function (seals supported surveys, while surveys provided a vehicle for distributing educational material), and each, in turn, stressed the importance of the other. As people became more aware of the anti-tuberculosis campaign, they purchased more seals; and as they purchased more seals, they became more aware of the campaign. By 1946, the CTA had two full-time staff employees as directors of the seal sale and health education respectively, and with the development of the provincial associations (particularly in Ontario) the seal sale alone had become a year-round operation.[136]

Because the seal sale had become so valuable, it was jealously guarded. Although they could not obtain a copyright for it,[137] tuberculosis campaigners did everything possible to prevent the use of a stamp or seal by other fund-raising groups, local or national.

The other function of the executive office was, as always, education. The federal government grant of $20,250 had been used to cover the cost of staff salaries and educational material in the past, but when demand increased, the CTA introduced a uniform policy in 1948 for all provincial associations, according to which the associations were charged cost-price for all supplies and materials issued from the national office. In 1944 alone it distributed more than 936,000 educational pamphlets across the country. In sum, reported the president in 1950, the CTA was the *federal* division of tuberculosis control that the Dominion government had never established.[138]

The CTA also continued its role as an influential intermediary, distributing CLIOA funds for tuberculosis work. After the establishment of the Quebec committee, the CTA had suggested that CLIOA provide the capital to improve education in the provinces, increase the national office staff, and organize provincial associations, which in turn would develop a program to increase the seal sale and thus raise more funds for preventive work. The insurance men approved and voted $10,000 a year in 1943, which was used toward salaries for provincial secretaries, a health education director in British Columbia, part of an x-ray survey in Quebec, and provision of pamphlets, a film, and staff education. By 1947, grants had been used to strengthen provincial programs in all the provinces. In total, from 1926 to 1945 CLIOA had pumped close to a quarter of a million dollars into the tuberculosis campaign, under CTA auspices, to encourage the development of government responsibility, proper treatment and prevention, and public awareness.[139]

But its involvement was coming to an end – with the introduction of federal grants, the dominion government assumed its role. "With the assistance now available from the Federal Government," wrote George Wherrett to J.K. Macdonald, chairman of the CLIOA public health committee, "I feel that further grants are unjustified." Nineteen forty-nine was the first year since 1926 that the CTA had not received CLIOA aid.[140]

In 1950, at the annual public health association meeting the senior medical health officer of Vancouver, Dr Stewart Murray, outlined three beliefs upon which postwar public health work in Canada was based: that public health services were for the whole public, not just for the poor; that the general state of public health depended largely on the degree of enlightenment of the citizens as a whole; and that compulsive legislation, unless it came from a convinced (that is, educated) electorate, was of limited use.[141] Universal education had always been a desired goal, but it achieved more prominence as a function of voluntary societies as governments took over other facets of the campaign. In addition, the provincial associations, Christmas Seal letters sent to almost two million homes, and mass surveys provided unprecedented opportunities for informing the people. Specialists were well aware, as they always had been, of their position as leaders and molders of public opinion: "Our knowledge and our efforts," proclaimed one expert somewhat arrogantly, "have to act on the mass like a tiny portion of yeast."[142] Efforts over the years were beginning to pay off. "So well, in fact, have people been indoctrinated about the benefits of sanatorium treatment," observed a *Bulletin* writer bemusedly, "that the problem today has become one rather of persuading them that tuberculosis is still a menace, ever waiting, ever ready – like the cost of living – to spiral up again once the controls are lifted."[143]

## The Changing Role of Volunteers

To accommodate the growing specialization in the tuberculosis campaign, medical advisory boards were established. Their function was, ideally, to maintain close cooperation between professional and lay workers. In fact, they probably provided another venue for the professionals to execute their ideas and influence policy. By the early fifties the provincial associations in Nova Scotia, Ontario, Manitoba, and British Columbia, along with the Montreal Anti-Tuberculosis League, had all established advisory committees of medical people.[144]

This development was but a mild symptom of the growing general concern by the end of the decade over the role of voluntary societies. The increasing involvement of various levels of government, the ever-expanding number of societies and causes clamouring for a share of the public's purse, and the substantial amounts they were raising for sometimes dubious causes led many individuals to wonder, first, what role, if any, voluntary associations should play in Canada and, second, whether they should be regulated – and if so, how. Some, like J. Limerick, one-time director of the New Brunswick Tuberculosis Association, echoed Rockefeller Foundation-type thinking, and thought tuberculosis work should be placed "on a sound, business-like basis, under one management, and with one source of funds" – the government.[145] In other words, a successful volunteer association, by pioneering various health programs and stimulating state responsibility, eventually rendered itself obsolete. But even the supporters of voluntarism queried the role the volunteer association was now playing. In Ontario the CTA participated in a federally funded study of the respective roles of voluntary and official effort in the tuberculosis program, which resulted in a reorganization of the Ontario Tuberculosis Association.[146] In keeping with the spirit of postwar regulation and organization, the *Canadian Journal of Public Health* recommended that peacetime legislation should be passed along the lines of the Federal War Charities Act, which had required all war charities soliciting public support and financial aid to be registered and their activities scrutinized, to avoid duplication of effort as well as exploitation.[147] Another alternative was a National Information Bureau, similar to one existing in the United States, that would obtain objective information on all health and welfare organizations, enumerate some general principles as to what features were or were not desirable, and make the information available to the public to evaluate and judge. It was this last position that the CTA executive supported, arguing that the right of voluntary associations to operate and appeal for funds was "part of the democratic system."[148]

By 1950 the issue of "federated appeals" had arisen: federation was suggested by some advocates as an efficient centralized solution to the burgeoning number of voluntary agencies and causes. With the *Financial Post* spearheading a press campaign against organized charities, especially the March of Dimes, it was hardly surprising that Ontario passed legislation enabling any appeal to be investigated.

In the space of just a few years, several changes in the tuberculosis campaign had followed quickly on one another, with almost bewildering speed. Mass surveys not only initiated a new era in case-finding but, with over 2 million people x-rayed by 1950, boosted public awareness and education. Beginning in 1948 federal health grants pumped three to four million dollars annually into the campaign and, along with wartime experience and federal construction grants, encouraged the provinces not only to fill in the gaps in their existing programs – to standardize and even accelerate them – but to branch out in new directions: into rehabilitation and x-ray examinations of general hospital admissions (as a more fruitful case-finding activity). In only a five-year period (1945 to 1950) treatment facilities increased approximately 50 percent, to a total of 17,000 beds in the country.[149]

And above all there was the long-sought specific: streptomycin, quickly followed by PAS and INH. Paid for with federal grants, they were soon distributed to all who might benefit and supposedly introduced the final phase of the conquest of the disease. At long last, using these drugs in combination with surgical resection, specialists could talk of the *cure*, not simply the control, of tuberculosis. The death rate, declining steadily but slowly since the beginning of the century, plummeted: from 1947 to 1953 it was cut by two-thirds in all the provinces.[150]

Tuberculosis, once so lethal, was fast becoming a disease of the elderly. By 1951 as many Canadians were dying of it over the age of forty as under, while in Saskatchewan even the rate of infection had fallen in school children to less than 1 percent per annum.[151] It was no wonder, then, if the specialists, seeing the spectacular decline in mortality and seeing mass surveys increasingly uncovering a greater percentage of other debilitating conditions and a smaller percentage of active tuberculosis, were optimistically looking ahead and discussing other uses for empty beds, and it was no wonder that the public, impressed with the effect of antibiotics, believed the disease to be well on its way to being eliminated.

Not quite. Although the death rate fell precipitously, the incidence of disease did not keep pace – in Ontario, although the former fell an impressive 70 percent from 1943 to 1952, the latter declined only 13 percent.[152] So the specialists who had been trying to convince a dubious public for years that tuberculosis was a curable, preventable, and even eradicable disease now ironically found themselves preaching caution: drugs were not a substitute for sanatorium treatment or a sure-fire cure; relapse was all too possible, and accelerated case-finding was essential if existing pockets of disease were to be eliminated. And with over ten thousand new cases reported in 1953 and treatment costs in nonfederal sanatoria alone close to $30 million, the campaign was far from over.[153] The specialist's position, reported George Wherrett ruefully, was "rather like that of an army which has had victory in the field after a long, hard battle. In their elation over success against the shock troops it is understandable if they rather forget that the enemy isn't down and out, that, in fact, it has a vigorous guerilla force seeded through the country, unconquered and capable of carrying on a sniping campaign. More than ten thousand killed and wounded in a year is a degree of success which a warlord might envy."[154]

Nevertheless, the back of the disease seemed to be broken. Accommodation peaked in 1953, and then the number of sanatorium beds occupied fell rapidly. Pockets of infection remained, notably in the native peoples, but the specialists began to move on to other chest conditions, and the president of the national association confidently predicted that the word "sanatorium," which had frightened so many in the past, would soon be replaced by "clinical centres for respiratory diseases."[155] By the end of the decade, sanatoria were either shutting their doors or converting their facilities to accommodate other chronically ill or diseased patients. The White Plague, once so feared, was reduced to a minor cause of death for Canadians – it seemed only the mopping-up process remained. The public turned its attention to other concerns: heart disease, cancer, mental illness.

In 1960, the Muskoka Hospital for Tuberculosis, the first sanatorium in Canada, was sold to the provincial government for use as a mental hospital.

# 9 The Disease and the Campaign: A Reflection of Twentieth-Century Social Philosophy

It is within the power of man to cause all germ diseases to disappear from the Earth.                                                   Louis Pasteur

The infectious diseases replace each other, and when one is rooted out it is apt to be replaced by others which ravage the human race indifferently whenever the conditions of health are wanting. They have this property in common with weeds and other forms of life, as one species recedes another advances.                                                   William Farr, 1873

It is seldom recognized that each type of society has diseases peculiar to itself – indeed, that each civilization creates its own diseases.    René Dubos

The tuberculosis campaign did not exist in a vacuum. A disease such as tuberculosis is inextricably interwoven with society, and Canadian society changed profoundly from 1900 to 1950. In 1901, 40.3 percent of the labour force was in agricultural occupations alone; this figure fell to 28.6 percent in 1931, and 15.7 percent in 1951. In 1941, 30.5 percent of workers were involved in primary occupations, but during the period of rapid industrialization after World War 2, this percentage declined to 12.8 (in 1961), while the percentage in man-ufacturing, mechanical, and construction jobs rose to 21.3. In addi-tion, the white-collar group, which had made up only 15.3 percent of the labour force in 1901, increased to 37.9 percent by 1961, emerging as the largest group in the decade from 1941 to 1951. Canada had become urbanized.[1]

Even these percentages do not tell the whole story, for more sophis-ticated technology had ushered in a "machine age." Machines in construction and other blue-collar work, in agricultural and primary industries, replaced men wielding shovels, picks, and axes. Cement was mixed, cows milked, trees chopped, and fields ploughed, all by some new mechanical device. This change not only affected rehabilitation and enhanced employment opportunities for former sanatorium patients; it also lessened the physical strain on Canadians in general. Some of the worst abuses of industrialization were dealt with, working conditions were improved, and social legislation was implemented, so that by 1950 tuberculosis no longer spelled financial ruin for a family hit by the disease. Free treatment was extended; and veterans' allowances, aftercare allowances, mothers' allowances, family allowances, and relief all offered some limited aid to afflicted individuals and their dependents.

Both treatment and preventive measures were affected. The movement from rural areas to urban centres with small houses or apartments that had no room for the chronically ill or aged caused the latter to fill crowded hospital wards and aggravate the nursing shortage in the 1940s.[2] The radio made extended bed rest more tolerable, and brought the Christmas Seal campaign into the home. Improved roads and automobiles enabled specialists to start travelling clinics for previously isolated areas.

Opportunities for infection lessened and general sanitation improved. The number of flies diminished, due both to better sanitation and to the use of the automobile, rather than horse, for transportation. The common drinking cup fell out of favour; spitting declined. The invention and general use of vacuum cleaners, detergents, washing machines, easily cleaned linoleum, and plastics made disinfection and higher standards of sanitation easier to achieve, with less individual effort.

## Accounting for the Decline of Tuberculosis

### Improved Living Standards

Scholars such as Thomas McKeown and René and Jean Dubos have attributed the decline of tuberculosis to improved sanitation, improved personal hygiene, and higher living standards that occurred as a result of a humanitarian movement for social reform beginning in mid-nineteenth century England, rather than to bacteriology and the germ theory.[3] McKeown, examining the price of food, argues that it was better nutrition, resulting in increased resistance, that accounted for the fall in death rates. Another writer went even further. "The public health movement," he insisted, "has not experienced a consistent and organically sound development ... the dominance of bacteriology in public health represents not a straight line advance, but rather a lateral deflection, if not an actual defection."[4] From this perspective, the most effective fight against tuberculosis in Canada was waged in the social reform period prior to World War 1, when anti-tuberculosis campaigners, lacking the medical technology they acquired later, not only attacked the germ, but attempted to improve living standards and build up "natural resistance."

Although the Dubos-McKeown hypothesis, by providing an explanation both for the association of tuberculosis with poor socioeconomic conditions and for the decline of the disease in the nineteenth-century Europe, has enjoyed considerable popularity, it is not without its detractors. The historian Leonard Wilson has argued that the placement of consumptives in workhouses and Poor Law infirmaries effectively isolated them from the population at large and so restricted the spread of the disease. The growth of sanatoria in the twentieth century continued the trend.[5] A subsequent study of various immigrant groups in Minnesota supported the same conclusion.[6] Moreover, studies of modern TB control programs, emphasizing identification, isolation and treatment of cases, have shown them to be effective – even among those developing nations with documented poor socioeconomic conditions.[7] And, as Sidel, Drucker, and Martin have observed, there is no evidence that the steady decline of tuberculosis documented by McKeown would have persisted without the introduction of anti-TB campaigns – "it is equally plausible that the decline would not have continued and that while improvements in socio-economic conditions may have caused reduction in tuberculosis up to a point, in the absence of public health interventions, tuberculosis rates would have plateaued."[8]

*Disease Cycles*
Another school of thought argues that much of this discussion is irrelevant; that diseases go in cycles, starting with an acute stage when the most susceptible individuals are killed, then passing to a more chronic form as those surviving have or develop some natural resistance, and then to a decline, as foci of infection diminish. Humans and microbes adapt to each other, and only a disturbance in the internal or external environment will lead to lower resistance and a fresh outbreak of disease. Dubos points to outbreaks in Europe that raged and then later faded – leprosy in the fourteenth century, plague in the fifteenth, syphilis in the sixteenth, smallpox in the seventeenth and eighteenth centuries, and scarlet fever, measles, and tuberculosis in the nineteenth century – as partial evidence.[9]

The history of tuberculosis among the Qu'Appelle Valley Indians lends credence to this evolutionary theory of disease. Before 1900, acute forms of tuberculosis were common; as the more susceptible individuals died, by 1921 the disease began to localize in the lung, assume its more common chronic form, and continue its decline.[10]

In 1945, in an effort to explain the uniformity in the rate of decline of tuberculosis in Ontario after 1900, N.E. McKinnon argued that a decline in infection had probably occurred "a considerable time" before 1900, which influenced the balance between sources and susceptibles "to give a self-propagating, progressively declining trend."[11]

Bates and Stead have noted that a TB epidemic in a given population typically peaks within 50 to 75 years after onset, then declines slowly, with the incidence decreasing 1 percent to 2 percent per year, as the more naturally resistant survivors reproduce.[12] Such "natural selection" has been suggested as an explanation for the relative resistance of Jews of Eastern European descent: their forced urbanization, undiluted (as other ethnic groups were) by rural immigration during the peak of the TB epidemic, led to a more vigorous selection of a resistant population.[13]

Individuals interested in public health had long noted and argued the implications of this theory. A 1924 editorial in the *Canadian Medical Association Journal* pointed out that tuberculosis had been declining for three-quarters of a century and questioned how much of this had been due to human efforts. If the disease acted as a selective agent, eliminating unfit "stock" and preventing their reproduction, "[i]t would follow, therefore," the writer reasoned, "that efforts directed towards improving the tuberculous individual's health would conflict with the efforts of natural selection."[14] In 1940, H.E. MacDermot of the Royal Edward Institute presented this argument again in a *Notes on Tuberculosis* article, quoting another specialist: "It may be a bitter pill for mankind to swallow when we suggest that natural selection may have done more for racial health in this matter than medical science."[15]

Recent work in immunology has added a more sophisticated perspective, without the eugenics flavour. Resistance to infection with *M. bovis* in a mouse model has been linked to a specific gene, while numerous family and twin studies have suggested not only a genetic predisposition to TB but an association with specific inherited immunological markers (that is, the HLA-DR allele). These, in turn, have been linked to specific ethnic groups.[16] It was the American Esmond R. Long who reflected an optimistic faith in the future and in medical science that was probably more common among the specialists: "If in the long run it must be admitted that our campaign preserves physiologically susceptible stock, steadily wiped out by the disease in former eras, presumably the advance of knowledge will enable us to deal with this fact in future."[17]

If the general decline in tuberculosis was primarily due to the evolutionary progress of the disease, then with the elimination of susceptible human stock, the increasing resistance of the remaining populace and a resulting, self-prorating decline in infection combined with improved sanitation and better working and living conditions (which, one might assume, eliminated the worst abuses of the Industrial Revolution and enabled Western Europeans and North Americans to adjust to a new urbanized, industrialized society), then the effect of the expensive, bacteriologically oriented campaign that came into its own in Canada after the World War 1, was perhaps negligible. "When the tide is receding from the beach," Dubos observed cynically, "it is easy to have the illusion that one can empty the ocean by removing water with a pail."[18]

*Socioeconomic Changes*

"Tuberculosis," commented David Stewart in 1930, was "a disease of the early mistakes of civilization. And it can be eradicated, as the weeds of dirty prairie land can be, only by the science and culture of a still higher type of civilization."[19] In his *Dreams of Reason*, Dubos stated the same fundamental concept somewhat differently: "each type of society has diseases peculiar to itself ... each civilization creates its own diseases."[20] According to this view, the epidemic of tuberculosis was brought about by the abuses and excesses of the Industrial Revolution; as soon as these excesses had been adjusted, it declined. Human beings might adapt and modify their environment so that the conditions favouring the development of one specific disease – tuberculosis, for example – will be eliminated; but in so doing they create new conditions to be adapted to, new problems to be resolved, and they foster the development of new diseases: cancer, heart disease, and mental illness.

Changes in twentieth-century North America appeared to bolster this argument. New technology had helped reduce infection by eliminating horses and stables, thereby eliminating a breeding ground for flies; new technology also virtually eliminated physical strain for the individual worker, while new synthetic materials were easier to clean and detergents made that cleaning easier. At the same time, increased use of the automobile caused air pollution and traffic accidents; automation alienated the individual worker, and caused mental, rather than physical, stress and frustration; while the new synthetics and detergents provoked allergies.[21] In Canada, as tuberculosis fell, cardiovascular/renal disease and cancer increased by 38.3 percent and 51.5 percent respectively from 1930 to 1964. And while the life expectancy at birth was 60 for men in 1931 and 66.33 in 1951, life expectancy at forty was, disappointingly enough, roughly the same: 31.98 and 32.45 respectively.[22]

Proponents of McKeown and Dubos have argued that the bacteriological approach probably did not have a great effect on the *general,* overall history of tuberculosis in Western Europe and North America. Instead, the concentration of public health workers on this method, although it may have accelerated a declining trend, increased the cost of health care, most of which was for treatment, and did nothing to build up a "religion of health living"[23] to prevent other debilitating diseases.

Yet, despite the flaws in the bacteriological approach to preventive medicine and health services, one should always remember that the specific techniques and methods developed, including surgery and antibiotics, undoubtedly saved thousands of individual lives. In the long-term epidemiological pattern of the disease this might not have been very important, perhaps; but for individual patients and their families, it was of very great significance. Moreover, on a local basis, it was most likely the organized campaign against the disease that was the major factor *accelerating* the *already declining* mortality and morbidity rates. Proof of this is demonstrated in the varying provincial rates – although here, again, it is impossible to isolate and measure exactly any one cause. Saskatchewan, the "model" province, was also the most rural; and tuberculosis was preeminently a disease of industrialization. Yet Saskatchewan was also the first to institute free treatment, have enough beds, and run mass community surveys.

More obvious is the influence the campaign against tuberculosis had in altering the pattern of health care and Canadians' attitudes toward government responsibility. It was the first costly, chronic disease with which the country had to deal; and the way in which responsibility was assumed, and authority determined, set the pattern for Canadian health services in general.

## Philosophical Changes: Plausibility, Not Proof

"Medical advances," Dubos states, "do not arise in a social vacuum. They are products of the sparks between the scientific knowledge of the time and the demands of the community."[24] And, as the British historian E.H. Carr once shrewdly observed, "Every society is an arena of social conflicts, and those individuals who range themselves against existing authority are no less products and reflections of the society than those who uphold it."[25] So it seems germane not only to ask *why* public health specialists – from turn-of-the-century reformers to end-of-the-century advocates of the views of Dubos and McKeown – were first enchanted and then ultimately disillusioned with the bacteriological focus, but also to ask what accounted for such a development in preventive medicine in general? In other words, what underlying *philosophical* changes in attitudes occurred as a response to the dramatic and often bewildering social, economic, scientific, and technological developments in North American society and how were these reflected in the public health movement and anti-TB campaign?

In his recent work, *Science and Religion in the Era of William James*, Paul Jerome Croce argues that Darwin's *Origin of the Species* "ignored the claims of religion ... and relied more on the *plausibility* of explanations than on the *certainty* of proof." As a result, "Darwin created equal controversy in religious *and* scientific circles for both the *content* and the *method* of his science."[26].

Specifically, Darwin's theory lacked proof in two ways: the emergence of a new species had never been observed and so was strictly conjectural, and any agent causing the variation posited by his theory was also unknown and therefore unproven. As such, his theory not only challenged traditional religion, as has been long recognized, but it also signalled a new approach to science: it was based on *plausibility and probability* rather than proof, and so challenged nineteenth-century scientific certainty. It was *this*, Croce observes, that was the "true Darwinian Revolution," and it at least justified – if it did not encourage – the application of "scientific methods" and statistical analysis to philosophical and social questions in the twentieth century. Paradoxically, Darwin's challenge to philosophical certainty in both the religious and scientific spheres would stimulate a quest for control and a "hunger for assurance" that would be assuaged by the secularization of society and the substitution of scientific methods, social engineering, and statistical probabilities for the old religious authority of spiritual truth.[27]

The philosophical change from the ideal of scientific proof to science as plausible explanation permitted the application of "scientific thinking" to social concerns in a much broader, less vigorous way. The advantage of studying probabilities was, of course, that probabilities provided insight into the underlying causes of social misfortunes; the disadvantage, not often recognized, was that such an approach (unfettered by rigorous concrete criteria for proof) could justify unacknowledged prejudices about specific classes, races, or habits. Reformers could see what they looked for, masking their meddlings with a patina of respectable statistical explanations. The Progressive Era is replete with examples of both consequences.

### Social Engineering and Scientific Management: A New National Class

If Darwinism liberated social and scientific theory from the burden of certain proof, turn-of-the-century advances in scientific knowledge and engineering triumphs seemed to justify the notion that scientific methods could solve social problems in the same way engineers solved technical ones. Using an engineering model – a practical application of the physical sciences well-suited to the results-oriented pragmatism peculiar to North American society – reformers and social thinkers adopted what John Jordan has termed a "machine-age ideology" that substituted an allegedly "scientific" rationalism for a religious one, appropriating the premises of engineering: "a supposition of objectivity, a stress on method, a belief in knowledge and predictable laws, and a linkage of knowledge to control over one's world."[28] Engineering methods would ensure efficiency, organization and predictability in an uncertain world, while expert-led scientific management would establish a new, rational society free of the tensions of class, race, and economics.

There was an unacknowledged dark side to that idealized view of a scientifically managed, expert-led, organized and centralized society: it was profoundly undemocratic. With an engineering model, it was assumed that, if all facts were known, expert, educated opinion would arrive at the one, best solution: there was little difference between solving the social problem of urban poverty or the rise of tuberculosis and building the Hoover Dam or manufacturing steel. A "morality of presumed objectivity" was substituted for the traditional morality of ethical opinion; reformers, managers, academics – the new intellectual elite in an increasingly secular society – were able to disavow self-serving behaviour as "disinterested benevolence."[29]

And if there was no need for inefficient, counter-productive, scandal-plagued, parochial politics and backroom deals, there was equally no role for democratic give-and-take brokering of compromise and consensus-building between competing political interests. In fact, as Jordan points out, many reformers argued that "old style" politics was outdated: "scientific management" would provide the one correct solution with a "nonpolitics" of administrative competence; and "because expertise transcended the self-interest of traditional class conflict, middle class experts could control both urban ethnic masses and plutocratic elites with power based in knowledge."[30]

As a result, a method of management – standardization and centralization, efficiently organized and controlled by a new administrative class of experts – became an end in itself. World War 1, with its various boards, helped entrench the technocratic administrators in North American political culture, giving rise to a coalition of social scientists, engineers, journalists, and foundation representatives who pursued an agenda of "rational reform" in the twenties.[31] Rarely did any of the intellectuals who seemed to move effortlessly among universities, foundations, and government advisory boards in the twenties and thirties ever question whether such wholesale application of methods appropriated from engineering and the natural sciences to social problems was beneficial – or even logical.

One important philosophical and political aspect of such developments was that it crossed traditional political lines. Proponents of expert-led scientific management and social engineering could – and did – range across the political spectrum, from John D. Rockefeller to Samuel Gompers. Conventional and misleading "left-right" distinctions obscured their common beliefs and assumptions. In a sense, the important conflict was not left versus right but old versus new: a traditional, individually based, somewhat parochial worldview premised on personal responsibility in a democratic society, frequently with strong links to religion, versus an expert-led, efficiently managed global worldview. This development was equally evident in medical science. As Paul Starr noted in his historical study of American medicine, "socialists and the Rockefeller philanthropies were equally committed to the extension of scientific medicine ... The assumptions of radicals, reformers and conservatives reflected the more general decline of confidence in the ability of the laymen to deal with their own physical and personal problems."[32]

At least two historians, Robert Wiebe and Christopher Lasch,[33] have addressed such social and intellectual changes in twentieth-century American society, noting the deleterious effects on participatory democracy. In *Self Rule* Wiebe posits that three classes emerged with the industrialization of the United States at the turn of the century: a new, largely urban national class, geared to national institutions and policies; a local middle class; and a lower working class. In contrast to the elites of the nineteenth century, who were often defined by their geographical identity (Boston Brahmins, Chicago Merchants), the new national class that emerged between 1900 and 1925 obtained its power and influence from nationally based corporate consolidation and finance, supported by interrelated specialties. As significantly, its focus shifted from the nineteenth century's emphasis on the democratic concept of "character," which, Wiebe observed, was defined by universal traits such as honesty or thrift and could therefore be judged by anyone, to knowledge and expertise requiring specialized training. As a result, Wiebe notes, the national class saw itself as the rightful leaders of ordinary citizens – for only other specialists and experts were qualified to judge experts.

The traditional, locally-based middle class – retailers, professionals – recognized and resented their loss of authority to this new group. Frequently the interests of the two were antithetical: large-scale "efficiency" for a national business meant price-cutting and the threat of bankruptcy to a small local firm. Loyalty to community, church, and family had no place in national policy. While the national class founded professional associations, the local middle class established service clubs – as Wiebe defines it, it was a battle for cultural control in which the national class "wrapped their own values in a mantle of science" and equated local America with an oppressive Protestantism, peopled by boorish, bigoted Babbits. 34

Like Jordan, Wiebe notes the fundamentally antidemocratic character of a centrally controlled, specialized system managed by professional administrators who used science and statistical studies to enhance their impartial image: "reforms that originated in a desire to make governments more responsive to people's needs ended up making them less responsive to people's voices."35 It was no accident that a national bureaucracy, spawned in the progressive era, divorced from traditional moral, religious, and cultural imperatives, achieved its modern form in the twenties as the government changed from one "expected to enact the People's will" to a modern state that was "supposed to look after the people's needs."36

In *The Revolt of the Elites and the Betrayal of Democracy*, Christopher Lasch supports much of Wiebe's argument. Gilded Age scandals had given politics a bad name; as a result, educated individuals began to demand the "professionalization of politics" with a civil service of trained experts free of tainted political party control. This demand became entrenched in the progressive era, with its reform demands for efficiency and scientific management and with government functions increasingly delegated to appointed commissions headed by specialized administrators. "Recognizing that political machines were welfare agencies of a rudimentary type, which dispensed jobs and other benefits to their constituents and thereby won their loyalty," Lasch notes somewhat cynically, "the progressives set out to create a welfare state as a way of competing with the machines."37 Public opinion was considered uninformed and therefore unreliable. Disinterested scientific inquiry with decisions by knowledgeable administrators obviated the need for discussion – as the American journalist Walter Lippmann opined, reflecting a view current in the new ideology, information made argument unnecessary.38

More critical than Wiebe, Lasch notes the scorn, even hostility, of the educated national class for the traditional nineteenth-century values of religion and individual responsibility. Government and university experts together would solve social problems without the nuisance of public debate. "They liked to contrast the scientific expert with the orator, the latter a useless windbag whose rantings only confused the public mind."39

In sum, a profound change occurred in North American society at the turn of the century. Philosophically, the ascendancy of Darwinism challenged not only traditional religious beliefs but conventional scientific tenets as well: plausibility and probability became acceptable scientific "proof." The astounding growth in knowledge in the natural sciences together with obvious concrete industrial and engineering achievements presented a seductive paradigm for the solution of seemingly intractable social problems. With the proper approach, it should be no more challenging to eliminate slum poverty than to dam up the Colorado River, while statistical probabilities provided a "scientific" justification for social policies and self-serving agendas. A new class of administrators and managers evolved that Wiebe calls a "national class" and Lasch terms an "educated class," and that Jordan traces back to an engineering paradigm and links to the growth of "liberalism" as we define it today. This new class was defined by attitude and social imperatives more than by traditional geographic or political alignments; it was in the ascendancy and promoted new "virtues" of efficiency, organization, standardization, centralization, and social engineering. Indifferent, even hostile, to the traditional values of religion, family, individual responsibility, and civic virtue, members of this class scorned the beleaguered members of the traditional middle class – the local, small-town businessmen and professionals – for their parochial, hidebound attitudes. By the 1920s the political and cultural agenda of this elite group of intellectuals was so firmly entrenched that Sinclair Lewis' Babbit would enter the cultural lexicon as an example of everything that was wrong with traditional small-town America – an attitude that would go largely unchallenged until the end of this century.

Much of this analysis has obviously been predicated on historical trends in the United States, and it is still unclear to what extent such developments influenced Canadian society. Certainly, as many historians have noted, the themes in the turn-of-the-century American Progressive era were similarly expressed in prewar Canadian society, while the development of large-scale centralized, increasingly American-dominated industry – mining and steel, hydroelectricity, pulp and paper – and its threat to small businessmen has been long discussed. Moreover, Canada's political and cultural traditions may fit even more comfortably with a "national class" ideology: "peace, order, and good government" is more suited to scientific management with centralization, standardization, and an efficiency-based society led by expert administrators than the often contrary and individualistic ideal of "life, liberty and the pursuit of happiness."

*Public Health and the Universities vs Private Practice*

Certainly awareness of such fundamental changes in North American society in the late nineteenth and twentieth centuries is fundamental in understanding the development and direction of public health and the anti-TB campaign. Neither operated in a vacuum; and the divisions and tensions in society at large were, unsurprisingly, faithfully reflected in the ostensibly impartial world of medical science and public policy. To assess the campaign – its principles, methods, and goals – independently of this context is not only unfair but misleading. For example, though both may be considered "capitalists," the distinction between large corporations and small businessmen has long been recognized. Less frequently acknowledged is that a similar division exists in the medical profession – although all may be physicians, the goals and attitudes of urban, university-based specialists and researchers and public health officials may be vastly different from small-town or suburban community-based doctors.

Reminiscent of the situation in the business world, university-based, research-oriented specialists and public health officials were analogous to and probable members of the new educated "national class" of administrators and corporate managers. Just as John D. Rockefeller had pioneered new, systematized "big business" policies, so his foundation, among others, actively promoted the development of North American medical schools patterned after Johns Hopkins University: university-linked institutions committed to research, with full-time academic professors and associated with teaching hospitals and a full complement of laboratories. As the expert dominated business and government in the social reform era, so the expert – the full-time academic professor – would manage medical education. In the 1890s, most North American medical schools used practising physicians to teach courses in fundamental sciences; less than twenty years later, most did not.[40]

The appointment of full-time staff threatened existing practitioners not only with a loss of status when they were replaced as clinical instructors but sometimes with a loss of income, when they lost admitting privileges at the university teaching hospitals. Such town-gown tensions were exacerbated by the fact that many full-time instructors were imported from distant institutions – they had closer links with other experts in their fields than with local private practitioners.[41] It was an indication of the academics' cultural authority that many of their beliefs – that teaching hospitals provided better care, that full-time professors were more effective teachers than practitioners – were adopted with little proof.[42] By the 1920s, medical schools, like other modern industries, had standardized their "methods of production," assuming a corporate form with their own experts, administrators, and bureaucracies. With their ever-expanding budgets, they had become big businesses.

There is no reason to expect that the private practitioners, displaced and condescended to by the new academic physicians, would react with any less hostility than small-town businessmen threatened by the encroachment of national corporations and trusts – and they did not. They resented the school medical health officers and dispensaries that were exploited by the specialists for training and research as a threat to their livelihood; they complained that government manufacturing of anti-toxins was an unfair business practice; and they opposed compulsory notification as a breach of doctor-patient confidentiality.[43]

In Canada these themes were played out most dramatically in Toronto. The 1902 federation of Trinity College and the University of Toronto had created a single medical faculty in that city, and, as Michael Bliss notes in his biography of Sir Joseph Flavelle, that Canadian millionaire and proponent of big business worked to establish, with provincial support, a new general hospital that was not only closer to the university but also exclusively a teaching hospital. Moreover, the faculty of medicine staff demanded it contain only free public wards under their control. This demand was strenuously opposed by the city councillors, who allied themselves with the threatened private physicians, supporting patients' right to choose their doctor.[44]

Flavelle and like-minded citizens envisioned the new hospital as having a dual purpose: intended both to treat the sick and advance the study of medicine, it would be administered by a new, efficient board of appointed trustees. Flavelle's philosophical support of their goals did not, however, blind the usually shrewd businessman to the characters of some of the academic physicians. "I cannot remember ever having had such a difficult lot to fight for," he wrote. "They have few friends, they have many enemies, and they are self-satisfied, or at least the reputed clique who lead them are."[45]

By 1919 Flavelle was supporting a plan to centralize clinical services – a plan at least partly put into place to meet the terms of grants from Eaton's and the Rockefeller Foundation.[46] Again there was strenuous protesting from private physicians who lost privileges and prestige – the hospital and faculty had become a "big business machine" because the university wanted "Yankee money."[47]

Closely allied and at times overlapping with the university academic physicians were those involved in public health. Like the faculty doctors, these, too, tended to have a national, rather than a local community, perspective, having more in common with each other than the private physicians in their area. For example, Charles Hastings, the Toronto medical officer of health from 1910 to 1929, reflected the biases of both the progressive era and Wiebe's national class when he transformed the department into a modern bureaucracy with new divisions organized under "scientific management." He, too, had a distrust of parochial machine politics, maintaining that experts should manage municipal services without political interference – an attitude that sometimes led to conflict with the city council.

By 1912 the university had awarded the first diploma in public health – and that same year the Public Health Act made a diploma a prerequisite for employment.[48] It was the advent of the career public health officer, the trained administrator who moved *not* back and forth from private practice to public health but in a *parallel* course among governments, appointed commissions, and voluntary associations. J.A. Amyot was director of the Ontario Board of Health Laboratory from 1900 to 1918 while he served as a professor at his alma mater, the University of Toronto, before becoming director of the quarantine branch of the new federal Department of Health in 1919.[49] Grant Fleming, Hastings' second deputy minister of health, moved on to become director of the Montreal Anti-Tuberculosis and General Health League, while several years later Robert E. Wodehouse would leave his position as secretary of the Canadian Tuberculosis Association to work as federal deputy minister of pensions and national health and, while doing so, would serve as president of the Canadian Public Health Association in the late thirties.[50] During the depression, the Dominion Council of Health, whose membership consisted of the senior provincial health officers together with five lay members, devised a special survey, for which it petitioned Rockefeller Foundation funds, not only to assess health activities in Canada but, as Wodehouse wrote to Dr John A. Ferrell of the foundation in 1936, to provide work for Dr A. Lessard, the Quebec council representative "who has been let out of the Quebec government employ ... and is really in need of the opportunity for employment."[51]

By the twenties, district medical officers of health were encouraged to complete Toronto's diploma program, since their positions were seen as a "springboard" to other positions in government health bureaucracies and large charities.[52] Johns Hopkins University had created the first Rockefeller Foundation-funded school of hygiene in 1916; by 1924 the University of Toronto had obtained Rockefeller money to open a similar school in 1927 that had a close, if not incestuous, relationship with the Toronto health department: not only did its senior staff teach health administration at the new institution, but the Canadian Public Health Association had its head office at the school of hygiene until 1963. By 1920 the Toronto health department was considered such a model of centralization, specialization, organization, and efficiency that the ubiquitous Rockefeller Foundation sponsored international students at the University of Toronto so that they could do field work with the municipal department.53

With the universities and health departments so closely aligned, it was not surprising that private practitioners were often as resentful and suspicious of public health officials as they were of academic physicians, and for much the same reasons: loss of prestige and threats to their livelihood. Throughout the second and third decades of this century they protested any potential infringement of their practices by the introduction of large-scale vaccines or school inspection. They resented "sharing" the supervision of their patients with the government officials and objected to public health nurses "undermining" the family doctor, who had to "struggle alone" to build up his practice.54 They supported their patients' resistance to notifications and isolation – for their bias and loyalty was to the individual *patient*, not society at large. In this respect, they were in direct opposition to public health advocates, as Charles Hastings spelled out clearly in a 1919 address on compulsory vaccination during a smallpox epidemic:

practically every activity of the Board of Health and the Department of Health means depriving some of our citizens of their personal liberty and the individual right to do so as they please, ofttimes compelling them to do the very things they do not want to do. That is why Departments of Health are unpopular, just in proportion to the efficiency with which they discharge their duty. Why all this interference with personal liberty and individual rights? Because British justice, properly interpreted means that when the liberty and rights of the individual are not in the interests of the welfare of the masses, the rights of the individual must yield."55

Like the service clubs and the small businessmen, the private practitioners were individualistic, self-supporting adherents of traditional civic virtues whose status and income were intrinsically a part of their local society; public health and academic physicians, in contrast, reflected a broader, more national perspective, like the new large corporations, foundations, and government advisory boards – their status relied on their place in their *profession*, rather than in their local community; their focus was *societal* rather than individual, and they valued new virtues of expertise, efficiency, organization, and standardization, all under the sometime nebulous rubric of "scientific management." And, as the century progressed, the gulf between the two groups would only widen.

It is difficult to say whether the field of public health was peculiarly well-suited, both philosophically and practically, to the changes occurring in turn-of-the-century North American society or whether it developed in the manner it did in order to adapt to such changes. Perhaps both views are true. In any event, public health advocates fortuitously and shrewdly accommodated and exploited concurrent developments in the natural sciences and society at large to transform a part-time profession into a career and a movement.

The public health movement drew both credibility and support from ongoing developments in scientific knowledge and the new Darwinian-justification of probability as proof. Late nineteenth- and early twentieth-century bacteriological discoveries – diphtheria toxoid, the tubercle bacillus – were extraordinarily well-suited to an expert-led, mechanistic engineering paradigm in which the problem, the disease, could be identified and the solution, a vaccine or a cure, found. Moreover, such discoveries mandated new laboratory-based knowledge and confirmed the value of experts. Equally importantly, the new reliance on probability and plausibility to account for developments in the natural sciences could be extended to medicine and public health, and it fueled support for "crusades" against a myriad of underlying "causes" of specific diseases: alcoholism, long hours of work, poor ventilation.

Without financial support, of course, these new philosophical attitudes might have had only limited influence – and it is here that the foundations, notably the Rockefeller institutions, played a key role. Between 1902 and 1934, nine major American foundations invested an impressive $154 million in medical education and research, which was almost half the total amount they spent on all other areas.[56] Like the public health movement itself, the Rockefeller and Carnegie foundations derived their organizational style and focus from an amalgam of Protestant missionary work and the oil and steel trusts.[57] Charles Rosenberg has demonstrated that a certain number of mid-nineteenth century pioneer public health advocates were motivated by a religious commitment to improving the sanitary environment of the more unfortunate by an "assumption that an intimate relationship existed between environment, health, and morals";[58] by the turn of the century, the Baptist-educated, social-gospel-inspired Rockefeller appointee Frederick Gates not only saw science as a secular religion but tellingly described the Rockefeller Institute for Medical Research as "a sort of theological seminary," so that medical research "will find out

... new moral laws and new social laws."[59] In such an effort the foundation funded research, schools of public health, and demonstrations, to rationalize and manage public health efficiently – which meant, practically, promoting larger, stronger institutions at the expense of the weaker, and using, as we have seen, a new administrative class of managers, analogous to those in large corporations. For example, only provinces with medical schools were eligible for Rockefeller Foundation funding of health units, which disqualified both Prince Edward Island and New Brunswick.[60] And with the decline in traditional religion, it would not be surprising if experts in charge of such a "secular religion" – public health – saw themselves as moral leaders, assuming the role of the traditional clergy; exploiting the tools of organization, management, and scientific knowledge for the common good; and also, by implication, transcending self-interest.

### Biases in the Campaign against TB

As a specific subset or representative of the public health movement, the anti-tuberculosis campaign – and those who led it – reflected the same themes. From its inception, the campaign was fashioned, managed, and led by an educated "national class": the career public health workers, like Wodehouse, Fleming, and Hastings; the large-scale industrialists and manufacturers (Adam Beck, Sir William Gage) who monitored public opinion and supported the movement and the sanatoria; and the academic physicians – Edward Archibald, Alan Brown, George Adami.

Unsurprisingly, the campaign reflected their biases: it favoured organization, standardization, efficiency. In keeping with such an outlook, the anti-TB campaign and its leaders were intimately allied with government functionaries and universities. By the 1940s, the national association had even become a self-described "federal division of tuberculosis control." If public health in general was a career – which, after the turn of the century, it became – it was accepted that public health physician-administrators would move seamlessly between government, universities, foundations, and advocacy groups. Robert Wodehouse would be "promoted" from secretary of the CTA to federal deputy minister of health; Grant Fleming would move from the Toronto health department to running the Montreal General Health and Anti-TB League; and J.G. Adami, a McGill professor, would become president of the Canadian Association for the Prevention of Tuberculosis. Although a public health, university, voluntary association, and government bureaucracy clearly evolved as the century progressed, there seemed to be little overt awareness or acknowledgement among the health bureaucrats that they were a special interest group with their own personal agenda for influence and authority.

Again, this is probably unsurprising: the general societal emphasis on expertise and scientific management, with its presupposition of a hierarchy of knowledge and skills and an assumption of one best answer, precluded such self-analysis. In this regard, public health advocates were merely following a specialized subset of a generalized ideology of social planning and management for the greater good.

The national-class ideology is evident again in the fairly constant tension that seemed to exist between the professional anti-TB workers and the physicians in private practice. Again, their philosophies and biases were frequently antithetical: while professional anti-TB advocates demanded a *communal* bias for the "greater good," with notification and isolation of the tubercular, the physician in private practice was loyal to the *individual patient* – and this loyalty sometimes meant fudging the death certificate or failing to report the disease to protect the livelihood of the victim and the victim's family. There was therefore little movement between the separate spheres: a physician in private practice tended to stay there, while a public health specialist may have focused on one disease or another or found employment in a government position, voluntary association, or university, but he would be very unlikely to move back into the role of an individual doctor caring for individual patients. As the century progressed, the gulf between private-practice patient care and administrative public health became increasingly too great to bridge.

With the anti-TB campaign therefore led and managed by representatives of Wiebe's national-class ideology, it would be expected that there would be frequent tension with representatives of more traditional values in Canadian society. In health care such values were best personified by individual, private-practice physicians, together with members of the service clubs. It was the service clubs – the Rotary Club, Kinsmen, Kiwanis, and Associated Canadian Travellers – who were the backbone of the campaign, with their running of the Christmas Seal sale; and yet it was the service clubs, with their fierce independence and parochialism, who too often "wasted" their fundraising on "inappropriate" food baskets, welfare handouts, and civic projects. Throughout the twenties, thirties, and forties, the national leaders lamented such "inefficiency" and struggled to organize these representatives of traditional values: provincial organizations and TB divisions were created; case-finding (rather than individual patient care) was promoted and rationalized. From the national perspective, the service clubs were too often almost a necessary evil: they did good work, yet they were unmanageable – intractable, and defiantly so.

## The Role of the Sanatoria: Straddling Both Worlds

Perhaps because of the nature of the disease and its protracted cure – its social consequences, chronicity, tedious treatment of months to years in bed – the successful sanatoria and their directors were forced to straddle both worlds. As specialists in charge of the bedrock institutional "treatment" of the disease, their bias was initially national: they had more in common with other TB professionals and public health professionals than local doctors, and they may have been salaried, with a community, public health focus. Yet, despite their university ties and the CTA's attempts to encourage research, they were often geographically isolated, so that individually they had closer links with local communities and service clubs. Moreover, as sanatorium physicians, they tended to treat their tuberculosis patients over an extended period of time, and so might come to view them as individuals as much as "cases." Certainly their record of research – increasingly significant as a marker of academic success – is, with the exception of R.G. Ferguson, mediocre. The sanatoria may have been centralized, specialized, provincial hospitals, but they were very poor cousins to the research-oriented urban centres attached to the medical schools.

Ironically, it may have been this characteristic that contributed to their success. Certainly, in the case of Saskatchewan it was George Ferguson's standing as an individual in his prairie community – his personal ability and integrity – that permitted the continuation of sanatorium funding during the depth of the depression and that permitted his continuing efforts to accommodate and support the family doctors. [61] According to his biographer, C. Stuart Houston, in other parts of Canada he was "sometimes the butt for his failure to enlist a field nursing staff," but he responded: "We can't go over the heads of family doctors. What we need is patients, and who will find them but the doctors? So we'll play ball with the family doctors."[62] A member in good standing of the local Rotary Club, a devoutly religious man and teetotaler who had once considered becoming a Methodist minister, he preached traditional, middle-class values for success – stay out of debt, acquire an education, work hard, and never lose faith. The difference between the two attitudes, new, or "national," and traditional, and Ferguson's alignment with the latter, was unwittingly spelled out by G.J. Wherrett: "His natural inclination to excuse the failings of others made some of us wonder if at times he put a premium on mediocrity and inefficiency. Later we were to realize that this was the secret of his success."[63]

## Changing Attitudes to the Campaign against TB

To criticize the regimentation and impersonality of the "science" of medicine, particularly as it applies to the anti-TB campaign, may be unfair. For such philosophical and sociological emphases and divisions in medicine merely reflected trends in society in general. If the anti-TB campaign was hierarchical, mechanistic, expert-focused and expert-led, and at times fundamentally undemocratic, with its underlying premise of social engineering, so were the ascending intellectual attitudes in North American society in general. Critiques of the campaign then, must be seen in the context of a struggle between "conventional" public health advocates and bureaucrats, such as Thomas McKeown, whose arguments owe much to national-class ideology, and those who are beginning to question the utility of the scientific management paradigm.

The new turn-of-the-century discoveries in bacteriology – the TB bacillus, diphtheria toxoid, the Wassermann test – and the important role infectious diseases such as TB, VD, and polio played in society had lent themselves to a mechanistic, scientific engineering approach to health: identify the cause and find a vaccine or cure. However, by the fifties, as the major infectious diseases – notably TB and polio – were brought under control, it became increasingly clear that tackling the new major killers in North America would not be as straightforward: cancer and heart disease, for example, did not appear to be caused by a germ in the way TB was. Instead, using an approach popularized in the social reform era and justified by Darwinism, plausible and probable causes were singled out – and lifestyle medicine was born.

The significance of this approach to the anti-TB campaign is largely historical and possibly tangential: it could be argued that the popularity of Thomas McKeown's thesis that the nineteenth-century decline of TB in Britain was due to improved nutrition is particularly seductive to a society in which specific causes of the most feared diseases – cancer, heart disease – have yet to be identified. Such historical revisionism, by denigrating the role of scientific and bacteriological triumphs, not only minimizes any concern we might feel regarding our ignorance but, perhaps more importantly for public health experts and intellectuals uncomfortable in and untrained for pure laboratory research, promotes lifestyle factors and preventive medicine to a pivotal role – and thereby enhances the authority and status of those who espouse and promote preventive medicine.

The irony, then, is that the initial conquest in North America of, first, TB and then polio, in concert with the development of a burgeoning bureaucracy, led to the entrenchment of professional "vocational meddlers" as Charles Edgley and Dennis Brissett somewhat cynically label professionals in the "helping professions":

operating on the belief that the presence of rules and regulations produces safety, security, and assurance, [they] attempt to extend their own sphere of influence while claiming the noble justification of protecting the innocent...

... Reforming the morals of others is clearly one way in which groups act to preserve the dominance and prestige of their own lifestyles ... meddling offers the promise of reaffirming a sense of efficacy and credibility in a world that seems so often to be totally out of control.

"Our belief," they conclude in a tone reminiscent of Wiebe or Lasch,

in the promise of a trouble-free life seems preserved and rationalized by the persistent identification of those persons who would make trouble for the rest of us. Nirvana is within our grasp, we seem to be saying, if only we could educate, rehabilitate, or treat these troublemakers. So we meddle, seemingly oblivious to the possibility that life may be just that proverbial "vale of tears," or at the very least, an imperfect juxtaposition of human frailty and power.[64]

If the anti-TB campaign was the first national, socially engineered and specialized public health crusade against a specific disease, it may also have been – with its intractable demand for notification, isolation of the infectious, and mass case-finding – an equally telling example of the meddling impulse, an impulse transformed through bureaucracy and technology into a movement that would set the tone for future self-appointed institutional "health police" to badger and hector the rest of us.

# 10 Conclusion

Gatsby believed in the green light, the orgiastic future that year by year recedes before us. It eluded us then, but that's no matter – tomorrow we will run faster, stretch out our arms farther ... And one fine morning –
So we beat on, boats against the current, borne back ceaselessly into the past.
F. Scott Fitzgerald, *The Great Gatsby*, 1925

As one pioneer medical health officer observed, the campaign against tuberculosis in Canada developed from the "incoherent, isolated and individualistic"[1] efforts of urban social reformers armed with "enthusiasm, determination and persistence"[2] – but woefully little else – into a specialized, organized, and businesslike multimillion dollar operation that profoundly altered the pattern of health care in Canada.

Studying the campaign in isolation, it appears that World War 1 was the ostensible watershed mark. Prior treatment had consisted of little more than Osler's "fresh air, good food, good houses and hope"; for tuberculosis, idealistic social reformers firmly believed, was a disease of civilization, to be eradicated along with all other evils associated with industrialization and urbanization: low wages, poor housing, alcoholism, and poor working conditions.[3] Local associations sprouted across the country promoting the construction of primitive sanatoria of shacks and tents, improving sanitation and hygiene to reduce infection, and working tirelessly to eradicate *all* social conditions predisposing an individual to the disease. "Since the sparks of infection would always fly," reflected David Stewart in retrospect, "the only worthwhile protection was fire-proofed houses."[4] Propelled by idealism and enthusiasm, they grappled with a disease that they perceived to be a symptom of the mistakes of civilization. Tuberculosis was preeminently, as Osler decreed, "a social disease with a medical aspect."

The war appeared to change this attitude and approach. The federal government poured previously undreamt-of funds into building up existing facilities and pioneering new treatment and diagnostic techniques. By 1920 most sanatoria were more closely akin to hospitals than to rural camps, with x-ray facilities, occupational therapy, laboratories, a budding use of surgery, and an increasing emphasis on rest as the fundamental cure.

Provision of care for soldiers in civilian sanatoria led inevitably to an extended and improved service for all Canadians. More important than the concrete results of spending by the Military Hospitals Commission and the Department of Soldiers Civil Re-establishment was a change in attitude – now health was demanded as a right of all Canadians, and it was considered a responsibility of the state.

The establishment of the federal Department of Health symbolized the acceptance of this concept of state responsibility for health care, something public health workers had demanded since the turn of the century. It also established the way in which government responsibility would be allocated in the future; for the federal government, which had spent $3.5 million on capital account alone to deal with the tuberculosis problem,5 moved with almost unseemly haste to relieve itself of any further responsibility for maintaining the facilities it had just erected or continuing for civilians any of the programs (such as occupational therapy) it had initiated for soldiers. Voluntary associations lacked the means to support these vastly expanded programs, leaving the provinces and, to a lesser extent, the municipalities, to assume the burden – in many cases, rather reluctantly.

If the war had improved tuberculosis facilities, it also demonstrated just how unhealthy "the fittest and finest" – Canadian youth – actually were. The influenza epidemic confirmed what many public health workers were beginning to suspect: existing health services, particularly in rural areas, were either inadequate or nonexistent. With a premium placed on health and many of the worst urban abuses corrected, tuberculosis workers focused their attention on the countryside – and since rural municipalities were almost invariably either incapable of or indifferent to establishing local health services, provincial responsibility again increased. Health units and travelling diagnosticians, operating out of both the sanatoria and the departments of health, were established.

Tuberculosis became "big business" in the twenties – and consequently, better organized. The role the federal government had pioneered with its wartime activities – stimulating provinces to assume more and more of the burden of tuberculosis care by funding capital expenditures and new ventures – was assumed by three organizations that, although "volunteer" in name, were professionally run with substantial funds, unparalleled in the prewar era, at their disposal: the

Red Cross, the Rockefeller Foundation and CLIOA. Under the auspices of the CTA, which, in turn, increased the national organization's influence in the campaign, they financed surveys, to take stock of the situation, demonstrations to set an example of health care, and health units to deal with the rural problem.

With the interwar political climate generally fostering the growth of provincial rights, the provinces, forced by the federal government's abdication of responsibility and encouraged by the limited "carrot-stick" financing of these new businesslike volunteer organizations, in turn assumed a growing percentage of both maintenance costs and capital expenditures. As specialized, bacteriologically oriented techniques such as heliotherapy and surgery were used more often and the period of mandatory rest was extended, it became obvious that neither the vast majority of patients nor the volunteer associations could afford to pay the hospitalization costs or erect expensive hospital-like sanatoria unaided. It was, of course, somewhat of a chicken-and-egg situation: without public demand for state support and the assumption of the economic burden by the provinces, sanatoria would have been incapable of financing new techniques, no matter how helpful. Municipalities were, in theory, responsible for the maintenance costs of their indigents, but with most avoiding it wherever possible and isolation of infectious cases now being seen to be an important preventive measure, tuberculosis workers were persistently demanding free treatment. In 1929 Saskatchewan, which had pioneered defining the situation with comprehensive surveys, became the first to initiate free sanatorium care for all its residents. It was an act as important for what it *represented* as what it did; for it symbolized the assumption of responsibility on the part of the provinces for treatment costs for *all* residents.

The growing specialization in treatment methods was mirrored in a growing specialization among volunteers. Before the war, lay urban reformers, *together* with public health specialists, had run the campaign. Now, specialists, working either for departments of health, sanatoria, or voluntary associations such as the CTA or the Saskatchewan Anti-Tuberculosis League, were in control. Many local associations that had been formed with the sole purpose of erecting a sanatorium either folded, attached themselves to the sanatorium as an auxiliary body, or amalgamated. With the treatment and diagnosis of the disease now requiring specialized training and technical knowledge, lay volunteers were not equipped to direct the campaign or help with the cure in the same way they had in the past. Instead, they funnelled their energies through women's groups and service clubs – notably the Rotary Club, the Kiwanis, and the Kinsmen. These became the grassroots support of the campaign – often, like the old local associations, parochial and stubbornly individualistic, but nevertheless fundamentally important in raising funds for preventive work and pioneering new ventures and community education. Specialization, organization, cooperation, and education became key themes of the postwar era.

With infection no longer universal and with the development of more specific medical techniques to deal with the disease, notably artificial pneumothorax and thoracoplasty, specialists shifted their focus. The elimination of the *germ*, rather than poor social conditions, became the most effective way to eradicate the disease. Again as a result of the war, the community, rather than the individual, was of paramount importance. It was a crucial change in attitude, one on which the subsequent campaign would be based. David Stewart reflected this altered approach among his associates when he observed in 1930 that

Twenty years ago or more the first question was, *what* made this man tuberculous – dingy house, foul factory, late hours, dust, drink, bad environment generally? Now the first questions are likely to be: *who* made this man tuberculous? Where has he already scattered his disease? What circle of contacts is he infecting? Then we thought first and foremost of the diseased person, but now usually first and most of the infected community ... Cure for the sick man – compassion first – may make the stronger appeal, but cure for the infected community – safety first – pays the bigger dividends.[6]

"Tuberculosis makes poverty, and poverty makes tuberculosis," he now maintained – but "there is nothing so wasteful as to treat poverty merely as poverty. When a focus of tuberculosis is healed a focus of poverty is cleared up, and in the best way, by removing its cause."[7]

It was an almost complete reversal of prewar social reform doctrine, most evident, ironically enough, in the depression and the drought-ridden thirties. Instead of working to improve the standard of living, the specialists directing the campaign now used "preventive" methods such as travelling and stationary clinics, examinations of suspect groups, and isolation of all infective cases in an attempt to reduce infection. For the first time, the falling rate of tuberculin-positive school children made this strategy seem possible. Eliminating the aggravating or secondary causes, such as poor living conditions, no longer provided adequate protection, affirmed R.G. Ferguson – that strategy was a "minor preventive measure."[8]

Instead, welfare work was left to other specialists: the growing number of professional social workers, relief officers, and charities. The bacteriological approach was in the ascendant.

The thirties also demonstrated all too clearly how few Canadians could afford proper health care – by 1940, the director of public health services of the Department of Pensions and National Health, J.J. Heagerty, observed that while the minimum cost of sanatorium treatment was over $1,000 per year, over 90 percent of Canadians had an annual income of less than $2,400.[9] Free treatment, he maintained, reflecting the view of most specialists, was essential for adequate control. Encouraged by the success of free treatment in Saskatchewan and faced with the obvious incapacity of municipalities and individuals to assume the burden, most provinces instituted it in name or fact by the end of World War 2.

Lay volunteers, through service clubs and seal committees, became even more important during the forties. With mass x-rays of the armed forces and war industries providing the example and a cheap, miniature film providing the means, "prevention" took on a new meaning as mass surveys of whole communities were inaugurated. Once again, the bacteriological approach and a focus on community safety that had developed since the Great War were emphasized. Financed by voluntarily raised funds (from the Christmas Seals) and organized locally by volunteers through service clubs and women's groups, these surveys were not only a means of discovering early cases but also an effective form of community education. Lay volunteers were crucial to the success of these surveys, for it was on their shoulders that the responsibility rested for getting each and every individual in the community out to be x-rayed. Consequently, the CTA, whose importance as an organizing body had increased with the growth of the seal sale, insisted that they could no longer be left to meander along in whatever fashion they chose. With CLIOA aid, the CTA organized provincial secretaries and associations to standardize, coordinate, and stimulate the increasingly technical and specialized campaign.

The forties also saw the long-sought entry of the federal government into the health field, assuming CLIOA's role of stimulating provincial involvement in tuberculosis work by providing new facilities and pioneering new programs to be maintained later. The federal grants also financed the provision to all who could benefit of the specific researchers had hunted for since Koch had discovered the bacillus: streptomycin and, later, PAS and INH. By now the campaign centred so much on the germ, through medical treatment (antibiotics and resection surgery) to effect a cure, institutionalization to segregate all infectious individuals, and surveys to ferret out early cases, that the president of the Alberta Tuberculosis Association could report without a trace of irony in 1951 that "Formerly the patient had been looked upon as a pair of lungs. We have learned not to do this anymore, but rather to regard him as a total person. We are concerned now not only with his medical problems but also with his personal problems."[10]

It might momentarily appear that the tuberculosis campaign had come full circle, back to Osler's dictum that tuberculosis was "a social disease with a medical aspect." Not quite. In the interim, expensive treatment facilities had been erected and a less costly, but still expensive, case-finding program had been developed; various levels of government had moved into the health field, paying most maintenance and capital costs; and volunteers were financing preventive work. By 1953 roughly $45 million was spent annually on tuberculosis services in Canada, with the major part – $40 million – being spent for hospitalization.[11] It was a huge business, far too important, those leading the campaign believed, to be left to the untrained. Although still a cooperative affair, specialists of all sorts – radiologists, chest specialists, social workers, public health nurses, occupational therapists, rehabilitation directors, health educators, and provincial secretaries – were firmly in control. "In essence," observed G.J. Wherrett in 1954, "it is the change from amateur to professional methods. It is not that volunteers are no longer willing to work, but they are the product of the times and they want their job to be on something like professional standards. They are no longer satisfied with good intentions and enthusiasm."[12]

The answer, the specialists felt, was full-time, specialized staff on provincial voluntary associations: health educators, secretaries, and seal sale directors, to advise the local association committees. The old local associations became overlaid by an organized and compartmentalized structure on the provincial and national level, run by full-time staff who directed volunteer efforts, now primarily for education and research, while a similar battery of specialists, generally supported by the provinces, ran the treatment side of the campaign. Despite a glimmering interest in the individual patient's psyche and social environment, actual preventive and curative measures still focused primarily on the bacteriological cause of the disease and community safety.

The way in which the campaign against tuberculosis developed in Canada had an indisputable effect on both health care and Canadian society in general. This does not imply that it was necessarily either the most efficient or the most effective means of dealing with the disease in both the short and long term. Some results – such as the modelling of the Canadian Cancer Institute and the Canadian Arthritis and Rheumatism Society on the CTA – are obvious; others less so.[13]

Significant as these results might be, however, they reflect only a limited view of the anti-TB movement. For just as the campaign against the disease undoubtedly influenced social policy and medical attitudes, underlying philosophical and socioeconomic changes – in Canada and North America, and perhaps more than pure science – in turn determined not only medical attitudes but also the focus, justification, orientation, and importance of public health preventive medicine in general.

There is a sense of inevitability in the foregoing presentation of the evolution of the Canadian campaign that not only is illusory but also obscures important questions. Why did the sanatoria become the bedrock of the campaign? How and why did the "experts" come to lead it? More curiously, who were these experts, trendsetters, and opinion makers? Doctors? Academics? Bureaucrats? Businessmen? How did their attitudes about and roles in society in general translate into their involvement in the anti-TB campaign? When and why did "preventive medicine" become such an iconic catchword that its superior worth was indisputable? And finally, how did the underlying philosophical attitudes and focus of the anti-TB movement mirror, reinforce, and ultimately justify not only more general philosophical changes in North American society but also the influence of those who espoused them?

### The Role and Influence of Sanatoria

This last point has already been more thoroughly addressed in the preceding chapter. The role of the sanatoria, however, is as controversial. Increasingly expensive sanatoria soon became the bedrock of the treatment, and the number of available beds was consistently used to evaluate the efficiency of the campaign. But was the erection of hospitals, which were costing an impressive $40 million annually to maintain by 1953, the best solution? For at the same time, a mere $5.5 million was spent by voluntary and government agencies together on *all other* activities: case-finding, diagnosis, home nursing, and welfare services.[14] It could be argued that had even a quarter of the hospitalization costs been channelled into prevention, not only would the rate of infection have been reduced more quickly, but the treatment costs would only have been a fraction of what they were.

There are several reasons that, at least partially, account for this emphasis on sanatoria. First, the individuals spearheading the campaign, including many of the pioneer sanatorium superintendents, had generally taken the cure themselves or knew someone, often a close relative, who had, and they were staunch advocates of this method of treatment.[15] They, in turn, influenced other volunteers, often wealthy and influential – such as William Gage in Toronto and Adam Beck in London – who expended time, effort, and money in the same cause. More important, perhaps, was its popular appeal. Not only the small minority who had had some contact or experience with a sanatorium worked for its establishment; for a whole spectrum of lay volunteers the erection of a sanatorium provided a concrete focus for voluntary effort. Tuberculosis workers observed throughout the campaign that it was always easier to raise public subscriptions and support for capital expenditures than for maintenance costs – not only was there a visible, permanent result, but it did not interfere with the subscribers' own businesses or living. With postwar emphasis on the community, some sort of isolation facilities were demanded, and the already existing sanatoria easily fulfilled that requirement, making them even more "essential."

Paradoxically, increasing provincial involvement and responsibility in health care encouraged their expansion. When supported by volunteers in the early years they had, of necessity, been simple, small affairs; the addition of federally financed equipment and accommodation increased maintenance costs to the point that only the state could afford their upkeep. Volunteers, raising limited amounts of money and chronically short of funds, looked to the government to relieve them of the burden of maintenance costs, which, as well as being the most difficult to inspire public subscriptions for, were the most overwhelming. As the government began to assume this burden, it became correspondingly easier for the volunteers to demand increased facilities – in the main, they were not supporting them. Moreover, their campaign of public education in the growing climate of state responsibility after World War 1 precluded most governments from refusing support. Only in Prince Edward Island and Quebec were the federally expanded sanatoria handed back to volunteers to maintain.

It was understandable that if provinces were increasingly forced to support high treatment costs, most were reluctant to move wholeheartedly into the preventive field. There was not the same public demand – as Charles Hastings observed acutely, if somewhat cynically, in 1917. "One reason why advances in preventive medicine have been so slow," he stated, "is that prevention lacks dramatic interest. It lacks those tragic characteristics which always appeal to the masses."[16] It was always difficult to convince a dubious community or government that the expenditure of large sums of money for the rather unglamourous maintenance of health and prevention of disease was warranted – particularly if the means were vague and unspecific "better living standards" and "good nutrition." The necessity of treating the same disease was, on the other hand, all too evident. Prevention was therefore left in the domain of the voluntary associations. They raised the funds, mostly through Christmas Seals, and the specialists spent them. As a result, prevention remained a small part of the tuberculosis campaign: only $5.5 million of a rough total of $45.3 million in 1953 (which included home nursing and welfare services) was spent on prevention, with approximately $2 million raised by volunteers.[17] This volunteer involvement, however, probably made the preventive campaign more effective.

The development of provincial or local sanatoria hinged on regional and demographic variations. In the predominantly rural Maritimes and West, the population was too sparse and scattered for local municipalities to develop their own services. They therefore built central, provincial sanatoria. Ontario, with a denser, more urbanized population, had a base on which to develop local sanatoria, particularly in the southern part of the province, and so local institutions, erected and directed by local associations, became the norm. Ontario was the bastion of local autonomy and voluntary responsibility and direction, although the provincial government supported the facilities. Conversely, it was only natural that the Prairies, notably Saskatchewan and Manitoba, with a history of cooperative systems operating in the political and economic spheres, would organize "pools" to maintain health services alongside those in wheat, eggs, and poultry.

How successful the sanatoria were in reducing TB by isolating the infectious is controversial. Barbara Bates, in her study of TB in Pennsylvania, noted that Baltimore, when compared to Philadelphia, had fewer visiting nurses and a higher rate of institutionalization – and a lower death rate.[18] Thomas McKeown has garnered much support for his hypothesis, based on studies of England and Wales in the nineteenth century, that the decline of TB was principally due to changes in socioeconomic conditions in general and nutrition in particular, while medical therapies and the identification and isolation of sufferers had a negligible impact.[19] In rebuttal, Leonard Wilson has persuasively argued that the isolation of the sick in public hospitals and workhouse infirmaries in nineteenth-century Britain, followed by the sanatorium movement, resulted in the *de facto* isolation of the tuberculous and that this isolation was key in reducing mortality from the disease.[20] Further studies of TB in Minnesota after World War 1 also link the decline in mortality rates to identification and isolation of active cases, rather than the more nebulous improved living standards.[21] Certainly, contemporary experience with tuberculosis has demonstrated increased infection rates not only in immunocompromised individuals (HIV positive individuals, drug addicts) but also in institutionalized individuals. It is plausible, therefore, that just as housing together active cases with uninfected individuals results in spread of the disease, isolation of the infected individuals reduces infection. The extent to which the sanatoria successfully fulfilled this function, however, is unlikely to be determined definitively.[22] And the arguments propounded may have more to do with attitudes toward technology and science and disease, fueled by underlying tensions between different ideological proponents for intellectual supremacy and societal influence, than any objective theories about the effectiveness of sanatoria.

## The Culture of the Sanatorium

If the sanatorium's role in lowering the TB death rate is questionable, its function and purpose in other, less concrete areas is not. Barbara Bates has argued that the sanatoria had four main goals. Initially, there was a strong religious and moral element, in keeping with the social gospel – they would "correct the moral decay of an urban society and ... save the souls of the hopelessly ill." This religious element evolved into a more secular, medical focus in the twentieth century: the sanatorium segregated the infectious to prevent spread of the disease. Care of the sick evolved into care of the sick and eradication of the disease through research.[23] Ultimately, whether they intended to or not, those involved in the anti-TB campaign created "a system of care for the chronically ill."[24]

In doing so, they struck a bargain of sorts. As Sheila Rothman has noted in her study of the social experience of TB in the United States, the sanatoria promoted *societal* well-being by isolating the infectious, and *individual* well-being with treatment and the possibility of cure – "Inside it, fear met hope." If the sanatorium enabled TB workers and philanthropists to "rescue" unwilling TB victims and "restore them to a productive life," they were also isolated, often in rigid, disciplined – almost prison-like – emotionally charged institutions. Strict regulations promoted a distance between staff and patients, with an underlying philosophy that only those who obeyed the prohibitions and edicts would be cured. As Rothman points out, such a rhetoric of willpower and discipline made patients more compliant and not only simplified work for the sanatorium staff but also shifted responsibility for cure of the disease to the patients themselves.[25]

A sanatorium subculture developed, not only with patients bound by a common disease but also with enforced isolation, rules, and an omnipresent sense of mortality. Friendships and flirtations became mixed up with fresh air, sleeping porches, hemorrhages, and lung collapse, and they were defined by gossip and black humor. Lidded sputum cups were nicknamed "music boxes" that, when opened, played "Nearer My God to Thee."[26] To celebrate the discharge of a patient hospitalized for over a year from the Queen Alexandra Sanatorium in London, Ontario, he and his fellow patients staged a mock funeral procession to the bus with the "corpse" laid out on a stretcher, wrapped in a sheet, and accompanied by mourners and a "clergyman."[27] But underneath the jocular defiance was frustration, depression, and despair. As another anonymous London patient, "San Tan," who was treated for a total of ten years, wrote in 1940 on the eve of the discovery of streptomycin, in a poem titled "Spring Lamentation":

Must I stay in this big, bare room
When It is spring without?
Yes, spring without a doubt,
For the trees are wrapped in a veil of green,
and the crocuses are out.
Must I lie
In this narrow bed, in this dreamy room,
When the snowy trilliums are in bloom
And the days slip sweetly by?
Doctor, please let me go!
You, who are a city's son,
You can never know
Where foaming freshets run
And the first spring beauties grow.
If I must stay,
Then hoist the hostile windows high
And let me see a patch of sky,
For this is jail to such as I.
Ah me, it is too much to bear;
Next year, perhaps, I shall be there.[28]

For some there was tragedy in the forced isolation, the hopes and ambitions deferred, year after year, as one-time friends and relatives moved on with life, so that, paradoxically, the only home and family that remained was the sanatorium. When the long-sought discharge took place, they discovered that they were still outsiders, displaced and lonely, missing the camaraderie of the institution they had longed to escape. As one young Nova Scotia woman, caught between the two, yet belonging to neither, wrote on her return home one summer, in a poem titled "The Only Life":

There have been times when I cursed the only life,
The only life for one –

Who has to sleep out in the cool night air,
And spend his days in the sun;

Oh! There were times when I grew tired of this life,
When discontentment within me raged,
I wanted a life, another life,
With people who were not "caged."

I longed for a life, a carefree life
With ambitions materialized,
The nearest thing to a perfect life
There is no such thing, I now realize.

'Tis a change, I find, to live with those,
Whose lives I have wished were my own,
But their lives can't be mine, they never can be,
And it's harder to fight alone.

To live with those day by day,
With disappointments, even as I,
With all one aim – "to try and get out,"
And thinking we will – bye and bye;

Alike in troubles, alike in joys,
Sharing a life, lazy and free,
Where there's many things in common,
And the most common is – TB.[29]

For even when the cure had been taken, the isolation continued. Paradoxically, the sanatorium may have made the sufferer feel less of a pariah – for although sufferers may have been sequestered from the rest of society, they were able to find comfort and camaraderie among others similarly afflicted. Once back home, they were alone: expatriates who returned as resident aliens, never as citizens. As Elizabeth Mooney writes in her memoir of her mother's struggle with TB, in and out of Saranac Lake over half a lifetime:

For much of their life together my mother was an exile and my father alone, but they managed to make a life. There was, after all, nothing else to do, and the less said about it, the better. They lived in a time which feared even a whisper of the disease from which she suffered ...

"Don't come too near your mother," my father said to me all my life, and of course I never did. I leaned away from her when she stooped to pin my hem for my piano recital, frightened by the sound of the rattle in her lungs. I held my breath when she pointed over my shoulder at the wrong word in the crossword puzzle, refused the piece of candy she handed me from her fingers.

"I never did that before," she said, looking at me, blue eyes wide with surprise at her own temerity. "But I just washed my hands."

I only shook my head and drew away. No soap and water could wash away tuberculosis. I knew that. I was imprinted with the fear, she did not know how to reach across it, and when she died we were still only polite friends.[30]

The English novelist and playwright, W. Somerset Maugham, who had himself spent time in a sanatorium, made use of a short story of a seventeen-year resident in a North Scotland sanatorium to describe the acceptance and support that the sanatorium, despite its rigidity and regulations, undoubtedly provided for many long-term residents.

Time passes very quickly. I like it here. At first, after a year or two, I went away in the summer, but I don't any more. It's my home now. I've got a brother and two sisters; but they're married and now they've got families; they don't want me. When you've been here a few years and you go back to ordinary life, you feel a bit out of it, you know. Your pals have gone their own ways and you've got nothing in common with them any more. It all seems an awful rush. Much ado about nothing, that's what it is. It's noisy and stuffy. No, one's better off here. I shan't stir again till they carry me out feet first in my coffin.[31]

### The Influence of TB Treatment on Government Responsibility and Health Care

Tuberculosis was a chronic and, therefore, costly disease that very few Canadians could afford to deal with themselves. The extension of free treatment had more far-reaching consequences than the mere government assumption of that particular burden. It demonstrated quite clearly that residents of a province did not take unnecessary advantage of free health services – those requiring treatment might be more often hospitalized and at an earlier stage, but they were nevertheless ill. It reassured Canadians and timid provincial governments that the extension of free treatment and other health services would not be unduly exploited; and it thus paved the way for the adoption of medicare. It was no accident that Saskatchewan, the first to extend free treatment to the tuberculous, was also the first to extend free treatment to sufferers of other chronic and costly diseases. As Allan Blakeney, then Saskatchewan's health minister, commented in 1964, "The introduction of diagnosis and treatment of tuberculosis at public expense was one of the early and essential steps in developing a program of health services available to all."[32]

Carl Berger, in discussing imperialists at the turn of the century, quotes the American literary historian, Vernon Parrington, observing that time is not always a just winnower and that history is partial to success. Lost causes "have a way of shrinking in importance in the memory of later generations," and a historian must "go back to the days before their overthrow and view them in the light of their hopes."[33] Nowhere is this more apparent than in the role the federal government played in the development of Canadian health services. When the British North America Act was passed in 1867, the Fathers of Confederation could have had no knowledge of the costly treatment facilities that would mushroom in the twentieth century as a result of a bacteriological approach to medicine. In fact, medical services meant something quite different. Only three years earlier, Pasteur had disproved the theory of spontaneous generation. Koch had yet to isolate the tubercle bacillus. Medical knowledge was rudimentary, treatment relatively simple, and public health little more than sanitation and control of epidemics. The first provincial department of health was only established almost two decades after Confederation, and even when established its authority and financial support was limited.

When the anti-TB campaign began to take shape at the turn of the century, the political machinery the reformers had to work with was sketchy, while the few and unreliable statistics they had indicated a national problem of epidemic proportions. Even these optimists were all too aware of the immense amount of money required to erect sufficient sanatoria and clinics, hire nurses, and support patients while they took the cure. It was not simply that existing departments of health were inadequate – it was more that there was no machinery established to cope with such a problem, no precedent indicating who should assume the burden of such long-term and costly care. It was a new kind of health services tuberculosis reformers were demanding, and as such, some maintained, it was open to almost any level of government willing or, ultimately, forced to accept responsibility. This confusion is most clearly stated by Dr C.J. Fagan, secretary of the British Columbia Provincial Board of Health, in 1905. "The state should do something," he argued, reflecting the views of most anti-TB reformers, "but what is the state – the Provinces or the Dominion? Under the Constitution, it is argued that the subject of Public Health was exclusively assigned to the Provinces and that the Dominion is not bound – although it is not contended that it has not the right if it is so inclined – to do something to mitigate the evil; to minimize the scourge of the White Plague.[34]"

Many early reformers believed that the key to the issue of federal responsibility lay in Fagan's words "if it is so inclined." Because it did nothing before the war, the limits of its responsibility, tuberculosis crusaders maintained, had yet to be defined. It was the role the federal government chose to play in providing tuberculosis services for veterans and the way it established its Department of Health in 1919 that defined how it would involve itself in the provision of health services in the following decades. The government had spent a substantial amount of money and continued to pay pensions to invalided tuberculous veterans in the postwar period. This expenditure had pleased those interested in tuberculosis work – how much it pleased the provincial governments, who were expected to support these new facilities, was more doubtful. Prince Edward Island flatly refused to maintain its expanded sanatorium, and the Quebec government quickly sold the Laurentian Sanatorium back to the volunteers; but elsewhere public opinion would have been against such a wholesale refusal of responsibility for maintaining such "gift horses." The creation of a federal Department of Health that was "all dressed up" as Fielding acidly observed, and had "no place to go" merely stated the federal position more clearly.[35] It would finance short-term ventures of capital expenditures, but it refused to involve itself in heavy, long-term maintenance costs.

This position is not particularly surprising. Providing health services, particularly for sufferers of chronic disease, would have been costly and would have had no obvious political benefits to outweigh the expense. Had it so desired, it might have been able to shoulder a good part of the burden not only of tuberculosis care but also of health services in general, therefore increasing not only its responsibility but its authority. R.L. Borden had pointed out the specious nature of the argument that tuberculosis was the sole responsibility of the provinces (under subsection 7 of section 92 of the British North America Act), which he illustrated by pointing to federal involvement in railways. Fourteen years later W.S. Fielding noted the same thing in reference to public health in general.[36] The invocation of the BNA Act, therefore, might have been not so much a reason as an excuse – "an evasion of the issue," the CTA president termed it in 1924.[37] There was no more cause for the federal government to look after lepers than the tuberculous – in fact, there was less, for leprosy was not an epidemic disease, being both less contagious and more isolated. If the provinces needed assistance, it would obviously be in the case of the tuberculous – but the very magnitude of the problem made the federal government leery of involvement. Its only substantial assistance to Canadian health care in the twenties was with grants to control venereal diseases – and this contribution, too, was a result of the war; it ended for all practical purposes by the World War 2, and it was, furthermore, done for the most part under provincial auspices.[38]

Had the federal government retained control of the tuberculosis facilities it erected and established the aggressive, adequately funded department of health that public health workers demanded – rather than a token affair – the development of health services in Canada might have been quite different. Instead of discussing the BNA Act, historians would have observed that tuberculosis was a costly and chronic disease of immense proportions, one that the provinces, with a limited tax base, could not have afforded to deal with on their own (an argument borne out by the federal grants in the forties), and they would have argued that disease can not be limited by arbitrary provincial boundaries and is, therefore, a truly national problem. Had federal sanatoria been erected, their construction would have been justified under the "quarantine" responsibility of the dominion government. On the other hand, it is only fair to note that the argument in favour of public health falling under provincial jurisdiction under the terms of the BNA Act was very strong indeed and that, given the political climate of the interwar period, with the provinces jealously guarding their rights and authority, it might have been impossible for the federal government to step in, no matter how desirous it might have been of doing so. The Privy Council had, after all, ruled in favour of provincial rights and jurisdiction in the case of Bennett's New Deal.[39] Moreover, because it is able to deal with problems peculiar to local areas, provincial control, it may be argued, may have been more effective.

Indulging in "what ifs" is sometimes a dangerous and often a futile practice – in this case, however, it is useful to demonstrate that the government may have had a choice and that that choice may have been determined by economic, rather than constitutional, factors. Seen in this light, prewar reformers' demands for aggressive federal involvement, although ultimately doomed to failure, were both logical and possible.

With the abdication of federal responsibility, provincial assumption of the health care burden and thus authority over health services was, if not inevitable, at least predictable. The municipalities were too small and often isolated, with an inadequate tax base, to provide the services Canadians were beginning to demand; and the return of federal facilities to the provinces and local associations and the assistance of the Rockefeller Foundation, CLIOA, and the Red Cross all stimulated provincial involvement. Although, again, it is wise to remember that the Rockefeller Foundation was willing to aid *any* level of government in improving its health services, and, in fact, it financed surveys in Halifax and Vancouver to do just that.

Public health specialists were practical individuals. By the 1930s, the provinces were firmly in control, financing capital expenditures and most of the maintenance costs. Demands made of the federal government were now for annual grants to aid the provinces in establishing health services – health units, for example.[40] This changing attitude is set out in a 1928 *Public Health Journal* editorial, "Federal Responsibility and Health." "The government of Canada," it observed dispassionately,

for many years interpreted the British North America Act as placing the responsibility for health conditions within our borders directly upon the provinces. Whether this is an accurate interpretation of the Act is open to question; some claim that legally no such interpretation can be made.

Leaving aside the question as to legal responsibility, there seems to be every common-sense, practical reason why the Dominion Government should take an active interest in and assume responsibilities for the health of the Canadian people. This does not mean that provincial governments should be relieved of responsibility, but rather that they should be stimulated, encouraged and assisted ...

At the present time and in the past, the Dominion government has occupied itself with the live-stock and various phases of agricultural interests of the country; in roads, in housing and many other activities. Why should the health of the Canadian citizen himself be the one object that the Dominion Government feels to be outside its responsibility?

We believe that the Dominion government should, through the Provincial Governments, subsidize health activities.[41]

Tuberculosis treatment was a problem that absorbed a large percentage of the money expended for health services; but the established provincial basis of health care was seen to be basically sound, although often inadequate and sometimes requiring internal reorganization. Although the odd individual, such as J.W.S. McCullough, chief inspector of health of Ontario, staunchly maintained that "control of health in all its realms remains a duty of the Dominion Government," public health workers in general demanded, instead, federal support in the form of grants-in-aid to augment existing programs and standardize facilities across the country, but not federal authority or supervision.[42] A few specialists, such as R.J. Collins, might point out the weak logic in the federal body caring for lepers and the provinces caring for the tuberculous, given the terms of the BNA Act, but nevertheless, he, like the rest, generally approved of the status quo.[43]

By the forties, many public health workers had heard and used the federal government's constitutional explanation to account for provincial control for so long they believed it themselves: "It should be remembered that the British North America Act of 1867," pointed out one editorial writer of the *Canadian Journal of Public Health* in 1948, "placed all matters relating to the care of the sick and needy specifically with the provinces."44 The uncommitted tone of the editorial twenty years earlier was lacking. The past was interpreted in the light of existing circumstances and used to justify the present.

The importance of tuberculosis in this development was that, having reached epidemic proportions, it was, by far, the most important chronic disease at the turn of the century when the pattern of health care was still being determined; it was infectious, so had to be controlled, yet there existed no vaccine, as there did for smallpox and diphtheria. Whichever body assumed the burden of dealing with TB undertook an extensive, costly, and long-term responsibility that appeared to have few political advantages. And assuming this responsibility, in turn, set an almost inescapable precedent for dealing with other chronic diseases that arose as tuberculosis was brought under control – notably cancer and heart disease.

To what extent this development contributed to the growing provincial autonomy and power exhibited since the turn of the century is beyond the scope of this book. It is probably impossible to assess precisely. And yet health care is intrinsically bound up in the fabric of Canadian society, particularly in the case of chronic disease, which accounted for 75 percent of all deaths from disease by 1939, compared to 6 percent fifty years earlier.45 It would be surprising if this change did not affect Canadians' attitudes to their governments. George Wherrett nicely summed up the situation existing among the tuberculosis volunteers in a 1949 letter to the director of the National Committee for Mental Hygiene advising the establishment of provincial divisions for fund-raising purposes. "I am more conscious as the years go by," he reflected almost sadly,

of the underlying philosophy of Canadians, e.g., that we are a federation of provinces, rather than a nation, in the strictest sense of the world. I believe this applies not only to political questions, but to all others as well. I often wish it were not so, but I believe we have to accept it as fact.

There seems to be a pretty deep-rooted antipathy on the part of the provinces to raising funds and sending them to a central office in Ottawa or Toronto, even though they might have a good share of them returned to them. On the other hand, they like to feel that they are an important cog in the national machine and will support the national office [CTA] in its role of coordination and overall direction.46

What was true of the volunteers was true of the official side of the campaign and of health services in general; and despite the desire of the CTA to "coordinate and direct," it was the provincial and local associations, raising the funds, that ultimately decided, like their government counterparts, how the money would be spent. He who pays the piper calls the tune – in this case, the provinces. Some might find it ironic that the federal government, when it finally chose to become involved, had no alternative but to establish grants-in-aid, which, paradoxically enough, served yet again to increase and reinforce provincial authority and autonomy.

## Tuberculosis Services in Quebec

Another problem that the study of the tuberculosis campaign in Canada throws into sharp relief is the development, or rather the lack of development, of health services in Quebec, particularly in Montreal. Why were the tuberculosis facilities so meagre, for so long? The fact that both Montreal and the Maritimes had the worst record would lead one initially to an economic explanation – and this is what Terry Copp argues in *The Anatomy of Poverty*.[47] Undoubtedly economics was a factor – and yet economics does not fully explain why Montreal, the largest city in the country, was so far behind Toronto in providing even rudimentary health and sanitation services; nor does it necessarily explain why the tuberculosis rate among Montreal's Jewish population was so much lower than the rate among both the English and French-speaking residents of that city. The Royal Commission report in 1910, as Copp noted, indicated a high rate of disease among Jewish immigrants[48] – yet by 1926, the Montreal Health Survey Committee noted, this had declined to 32 per 100,000, compared to 95 for the English and 167 for the French.[49] Throughout the thirties and forties this discrepancy continued. Jewish immigrants did not form a wealthy segment of the population, so a simple economic explanation is inadequate.

Health care for the French-speaking majority in Quebec was the prerogative of the Catholic Church. As late as 1950 seventeen of the twenty tuberculosis institutions for the French-speaking population in the province were operated by a religious body; while at least one "lay" agency, the Bruchesi Institute, had been staffed by nursing sisters since its inception.[50] Moreover, the campaign against tuberculosis itself differed in several respects from that in the rest of the country and bolstered the argument that French-speaking Quebec doctors looked to France for inspiration and guidance.[51] The Grancher System, peculiar to Quebec, was invented in France: "Because of its essentially French tradition," enthused a Department of Health specialist, "the French Canadian medical profession could not fail to sponsor the adoption of a system of child tuberculosis prevention which has amply proved its worth."[52] BCG, which, as we have seen, was used more extensively and enthusiastically in Quebec than in any other province, was first developed in the "parent" country; the dispensary system, although pioneered in Edinburgh, was promoted in Paris; and even the Rockefeller Foundation's financing of health units had a French precedent in that organization's attempt to help deal with France's tremendous tuberculosis problem resulting from World War 1.

The diagnosis of tuberculosis highlighted again the rift between the American school of phthisiology and the French one. As Adrien Plouffe, assistant director of the Montreal department of health explained, the former school, with which the majority of English-speaking Canadian doctors aligned themselves, focused its attention almost exclusively on the use of x-rays, while the latter "insists first of all on a clinical examination of the lungs, a sputum examination and then a radiograph. That seems to be," he concluded, "the reasonable, logical and straightforward way of dealing with our patient."[53] English-speaking doctors would have reversed the order. The rift between schools also had extensive implications in preventive work – for while R.G. Ferguson and his associates enthusiastically and energetically endeavoured to x-ray every Saskatchewan resident, the Quebec department of health concentrated on the extension of BCG. Both practices were bacteriological attempts to prevent the disease, but the French school was more clinically oriented, preferring the technique of the French Laennec, the inventor of the stethoscope, to Roentgen's rays. Plouffe maintained this approach was "more eclectic, less exclusive"; Stewart and his English-speaking associates found it too vague and unreliable.[54] "Put not your faith in physical signs," the director of the Manitoba Sanatorium insisted, "an absolute necessity is the well-taken, well-read x-ray plate," for "the Laennec of the twentieth century is Roentgen."[55] If ideas had to gain acceptance in France before being adopted generally in Quebec, that might partially explain the difference in emphasis and lag in the campaign.

It must be remembered that these two positions were also influenced by the different state of the disease in Quebec and in the West. Quebec, which was closer to the old pre–World War 1 state of universal infection, tried to build up resistance with a limited vaccine; the others, from the twenties onwards, tried to eliminate infection. This difference in treatment still does not explain *why* the state of the disease was different in Quebec, but it does at least serve to highlight the attitude of the population: from the days of the 1910 Royal Commission report, tuberculosis specialists in Quebec, French and English alike, had raged against the fatalistic attitude toward the disease they witnessed among the French-speaking residents of the province. Whether this attitude was due to the Church's teaching that death from disease was the Will of God, to be accepted with equanimity, or whether it was an understandable result of the lack of preventive and treatment facilities and of hospitalizing cases at such an advanced stage that they generally died (why not be fatalistic when nothing could be done?) is debatable. Possibly the fatalistic approach to treatment was a result of the Church's teaching, and both attitudes reinforced one another.

## The Role of Volunteers in English Canada and Quebec

In any event, one thing is clear: the Church, usually through its nursing sisters, controlled and supported the tuberculosis services for the French-speaking majority. Unlike the English-speaking and Jewish minorities in Montreal, and unlike the campaigns in the rest of the country, the campaign in this group lacked a volunteer lay base; and this was an important determining factor in the development of tuberculosis services in both Quebec and Canada.

Lay volunteers were the bedrock of the campaign in English Canada. In some cases this is obvious – notably in Ontario, where independent boards, such as the National Sanatarium Association and the Hamilton and London health associations, built and actually ran, as late as 1953, twelve of the fourteen sanatoria, although the government paid the maintenance costs.[56] In fact, the CTA reported, at that time fully two-thirds of Canadian sanatoria were operated by independent voluntary boards.[57] The women's institutes mobilized public opinion in Prince Edward Island to establish a sanatorium and provincial health department, and sponsored the first health unit in British Columbia.[58] Except in Nova Scotia, where the government built the sanatorium, it was local volunteer associations across the country that first canvassed for public subscriptions and demanded government aid to erect sanatoria.

In the West, the grassroots voluntary influence was less obvious but, paradoxically enough, more pervasive. Both the Saskatchewan Anti-Tuberculosis League and the Manitoba Sanatorium Board, mainly lay and voluntary in their composition, organized all the facilities and programs for the diagnosis, treatment, and prevention of tuberculosis in their respective provinces. And preventive work, carried out under their auspices, was financed almost completely by Christmas Seals. As in Ontario, they rested on a volunteer base; unlike their counterparts in Ontario, they were organized on a centralized, cooperative basis, reflecting the same collective approach they had to political and economic questions. Their treatment facilities were government supported, but not government controlled.

The service clubs and local seal associations ran the sale and manned the surveys that were particularly essential after the World War 1. Even after provincial associations were organized or provincial departments used the funds they raised, they remained the basis of the preventive campaign. The surveys demonstrated most clearly how necessary voluntary associations were for community education, organization, and, ultimately, mobilization. As G.J. Wherrett wrote to K.L. Dawson of the Nova Scotia Tuberculosis Commission, Alberta provided a typical example of how a voluntary association both cooperated with and was directed by an official body in running a successful survey: "The provincial association bought the equipment with Seal Sale funds and the Department supplied the technical personnel to operate the machine. The provincial association arranges for the surveys and organizes local committees to interest the people to take full advantage of the survey. Where there is little interest there is about 50% participation, but where the local people organize the survey and arouse interest, participation goes up to about 90% or more."[59]

As the specialists recognized, volunteer associations had an influence far out of proportion to the amount of money they raised. And as the surveys demonstrated, they served as leaders and pioneers to educate, arouse, and mobilize the public; raised money to pioneer new programs; and stimulated government action. The pasteurization of milk, sanatoria, health units, and rehabilitation were all initiated by these groups. "Probably the greatest contribution which the twentieth century has made to the welfare of the race," opined Maude Abbott, "has been through the growth of community measures on a large scale for the preservation and prevention of disease by means of large volunteer organizations of representative citizens, under whose aegis investigations into sanitary and social conditions are carried out, legislation is influenced and reforms are recommended, welfare agencies administered and that form of instruction known as "health education" spread among all sections of the population. This is the ideal of the public health movement of the present day." J.J. Heagerty quoted Abbott, significantly, in a 1934 article on the development of public health in Canada.[60]

R.E. Wodehouse, as CTA secretary, was even more enthusiastic about the benefits of voluntary efforts. "In a sanatorium administered by a voluntary committee," he argued in 1931, "the administration has to be economical, efficient, humane, and present each year a report of stewardship which will attract not only the tuberculous sick to seek, without hesitation, the institutional treatment available, but the municipalities and public to give more and more towards the cost of construction and maintenance of the institutions. Enough beds will eventually be erected ... The voluntary committee will make it its business to urge the municipalities and the government for necessary legislation and financial assistance."[61] His successor, George Wherrett, was more cautious, however. In a 1962 Royal Commission report on Health Services in Canada, he noted that "There is evidence to show that these [voluntarily managed organizations] have operated at lower costs than institutions operated by government agencies. They have, however, in some instances, done so by maintaining salary schedules and superannuation rates below the level of other government agencies or private practice."[62]

Whether voluntarily run institutions were more efficient or economical than their state-run counterparts is a moot point; for the importance of volunteers and voluntary associations lay not so much in the amount of money they raised or even the work they did (although it was, nevertheless, very important) but in the community education and responsibility they inspired and mobilized. George Porter, an early CTA secretary, maintained in his autobiography that large audiences for tuberculosis lectures were due to the work of "some outstanding men or women," such as Janey Canuck, or "a good local committee."[63] Howard Holbrook believed the successful fight against the disease in Hamilton was due to that city's "community conscience" – inspired by the Hamilton Health Association.[64] And mass surveys were visible evidence of the necessity of volunteers in community education and action.

It was this grassroots lay voluntarism that was largely lacking in French-speaking Quebec.[65] In a sense, there was no obvious need for it – the orders of nursing sisters provided an already established outlet through which women with humanitarian interests could channel their energies; they were experienced at running hospitals and had the sanction of the Church and funds to support the work they did. And they were usually dedicated individuals doing valuable, if limited, work, which the English specialists in Montreal recognized.

The English-speaking community lacked the religious unity of the French-speaking majority in Quebec. Women and men with a humanitarian bent had no ready-made structures, like nursing sisterhoods, through which they could act; and the diversity of Protestant churches precluded any sort of religious organizations from being established through which everyone could funnel their charitable impulses. Those individuals interested in alleviating a particular social problem – infant mortality, tuberculosis, poverty, alcoholism – banded together of necessity in lay associations. The prewar social gospel inspired many with a sense of urgency and a rationale proving it to be their duty to eradicate poor social conditions; but with no single unifying theological explanation or organization to direct or assist them and being forced to act through lay associations, they could only turn to the community and its extension, the state, for aid in implementing their goals. In addition, the lack of the formal religious influence so pervasive in the French-speaking sector reinforced their emphasis on community responsibility. Disease was not an unavoidable result of God's Will but resulted from government inertia and irresponsibility, which stemmed directly from community apathy and ignorance. "French Canadians are fatalists," reported the Quebec Royal Commission in 1910; "they think that diseases are sent them by God, by Providence; that they themselves have nothing to do with it; that diseases are not avoidable. The result of looking at disease from this point of view is that as a rule they do not believe in the contagiousness of many diseases, especially of tuberculosis, which they attribute to heredity; they wait too long before getting their sick attended too [*sic*], and finally, they console themselves too easily for the loss of a relative or of a child, believing that his time has come."[66] In contrast, Charles Hastings expressed a fundamental difference in outlook when he condemned the municipalities, not the Lord, as the body which "Taketh away."[67]

When J. George Adami suggested that lay sisterhoods modelled on the French nursing orders be established in the English community,[68] he was acknowledging the valuable work done by these nuns in alleviating human misery. But he missed the point. These "lay sisterhoods" were not essential in the English community, because organizations had already developed that served the same function in ameliorating poor social conditions and administering aid: the women's institutes, the IODE, anti-TB leagues, health associations. and countless other middle-class groups. Unable to rely on a specific church, they acted as leaders themselves and turned instead to the community for support. Health became a grassroots effort.

To get financial support from a community for health facilities or programs, either through voluntarily donated or government funds, the community has to be educated to see the need of donating, subscribing, or approving the voting of these funds. There was often not this need in Quebec. Religious bodies ran the health services and built the facilities – community education and lay grassroots support was largely irrelevant. Moreover, as Marta Danylewycz notes in a study of turn-of-the-century nuns and feminists in Montreal, the relinquishing of control by lay women to religious communities marginalized and weakened the influence of the former further and confirmed Church control.[69]

Such a state of affairs was not limited to anti-TB work and was in keeping, generally, with the clerical-nationalist philosophy that saw the family as the fundamental unit and the Church as its agent in health and welfare work – and that believed any state involvement to be a threat to religious authority. Paul-André Linteau notes in his study of Quebec from 1867 to 1929 that the Taschereau government's 1921 Public Charities Act, which provided that the costs of hospitalizing indigents would be shared among an institution, a municipality and the province, not only met strong resistance but also led the Catholic bishops to demand the following year that the act be amended so that the government could not exercise any control over any funds paid to the institutions.[70]

With the Church in control and no lay associations to mobilize community demand, the government, which was usually leery of interfering in the Church's sphere of influence and which, like most, had no desire to take on added financial burdens unless it was politically expedient or beneficial, probably saw no reason to act. Instead, it moved only into areas in which the Church had set up no institutional health organizations – for example, health units in the rural areas. In this it paralleled the other provinces, who involved themselves in rural health because the local communities, the municipalities, were unable to cope. In more densely populated areas – notably Montreal – all levels of government preserved a "hands-off" policy.

Health services in French-speaking Quebec, then, were imposed from above, either by the Church or later the state, rather than as a result of grassroots demand. Consequently, they were not only sketchier but less effective – for a community that had not been educated and mobilized to demand them was less likely to use them when they were provided. This is demonstrated most clearly in the mass community surveys that had only a 30 percent turnout in Quebec, compared to over 90 percent in Western towns, and 70 percent in Nova Scotia.

The specialists in English Canada were well aware of this situation and operated with it, attempting even to exploit its advantages. G.J. Wherrett, writing to Grant Fleming in 1938, suggested that a nursing order, "such as the one operating the Sacred Heart Hospital, should be approached and encouraged to build a six-hundred-bed sanatorium at a suitable site," and he maintained that "If the government could be persuaded to give the same per diem grant as they are giving to the Sacred Heart Hospital, I believe that an Order could build and maintain the institution with very little, if any, help from the government."[71] There was no mention of the "community conscience" Holbrook considered so important. Nor was there any mention of local service clubs or volunteer associations when one sanatorium director outlined in great detail the organization of mass surveys in Quebec.[72] As late as 1948 G.J. Wherrett informed the chairman of the CLIOA public health committee that he was reasonably satisfied with the tuberculosis program in all the provinces, with the exception of Quebec, which had 45 percent of the total deaths, but only 29 percent of the population. "The organization in the province lacks the force that other provinces have," he noted. "There is not the unity of purpose found in the other provinces, resulting in wide gaps and even overlapping. The provincial organization is spread too thin."[73]

Under Duplessis, the support of the tuberculosis campaign passed to the province, which, in only two years, spent an impressive $26 million on expanding and maintaining tuberculosis facilities and services (1946–48).[74] But government agencies cooperated closely with the Church, and neither relied on community support. Funds raised through Christmas seals, for example, were not the essential they were in Saskatchewan. Dr Hugh E. Burke of the Royal Edward Institute summed up in 1950 the "circumstances which have made the tuberculosis problem in Canada what it is today." "Those provinces which have had the greatest measure of success in the field of tuberculosis prevention and control," he noted, "have had strong leaders and whole-hearted community backing and ... other provinces – ones that have not as yet had as great a measure of success in this particular field – have had to try to forge the tools with which to prevent and control tuberculosis without strong leaders, and particularly without whole-hearted community participation and support."[75]

### Accounting for Regional Differences

Saskatchewan's and Alberta's increases of 26.5 percent and 30 percent respectively in seal sale returns from 1936 to 1937 demonstrated the inadequacy of a simple economic explanation of the tuberculosis campaign's development, considering the crop failure and drought conditions then existing in those provinces. So did the mortality rate of the Jewish community in Montreal, as has been mentioned. The Royal Commission had noted in 1910 that "a great many Jews are also tuberculous because they work in small unventilated, dirty and crowded shops" – yet by 1928 their mortality rate was much better than the rates of the English and French-speaking population.[76]

Specialists were well aware of this discrepancy: in 1940, Dr Eugene Gagnon, assistant director of the Montreal department of health, noted that the tuberculosis mortality rate among the Jews in the previous twenty years had been only 40 percent of the rate of the entire population, and he outlined some possible causes. These included almost everything from the suggestion that since 60 percent were immigrants, they had been medically examined and the disease screened out (a dubious hypothesis, considering the manner in which immigrants had been examined, particularly before the war), to their working in "light manufacturing" (that is, the clothing industry) instead of heavy industries, associating primarily with one another (and so not subject to contagion from the more infectious Catholics and Protestants), and having a racial resistance.[77]

Edward Playter may have come closer to the truth fifty years earlier when he accounted for the lower rate in cultural terms (although his specific reason was suspect) – the Jewish population, he reported, took greater care in selecting meat.[78] Gagnon, too, noted the same phenomenon, "The Jew does sacrifice luxuries for the necessities of life," he generalized, "he allows himself a whole-some varied and abundant diet ... he is mentally inclined to take good care of his health and to seek early treatment for his ailments and those of his family."[79]

To what extent these statements are true is impossible to prove. The Jewish culture did emphasize personal hygiene; and, at least equally importantly, demonstrated a belief in community responsibility to a marked degree, probably because of a realistic awareness that if community members did not "take care of their own," no one else would. In any event, a community with 60 percent of its members foreign-born and not members of the economic elite had managed, as Gagnon noted, to have "more beds per caput in hospitals and sanatoria than any other group." The reason for that, he believed, was quickly apparent: "While their number represents only 6 percent of the total population, the amount of money subscribed by them for public charities exceeds 18 percent of the total of all subscriptions. The Jewish destitute are therefore much better provided for than any of the other groups of the population."[80]

It could be argued that with the community looking after the poor in a more responsible fashion, the chances of their breaking down decreased; and with contagious cases effectively isolated and treated, the foci of infection shrank, lessening the danger to the community at large. Since community responsibility was combined with a religiously based emphasis on health, it was not surprising this group's mortality rate was 40 percent below the average. On the other hand, this argument may be misleadingly simplistic and reflect preventive medicine biases more than scientific and epidemiological evidence warrants. Recent experimental data gleaned from animal models suggests that innate resistance or susceptibility to *M. tuberculosis* and BCG (as an infectious agent) is at least partially under genetic control, while human studies not only show a greater concordance rate of TB infection in identical (monozygotic) compared to fraternal (dizygotic) twins but have linked specific HLA genes to susceptibility. Moreover, different ethnic populations – particularly populations in North India and African and Mexican Americans – have been linked to specific genetic (HLA) markers associated with TB.[81] In fact, it has been suggested that some lysosomal storage diseases (for example, Gaucher's, Niemann-Picks, Tay Sachs) developed in those Ashkenazi Jews surviving tuberculosis epidemics in Eastern Europe,[82] while resistance of Eastern European Jews had been noted as early as 1912 by McCarthy in Boston, who had postulated that forced urbanization (undiluted by rural migration) during the peak of the European TB epidemic had selected out the most resistant.[83] The charitable impulses of the community, although admirable, may have been only minimally influential.

This issue of the better rate among the members of Montreal's Jewish community highlights yet again the problem of isolating and evaluating factors in accounting for morbidity and mortality rates. For the same or similar states of affairs in two communities is not necessarily the result of the same causes – both Quebec and Saskatchewan, for example, lacked rehabilitation programs by 1950. The former, still attempting to build adequate treatment facilities, had yet to establish a rehabilitation program; but the latter, with a predominantly rural population of patients who generally returned to the farm, treated most cases at an early stage and had a low rate of infection and an excellent preventive program, and therefore had passed the point of needing one.

Similarly, the high mortality rates in Quebec and the Maritimes may have stemmed from different causes. In 1942 J.J. Heagerty blamed high mortality rates in Quebec on an insufficient amount of money being expended on diagnosis and treatment and pointed out that while Nova Scotia and New Brunswick compared favourably with other provinces in regard to total capital expenditure for prevention and treatment, the incidence of disease was excessive, so that case-finding facilities and treatment beds were inadequate.[84] Wodehouse maintained that this told only part of the story – in addition to an increase in the number of treatment beds, the Maritimes, like Quebec, needed to institutionalize more indigents (largely the responsibility of the municipalities until the forties). He informed E.E. Reid of CLIOA in 1930 that it was "the most essential improvement necessary in the Maritimes, and the one particular feature in which they have dragged behind the rest of Canada."[85] He pointed to Nova Scotia where 75 percent of the patients in the, ironically enough, government-owned sanatorium at Kentville were self-financed. "Both of these factors" (the lack of beds and the insufficient number of cases from poor homes treated), he insisted dogmatically, "would have been corrected by greater voluntary effort and earlier education of the province and municipalities to pay for the upkeep of indigent cases."[86]

The situation was paradoxical. With the erection of a provincial sanatorium in Nova Scotia at such an early date (1904) and the donation of the provincial sanatorium in New Brunswick by Mrs Jordan, tuberculosis workers lacked the concrete focus other volunteer associations had used to build a campaign and get grassroots support. "No further stimulus was necessary to raise funds," a *Bulletin* writer (probably Wodehouse) argued, "and very little further stimulus developed for any other cause. Where financial requirements necessitate maintenance of active voluntary committees, the public is necessarily kept well informed and the doctors and public are wide awake to the advantages of early diagnosis and early institutional treatment."[87] The problem in Nova Scotia was compounded when the CLIOA-sponsored commission became mired in provincial politics (the provincial Conservative organizer for two elections was appointed the medical director), while the superintendent of the provincial sanatorium, A.F. Miller, ran it, an exasperated Wodehouse commented, "as a semi-private or private institution," always able to "have the policy of the Government concur with his own ideas."[88]

In 1941 G.J. Wherrett noted several other factors influencing the high mortality rate in the Maritimes. First, the difference in age of the population – if the rate was standardized for age, the rate increased for the Prairie provinces and lowered for the Maritimes (although the rates were still very different). Second, there was an economic factor that, in turn, demonstrated again the difference between the Maritimes and Quebec, although both had high rates. If tuberculosis rates varied according to the wealth of the community, the situation in the Maritimes could be explained more readily in simple economic terms than that in Quebec. For while the Maritimes had 9.7 percent of the population, according to the Commission on Dominion Provincial Relations, that region had only 6.4 percent of the wealth and 13.5 percent of the tuberculosis deaths. Quebec, on the other hand, had 27.7 percent of the population, 26.1 percent of the wealth, and 42.7 percent of the deaths.[89]

## Ethical Issues of Prevention

A final issue that the anti-TB campaign throws into sharp relief is the principle of prevention. Again, it is a common bromide that prevention is better than cure – certainly this was the focus throughout much of the campaign, and it is a public health axiom that is used even today to justify a range of programs from nutritional supplementation to vaccinations, some of which may involve substantial investment and even potential risks to the individual, for the "greater good."

It is BCG that demonstrates how troublesome such decisions can be. Ferguson's studies had indicated that it conferred a partial immunity – undoubtedly a benefit in "TB-soaked" communities such as those of the Western Canadian native peoples. Yet use of the vaccine rendered the tuberculin test useless as a case-finding tool because all who were vaccinated were positive, mandating, instead, the frequent and widespread use of x-rays to identify those who were infected. Moreover, as a recent study in the *New England Journal of Medicine* demonstrated, there are potential life-threatening hazards associated with use of the vaccine, particularly in the immunocompromised – the very class of patients most at risk for TB, patients who would be the preferential candidates for its use.[90]

The campaign against tuberculosis in Canada, with the problems it faced and issues it raised, has sobering parallels in health care today. With an objectivity engendered by time, it is both easy and tempting to criticize the emphasis placed and money spent on treatment and sanatoria, to the detriment of preventive medicine. Yet we make the same choices today, for much the same reason: compassion. When confronted with a heart attack or trauma victim in the emergency room, we immediately look for beds in coronary or intensive care units. Forced to care for an elderly woman with congestive heart failure for two or three days in a hospital hallway because there are no beds available on the ward, we, too, become frustrated and demanding. Long-term prevention – a low-fat diet, exercise, seat belts – may theoretically be healthier, but it offers no solution for the ill, suffering patient.

The emphasis on sanatoria and surgery also demonstrates the striking cost of what Lewis Thomas has termed "halfway technology" – "the kinds of things that must be done after the fact, in efforts to compensate for the incapacitating effects of certain diseases whose course one is unable to do very much about. It is a technology designed to make up for disease, or to postpone death." As such, it is both "highly sophisticated and profoundly primitive … the kind of thing that one must continue to do until there is a genuine understanding of the mechanisms involved in disease … It is a characteristic of this kind of technology that it costs an enormous amount of money and requires a continuing expansion of hospital facilities. There is no end to the need for new, highly trained people to run the enterprise … The only thing that can move medicine away from this level of technology is new information, and the only imaginable source of this information is research."[91]

In an age of incurable and chronic disease, the example of the anti-TB campaign warns us of the high costs ahead if we slight research in favour of humane arguments for treatment and intellectual demands for prevention. Costs for TB in Canada were beginning to spiral out of control by the forties. Harsh as it sounds, it was neither halfway "prevention" nor "treatment" but the discovery of antibiotics that contained the *economic* cost of the disease.

"People in general are hard to teach," observed David Stewart.[92] Throughout the campaign, enthusiastic and energetic anti-TB workers had run up against that fundamental problem. "It should not be difficult to interest people in the preservation of their own lives and those of their children," commented an exasperated and bewildered Duke of Connaught in 1912, "but the apathy and obstinacy of the mass of the population is a phenomenon which is an everlasting wonder."[93] Sixty-five years later, the face of Canadian society had altered almost unrecognizably, and tuberculosis had been virtually eradicated; yet the federal minister of National Health and Welfare, Marc Lalonde, voiced the same complaint: "people often put more time and care into the upkeep of ... a car than into the upkeep of their own bodies."[94]

Tuberculosis workers had much to be proud of – the campaign against the disease had been a success; by the fifties, it seemed only the mopping up remained to be done in Canada. And yet, it was a success tinged with defeat; for the utopia that the idealistic social reformers had so optimistically and confidently envisioned with the eradication of tuberculosis was still, disappointingly, far, far off. Perhaps Edward Playter, a Toronto physician, summed it up best in 1895. "Destroy and prevent the growth of the germs only," he warned with uncanny foresight, "and this pretubercular condition of the body will develop into something possibly worse than consumption – cancer, it may be, or other specific disease ... We cannot live unhygienic lives and by simply destroying the so-called disease germs retain good health."[95]

It is AIDS that shows how far we have come and yet how little we have learned from the fight against TB. Both diseases were at one time infectious and incurable. Issues once so heatedly discussed in the anti-TB campaign have again surfaced with AIDS: to what extent does a patient have a right to anonymity when suffering from a contagious disease? Should there be notification of AIDS patients, with incarceration of incorrigibles, the way there had once been with the uncooperative tuberculous? Is free treatment – particularly expensive, experimental medication – a right or a privilege?

Perhaps coping with AIDS can give us a humbling, visceral appreciation and understanding of the enormous task that confronted anti-TB reformers. Despite the rhetoric today, tuberculosis was probably more devastating than AIDS. In an era with minimal social assistance,

TB could mean financial ruin for a family, and the social consequences of isolation in a sanatorium for years on end could be as severe a psychological blow. Moreover, TB was both more widespread and contagious – a cough in the face from a careless consumptive might be enough to cause the disease. This is in stark contrast to HIV positivity which, in North America, is largely related to unprotected sexual intercourse, dirty needles, and contaminated blood products. Our morbid fear of AIDS is almost palpable; imagine, then, how much more understandable and forgivable "phthisiophobia" might be. And AIDS, like TB, raises the question of the price – individual and political, as well as economic – of prevention.

It is perhaps the ultimate irony, a cynical metaphysical joke, that AIDS, the most feared disease of the last decade of the twentieth century, has led to a recurrence of the most feared disease of the start of the century – tuberculosis. "Each generation," George Santayana once commented somberly, "breaks its eggshell with the same haste and assurance as the last, pecks at the same indigestible pebbles, dreams the same dreams, or others just as absurd, and if it hears anything of what former men have learned from experience, it corrects their maxims by its first impressions, and rushes down any untrodden path which it finds alluring, to die in its own way, or become wise too late, and to no purpose."[96]

That is an unnecessarily pessimistic note upon which to conclude, however. Despite the failures, humankind has made tremendous advances in knowledge in the last century. Perhaps one needs haste and assurance, absurd dreams, and the lure of untrodden paths to discover anything at all.

Nevertheless, we are all molded by our society – scientists and laymen, reformers and conservatives alike – and, paradoxically, only insofar as we understand that we are will we be able to transcend this fact. It is this that may be one of the most valuable insights an appreciation of the anti-TB campaign and its complex links to North American society can teach us: to approach our own moral crusades, especially those with a scientific veneer and an ostensible scientific rationale, such as the environmental and anti-smoking movements, with skepticism, detachment, tolerance, and humility. "Man's capacity to rise above his social and historical situation," remarked historian E.H. Carr, "seems to be conditioned by the sensitivity with which he recognizes the extent of his involvement in it."[97] Perhaps a solution for the future, then, lies in an awareness of the past, rather than an illusory objectivity, born out of ignorance, about the present. Otherwise, like Gatsby, we will "beat on, boats against the current, borne back ceaselessly into the past."

# APPENDICES

# Appendix One:
# Tuberculosis Institutions
# in Canada

Table A1

Sanatoria Established in Canada before 1920

| Institution | Year |
|---|---|
| Muskoka Cottage Sanatorium, Gravenhurst, ON | 1896 |
| Muskoka Free Hospital for Consumptives, Gravenhurst, ON | 1902 |
| Toronto Hospital for Consumptives, Weston, ON | 1904 |
| Provincial Sanatorium, Kentville, NS | 1904 |
| Mountain Sanatorium, Hamilton, ON | 1905 |
| Tranquille Sanatorium (King Edward Sanatorium), Tranquille, BC | 1908 |
| St Catharine's Consumptive Sanatorium (later Niagara Peninsula Sanatorium), St Catharine's, ON | 1909 |
| The Grace Dart Home Hospital, Montreal | 1909 |
| Ninette Sanatorium, Ninette, MB | 1910 |
| Queen Alexandra Sanatorium, London, ON | 1910 |
| Royal Ottawa Sanatorium, Ottawa | 1910 |
| Lake Edward Sanatorium, Lake Edward, QC | 1911 |
| Laurentian Sanatorium, Ste Agathe, QC | 1911 |
| King Edward Tuberculosis Hospital, Winnipeg, MB | 1912 |
| Jordan Memorial Sanatorium, The Glades, NB | 1913 |
| Brant Sanatorium, Brantford, ON | 1913 |
| Queen Mary Hospital for Consumptive Children, Weston, ON | 1913 |
| Mount Sinai Sanatorium, Ste Agathe, QC | 1913 |
| St John Tuberculosis Hospital, St John, NB | 1915 |
| Calydor Sanatorium (private), Gravenhurst, ON | 1916 |
| Fort Qu'Appelle Sanatorium, Fort Qu'Appelle, SK | 1917 |
| Laval Hospital, Quebec, QC | 1919 |

Table A2
Resident Tuberculosis Treatment Institutions of Canada, 1927

| Institution | Replacement Value ($) | Total Annual Government Grants for Upkeep ($) | Number of Resident Medical Staff | Number of Resident Nursing Staff | Number of Other Employees | Gross Cost per Diem ($) | Number of Beds Infirmary | Pavilion | Children's | Total | Number of Patient Days / Total Days | Average Number of Days per Stay Diagnosis | Treatment | Incipient Cases at Admission | Moderately Advanced at Admission | Far Advanced at Admission |
|---|---|---|---|---|---|---|---|---|---|---|---|---|---|---|---|---|
| **Nova Scotia** | | 243,112 | | | | | | | | | | | | | | |
| ns San. | 620,000 | | 4 | 24 | 100 | 3.18 | 113 | 184 | – | 297 | 75,713 | 10 | 121 | 42 | 63 | 137 |
| Halifax Hosp. | 150,000 | | 1 | 11 | 10 | – | 50 | – | 6 | 56 | – | – | 240 | – | – | – |
| **New Brunswick** | | 90,000 | | | | | | | | | | | | | | |
| Jordan Mem. San. | 250,000 | | 2 | 6 | 30 | 3.20 | – | 70 | – | 70 | 25,876 | – | – | 7 | 32 | – |
| St John Co. Hosp. | 250,000 | | 3 | 22 | 30 | 2.68N | 132 | – | 20 | 152 | 45,602 | – | 148.2 | 11 | 19 | 90 |
| **Quebec** | | 500,000 | | | | | | | | | | | | | | |
| Lake Edward San. | 200,000 | | 2 | 7 | 35 | 2.74N | 20 | 75 | – | 95 | 25,528 | – | 109 | 26 | 50 | 42 |
| Laurentian San. | 700,000 | | 2 | 17 | 83 | 2.25 | 90 | 160 | – | 250 | 82,077 | – | 300 | 66 | 108 | 41 |
| Laval Hosp. | 600,000 | | 5 | – | 71 | 1.25 | 44 | 156 | 60 | 260 | 93,075 | – | – | 127 | 105 | 122 |
| Mt Sinai San. | 60,000 | | 1 | 3 | 15 | 2.10 | 58 | – | – | 58 | 18,250 | – | – | 15 | 14 | 38 |
| Grace Dart Hosp. | 35,000 | | – | 4 | 7 | 2.08N | 46 | 24 | – | 70 | 8,267 | – | 79.5 | – | – | – |
| Sacred Heart Hosp. | 1,980,000 | | 2 | 47 | 229 | 2.45N | 300 | 300 | 60 | 660 | 106 | – | – | 83 | 182 | 433 |
| **Ontario** | | 2,014,846 | | | | | | | | | | | | | | |
| Brant San. | 119,000 | | – | 8 | 10 | – | 10 | 20 | 20 | 50 | 19,172 | 201 | – | 12 | 14 | 12 |
| Essex Co. San. | 200,000 | | 2 | 9 | 17 | 2.57N | 21 | 24 | 36 | 84 | 29,100 | – | 210 | 6 | 21 | 4 |
| Freeport San. | 191,000 | | 1 | 10 | 18 | 2.67 | 40 | 30 | 6 | 76 | 24,090 | – | 217 | 6 | 22 | 12 |

Continued on next page

Table A2 (continued)

| | | | | | | | | | | | | | | | |
|---|---|---|---|---|---|---|---|---|---|---|---|---|---|---|---|
| Mountain San. | 777,000 | | 6 | 44 | 116 | 2.57 | 120 | 185 | 75 | 380 | 112,203 | – | 181 | 35 | 37 | 124 |
| Muskoka Hosp. | 1,418,000 | | – | 30 | 103 | – | 210 | 96 | – | 306 | 112,626 | – | 321 | 90 | 106 | 148 |
| Queen Alex San. | 1,000,000 | | 6 | 25 | 130 | 2.65 | 182 | 130 | 30 | 342 | 100,027 | – | 273 | 43 | 54 | 159 |
| Royal Ottawa San. | 600,000 | | 2 | 20 | 38 | 2.44 | 60 | 45 | 35 | 140 | 33,626 | – | 166 | 12 | 13 | 50 |
| St. Catharines San. | 30,000 | | 1 | 3 | 5 | 2.20 | 20 | – | 1 | 21 | 6,166 | – | 176 | 3 | 2 | 13 |
| Toronto Hosp. | 986,000 | | 5 | 50 | 111 | 2.48 | 267 | 126 | 107 | 500 | 125,622 | 266 | – | 10 | 168 | 138 |
| Calydor San. | 200,000 | | 2 | 9 | 26 | 4.49N | 50 | 50 | – | 100 | 154,000 | 186.5 | 1 | 13 | 21 | 40 |
| IODE Preventorium | 200,000 | | – | 18 | 13 | 1.81N | – | – | 108 | 108 | 26,428 | – | 97 | – | – | – |
| Manitoba Manitoba San. | 800,000 | 52,000 | 5 | 19 | 97 | 3.009 | 100 | 100 | – | 291 | 101,392 | 1.2 | 347 | 10 | 23 | 171 |
| King Ed. Mem. H. | 150,000 | | 3 | 10 | 10 | 4.12 | 100 | – | – | 100 | 29,342 | – | 241 | 5 | 22 | 75 |
| Saskatchewan San. Fort. | 1,100,000 | 167,424 | 6 | 48 | 99 | 2.86 | 179 | 43 | 78 | 300 | 110,513 | 7.6 | 307 | 16 | 34 | 92 |
| Saskatcon | 600,000 | 72,700 | 4 | 31 | 42 | 2.70N | 155 | – | – | 155 | 56,881 | 1.4 | 374 | 25 | 16 | 93 |
| Alberta Cen. Alta. San. | 500,000 | | 4 | 16 | 68 | 2.87 | – | 50 | – | 50 | 65,015 | 205 | 268 | 12 | 34 | 116 |
| British Columbia Tranquille San. | 445,000 | 325,250 | 4 | 22 | 114 | 3.79 | 162 | 78 | 5 | 245 | 81,422 | – | 438 | 15 | 25 | 91 |
| Van. Gen. Hosp. | 200,000 | | 1 | 19 | 8 | 3.22 | 90 | – | – | 90 | 23,504 | – | 161 | – | – | – |
| Queen Alex. San. | 60,000 | | – | 6 | 5 | – | – | – | 45 | 45 | – | – | – | – | – | – |

*Source:* Canadian Tuberculosis Association, *Bulletin*, 7 (Sept. 1928), p. 3.
*Note:* N indicates that only net cost was given.

Table A3
Number of Beds in Tuberculosis Institutions, 1946 to 1953

| Province | 1946 | 1947 | 1948 | 1949 | 1950 | 1951 | 1952 | 1953 |
|---|---|---|---|---|---|---|---|---|
| Newfoundland | 430 | 433 | 433 | 435 | 435 | 784 | 788 | 785 |
| Prince Edward Island | 140 | 145 | 145 | 150 | 150 | 166 | 150 | 150 |
| Nova Scotia | 1,131 | 1,141 | 874 | 1,011 | 1,221 | 1,204 | 1,205 | 1,198 |
| New Brunswick | 758 | 958 | 913 | 926 | 908 | 1,004 | 1,016 | 1,025 |
| Quebec | 4,055 | 4,044 | 4,045 | 4,534 | 5,767 | 5,903 | 5,789 | 5,915 |
| Ontario | 3,999 | 4,023 | 4,308 | 4,262 | 4,476 | 4,480 | 4,412 | 4,577 |
| Manitoba | 938 | 1,153 | 1,253 | 1,259 | 1,287 | 1,294 | 1,279 | 1,263 |
| Saskatchewan | 851 | 803 | 871 | 883 | 883 | 881 | 828 | 867 |
| Alberta | 797 | 787 | 751 | 1,008 | 940 | 976 | 1,088 | 1,180 |
| British Columbia | 925 | 1,301 | 1,352 | 1,316 | 1,433 | 1,411 | 1,583 | 1,588 |
| Yukon and Northwest Territories | – | – | – | – | 239 | 304 | 363 | 429 |
| Canada | 14,024 | 14,788 | 14,945 | 15,784 | 17,737 | 18,407 | 18,501 | 18,977 |

Source: Canada. Department of National Health and Welfare, *Tuberculosis Services in Canada*, 21.
Note: Figures do not include beds for tuberculosis patients in mental institutions.

Table A4
Expenditures of Nonfederal Sanatoria in Canada, 1948 to 1953

| Year | Expenditures ($ millions) |
|---|---|
| 1948 | 17.0[1] |
| 1949 | 19.2 |
| 1950 | 22.1 |
| 1951 | 26.8 |
| 1952 | 29.2 |
| 1953 | 32.2 |

Sources: DBS *Tuberculosis Institutions, 1948 to 1952*; DBS *Tuberculosis Statistics, 1953*; Canada. Department of National Health and Welfare. *Tuberculosis Services in Canada*, 62
[1]Excludes Newfoundland.

Table A5
Revenue of Tuberculosis Sanatoria, in millions of dollars, 1948 to 1953

| Source | 1948 | 1949 | 1950 | 1951 | 1952 | 1953 |
|---|---|---|---|---|---|---|
| Provincial governments[1] | 11.2 | 13.0 | 15.7 | 17.6 | 20.4 | 23.4 |
| Municipal governments | 1.8 | 1.7 | 2.0 | 2.4 | 1.7 | 1.6 |
| Federal government | 1.7 | 1.9 | 2.1 | 2.3 | 2.8 | 3.0 |
| Paying patients | 0.6 | 0.6 | 0.6 | 0.7 | 0.7 | 1.0 |
| Workmen's compensation boards | | | 0.1 | | | |
| and other contracts | 0.1 | 0.1 | | 0.2 | 0.4 | 0.7 |
| Other operating revenue | 0.1 | 0.2 | 0.4 | 1.1 | 0.7 | 0.5 |
| Special revenue[2] | 1.4 | 1.4 | 1.4 | 1.7 | 1.7 | 1.9 |
| All sources | 16.9 | 18.9 | 22.3 | 26.0 | 28.6 | 32.1 |

[1] Includes payments made by province to sanatoria from federal grants allocated through the National Health Program.

[2] Includes income from investments, contributed services, Christmas Seal campaigns and other sources.

Source: DBS Tuberculosis Institutions, 1948 to 1952; DBS Tuberculosis Statistics, 1953; Canada. Department of National Health and Welfare. Tuberculosis Services in Canada, 63

# Appendix Two:
# Funding the
# Tuberculosis Campaign

Table A6
Federal Tuberculosis Control Grants, Provincial Expenditures, Fiscal Years 1948–49 to 1952–53 Inclusive

|  | Amount Available | Expenditures | Percentage Expended |
|---|---|---|---|
| Canada | $18,772,000 | $16,306,000 | 86.9 |
| Newfoundland | 824,000 | 681,000 | 82.6 |
| Prince Edward Island | 261,000 | 211,000 | 80.5 |
| Nova Scotia | 1,038,000 | 1,034,000 | 99.6 |
| New Brunswick | 847,000 | 770,000 | 90.9 |
| Quebec | 6,469,000 | 6,652,000 | 102.8 |
| Ontario | 4,515,000 | 3,186,000 | 70.6 |
| Manitoba | 1,108,000 | 642,000 | 57.9 |
| Saskatchewan | 1,030,000 | 928,000 | 90.1 |
| Alberta | 1,117,000 | 917,000 | 82.1 |
| British Columbia | 1,550,000 | 1,279,000 | 83.8 |

Table A7

Federal Tuberculosis Control Grants: Expenditures by Type of Program as a
Percentage of Total Expenditure, Fiscal Years 1948–49 to 1952–53

| Program | Canada | NF | PEI | NS | NB | QC | ON | MB | SK | AB | BC |
|---|---|---|---|---|---|---|---|---|---|---|---|
| Sanatoria | 41.3 | 57.8[1] | 29.7[2] | 64.9[1] | 53.0[2] | 45.3[2] | 16.7[2] | 30.1[2] | 28.4[3] | 80.3[1] | 35.3[2] |
| Drugs | 13.6 | 18.8 | 14.0 | 17.9 | 11.7 | 9.9 | 22.3 | 13.5 | 11.4 | 7.5 | 12.7 |
| Training of personnel[4] | 3.9 | 2.7 | 1.5 | - | 0.7 | 7.2 | 0.4 | 1.2 | 0.9 | 2.3 | 5.1 |
| Diagnosis and case-finding services | 36.5 | 15.7 | 54.8 | 17.2 | 34.5 | 30.2 | 55.0 | 55.0 | 54.1 | 9.9 | 46.5 |
| BCG vaccination programs | 2.7 | 5.0 | - | - | .1 | 5.5 | - | 0.2 | 3.6 | - | - |
| Research | 2.0 | - | - | - | - | 1.9 | 5.6 | - | 1.6 | - | 0.4 |
| Total expenditure | 100.0 | 100.0 | 100.0 | 100.0 | 100.0 | 100.0 | 100.0 | 100.0 | 100.0 | 100.0 | 100.0 |

Source: Canadian Tuberculosis Association, Annual Report, 1953, 126–7.

[1] Includes equipment, salaries of sanatoria personnel, rehabilitation services, maintenance of sanatoria patients.

[2] Includes equipment, salaries, rehabilitation.

[3] Includes equipment, salaries.

[4] Includes physicians, nurses, technicians

Table A8
*Expenditures under the Hospital Construction Grant,* Fiscal Years 1948–49 to 1953–54
Inclusive

| Province | Number of Patient Beds in Sanatoria | Number of Beds for Sanatoria Nurses | Number of Beds for Tuberculous Patients in Mental Institutions | Amounts Expended ($ thousands) |
|---|---|---|---|---|
| Newfoundland | 386 | 12 | – | 309 |
| Prince Edward Island | – | – | – | – |
| Nova Scotia | 200 | – | – | 22 |
| New Brunswick | 125 | 94 | – | 174 |
| Quebec | 2,208 | – | – | 2,278 |
| Ontario | 619 | 123 | – | 995 |
| Manitoba | 18 | 15 | – | 23 |
| Saskatchewan | – | – | – | – |
| Alberta | 488 | – | 264 | 278 |
| British Columbia | 264 | – | 581 | 682 |
| Total | 4,308 | 244 | 845 | 4,761 |

*Sources:* Department of National Health and Welfare, Research Division, based on data from Directorate of Health Services, Health Grants Administration; Canada. Department of National Health and Welfare, *Tuberculosis Services in Canada,* 12.

Table A9
Special Grants from Various Sources, 1920–45

| Year | Revenue ($) | Expenditure ($) |
|---|---|---|
| 1920 | 5,000 Red Cross<br>10,000 Dominion government | |
| 1921 | 10,000 Dominion government | |
| 1922 | 10,000 Dominion government<br>10,000 Red Cross | 1,000 to each province for school survey |
| 1923 | 15,000 Dominion government<br>10,000 Red Cross | 3,000 grants to provincial surveys |
| 1924 | 20,000 Dominion government<br>5,000 Red Cross<br>2,500 Sun Life Ass. Co. | 5,000 Three Rivers Demonstration<br>2,500 Three Rivers Demonstration |
| 1925 | 500 Red Cross<br>2,500 Sun Life Ass. Co. | 2,500 Three Rivers Demonstration |
| 1926 | 5,000 Dominion government<br>5,000 Red Cross<br>5,000 Sun Life Ass. Co. | 9,500 Three Rivers Demonstration |
| 1927 | 15,000 Can. Life Ins. Off. Ass.<br>5,000 Dominion government<br>10,000 Red Cross<br>5,000 Sun Life Ass. Co. | 20,000 Three Rivers Demonstration |

Continued on next page

Table A9 (continued)

| Year | Revenue ($) | Expenditure ($) |
|------|-------------|-----------------|
| 1928 | 1,000 Sun Life Ass. Co. | 1,000 Sun Life Scholarship |
|      | 15,000 Can. Life Ins. Off. Ass. | 15,000 Maritime Tuberculosis Educational Committee |
| 1929 | 5,000 Red Cross | 5,000 Three Rivers Demonstration |
|      | 15,000 Can. Life Ins. Off. Ass. | 15,000 Maritime Tuberculosis Educational Committee |
| 1930 | 18,000 Can. Life Ins. Off. Ass. | 18,000 Maritime Tuberculosis Educational Committee |
|      | 4,500 Sun Life Ins. Co. | 2,500 Quebec diagnosticians |
|      |  | 2,000 CTA printing |
| 1931 | 2,500 Sun Life Ass. Co. | 2,500 Quebec diagnosticians |
|      | 18,500 Can. Life Ins. Off. Ass. | 15,000 Maritime Tuberculosis Educational Committee |
|      |  | 500 CTA general expenses |
| 1932 | 18,000 Can. Life Ins. Off. Ass. | 18,000 Maritime Tuberculosis Educational Committee |
|      | 2,500 Sun Life Ass. Co. | 2,500 CTA general expenses |
| 1933 | 12,000 Can. Life Ins. Off. Ass. | 12,000 PEI |
| 1934 | 9,000 Can. Life Ins. Off. Ass. | 9,000 PEI |
| 1935 | 15,000 Can. Life Ins. Off. Ass. | 15,000 PEI |
| 1936 | 12,000 Can. Life Ins. Off. Ass. | 12,000 PEI |
| 1937 | 12,000 Can. Life Ins. Off. Ass. | 12,000 PEI |
| 1938 | 10,000 Can. Life Ins. Off. Ass. | 5,000 PEI |
|      |  | 5,000 Quebec |
| 1939 | 10,000 Can. Life Ins. Off. Ass. | 10,000 Quebec |
| 1940 | 10,000 Can. Life Ins. Off. Ass. | 10,000 Quebec |
| 1941 | 5,000 Can. Life Ins. Off. Ass. | 5,000 Quebec |
| 1942 | 5,000 Can. Life Ins. Off. Ass. | 5,000 Quebec |
| 1943 | 5,000 Can. Life Ins. Off. Ass. | 5,000 Quebec |
| 1944 | 7,500 Can. Life Ins. Off. Ass. | 933.88 Alberta |
|      |  | 600.00 British Columbia |
|      |  | 2,000.00 Quebec |
|      |  | 321.37 Saskatchewan |
|      |  | 2,311.20 Pamphlets |
|      |  | 930.70 Film |
|      |  | 402.85 Staff education |
| 1945 | 10,500 Can. Life Ins. Off. Ass. | 2,466.12 Alberta |
|      |  | 1,200.00 British Columbia |
|      |  | 2,000.00 Ontario |
|      |  | 500.00 PEI |
|      |  | 2,000.00 Quebec |
|      |  | 300.00 Saskatchewan |
|      |  | 1,300.00 Pamphlets |
|      |  | 733.88 Staff education |

Source: Wherrett, *Miracle of the Empty Beds*, 28–9.

Table A 10
Canadian Christmas Seal Campaign Returns, 1927–72

| Year | Returns ($) | Year | Returns ($) | Year | Returns ($) |
|------|-------------|------|-------------|------|-------------|
| 1927 | 141,312.75 | 1943 | 577,252.00 | 1959 | 2,533,379.00 |
| 1928 | 196,914.05 | 1944 | 729,753.39 | 1960 | 2,519,132.00 |
| 1929 | 223,344.60 | 1945 | 912,293.00 | 1961 | 2,536,242.00 |
| 1930 | 232,222.86 | 1946 | 1,218,224.00 | 1962 | 2,601,278.00 |
| 1931 | 179,223.01 | 1947 | 1,397,396.00 | 1963 | 2,755,303.00 |
| 1932 | 146,250.20 | 1948 | 1,488,515.00 | 1964 | 2,784,036.00 |
| 1933 | 135,535.41 | 1949 | 1,427,374.00 | 1965 | 2,924,276.00 |
| 1934 | 152,721.01 | 1950 | 1,355,954.00 | 1966 | 2,878,296.00 |
| 1935 | 156,251.00 | 1951 | 1,646,253.00 | 1967 | 3,059,777.00 |
| 1936 | 171,391.20 | 1952 | 1,823,496.00 | 1968 | 3,198,423.00 |
| 1937 | 191,495.17 | 1953 | 1,945,884.00 | 1969 | 3,112,325.00 |
| 1938 | 197,122.35 | 1954 | 1,961,533.00 | 1970 | 3,251,872.00 |
| 1939 | 219,677.47 | 1955 | 2,110,940.00 | 1971 | 3,385,027.00 |
| 1940 | 273,940.23 | 1956 | 2,255,970.00 | 1972 | 3,702,551.00 |
| 1941 | 327,265.13 | 1957 | 2,437,249.00 | | |
| 1942 | 431,179.28 | 1958 | 2,508,415.00 | | |

Source: Wherrett, Miracle of the Empty Beds, 31

# Appendix Three:
# Preventive Work and
# Tuberculosis Mortality

Table A11
Case-finding Activities in Canada, 1944 to 1953

| Year | Clinics | Mass Surveys | Hospital Admissions | Total |
|------|---------|--------------|---------------------|-------|
| 1944 | 314,618 | 439,610 | | 754,228 |
| 1945 | 432,767 | 526,413 | | 959,180 |
| 1946 | 444,739 | 917,482 | | 1,362,221 |
| 1947 | 538,033 | 1,292,306 | | 1,830,329 |
| 1948 | 522,882 | 1,613,496 | | 2,136,378 |
| 1949 | 545,904 | 1,745,546 | | 2,291,450 |
| 1950 | 514,579 | 1,888,145 | 306,347 | 2,709,071 |
| 1951 | 542,112 | 2,039,064 | 439,192 | 3,020,368 |
| 1952 | 582,371 | 1,932,700 | 489,824 | 3,004,895 |
| 1953 | 611,523 | 2,214,721 | 560,359 | 3,386,603 |

*Source:* Wherrett, "Recent Developments in Canada's Tuberculosis Services," *Canadian Journal of Public Health*, 46 (March, 1955), 97.

Table A12
Number of BCG Vaccinations in Canada, 1926–49

| | BC | AB | SK | MB | ON | QC | NB | NS | PEI | NF | Total 1926–50 |
|---|---|---|---|---|---|---|---|---|---|---|---|
| 1926–34 | | | | | | 6,192 | | | | | |
| 1934–42 | | | 2,400 | | | 48,732 | | | | | |
| 1942 | | | 178 | | | 10,104 | | | | | |
| 1943 | | | 364 | | | 13,054 | | | | | |
| 1944 | | | 364 | | | 17,309 | | | | | |
| 1945 | | | 364 | | | 18,881 | | | | | |
| 1946 | 1 | | 364 | 6 | 4 | 21,484 | | | | | |
| 1947 | 238 | 153 | 416 | 186 | 268 | 29,501 | 1 | 243 | 197 | 160 | |
| 1948 | 1,340 | 1,675 | 740 | 1,699 | 2,235 | 33,909 | 82 | 461 | 45 | 373 | |
| 1949 | 2,187 | 1,112 | 665 | 1,321 | 2,000 | 65,404 | 483 | 371 | 217 | 281 | |
| First three numbers 1950 | 272 | 183 | 100 | 202 | 37 | 25,628 | 22 | 71 | 6 | 30 | |
| Total | 4,038 | 3,123 | 6,155 | 3,414 | 4,544 | 290,198 | 588 | 1,146 | 465 | 844 | 314,515 |

Source: Canadian Tuberculosis Association, Annual Report, 1949, 23
Note: The figures for Saskatchewan are not exact and show only an extreme minimum.

Table A13
Deaths from All Forms of Tuberculosis, 1921–55

| | Canada | NF | PEI | NS | NB | QC | ON | MB | SK | AB | BC | YT | NT |
|---|---|---|---|---|---|---|---|---|---|---|---|---|---|
| 1921 | 7,698 | | 128 | 702 | 413 | 2,909 | 2,083 | 420 | 322 | 313 | 408 | | |
| 1922 | 7,664 | | 112 | 695 | 418 | 2,923 | 1,979 | 376 | 342 | 312 | 507 | | |
| 1923 | 7,847 | | 93 | 652 | 439 | 3,029 | 1,989 | 402 | 352 | 366 | 525 | | |
| 1924 | 7,675 | | 100 | 665 | 419 | 3,025 | 1,823 | 388 | 363 | 365 | 527 | | |
| 1925 | 7,469 | | 86 | 580 | 405 | 2,937 | 1,842 | 383 | 344 | 354 | 538 | | |
| 1926 | 7,929 | | 90 | 644 | 417 | 3,277 | 1,835 | 387 | 382 | 365 | 532 | | |
| 1927 | 7,814 | | 72 | 643 | 412 | 3,145 | 1,803 | 369 | 391 | 396 | 551 | 6 | 26 |
| 1928 | 7,914 | | 100 | 571 | 403 | 3,206 | 1,832 | 399 | 378 | 338 | 633 | 6 | 48 |
| 1929 | 7,808 | | 75 | 522 | 379 | 3,286 | 1,703 | 424 | 377 | 391 | 615 | 8 | 28 |
| 1930 | 8,149 | | 103 | 548 | 392 | 3,350 | 1,791 | 456 | 407 | 408 | 620 | 15 | 59 |
| 1931 | 7,645 | | 68 | 524 | 339 | 3,178 | 1,728 | 429 | 326 | 382 | 642 | 11 | 18 |
| 1932 | 7,198 | | 88 | 519 | 328 | 2,983 | 1,604 | 397 | 281 | 401 | 565 | 13 | 19 |
| 1933 | 6,983 | | 72 | 478 | 352 | 2,927 | 1,465 | 414 | 297 | 390 | 544 | 15 | 29 |
| 1934 | 6,474 | | 93 | 467 | 285 | 2,680 | 1,337 | 389 | 293 | 318 | 569 | 11 | 32 |
| 1935 | 6,664 | | 60 | 488 | 335 | 2,813 | 1,303 | 432 | 272 | 329 | 565 | 22 | 45 |
| 1936 | 6,846 | | 61 | 485 | 357 | 2,890 | 1,327 | 420 | 279 | 382 | 562 | 33 | 50 |
| 1937 | 6,728 | | 65 | 461 | 388 | 2,769 | 1,315 | 426 | 303 | 340 | 602 | 12 | 47 |
| 1938 | 6,172 | | 81 | 415 | 342 | 2,616 | 1,237 | 349 | 271 | 280 | 535 | 17 | 29 |
| 1939 | 6,044 | | 63 | 428 | 286 | 2,680 | 1,085 | 367 | 233 | 283 | 552 | 18 | 49 |
| 1940 | 5,845 | | 56 | 415 | 295 | 2,503 | 1,011 | 369 | 241 | 321 | 578 | 4 | 52 |
| 1941 | 6,157 | | 70 | 429 | 314 | 2,685 | 1,100 | 328 | 284 | 329 | 533 | 11 | 74 |
| 1942 | 6,061 | | 43 | 379 | 330 | 2,719 | 1,093 | 336 | 251 | 271 | 558 | 18 | 63 |
| 1943 | 6,263 | | 42 | 417 | 225 | 2,842 | 1,101 | 384 | 250 | 294 | 613 | 14 | 81 |
| 1944 | 5,853 | | 58 | 357 | 238 | 2,624 | 1,068 | 348 | 223 | 291 | 517 | 27 | 102 |
| 1945 | 5,694 | | 42 | 338 | 266 | 2,555 | 1,015 | 315 | 227 | 263 | 525 | 21 | 127 |
| 1946 | 5,941 | | 55 | 382 | 277 | 2,628 | 1,054 | 324 | 223 | 302 | 576 | 19 | 101 |
| 1947 | 5,577 | | 63 | 309 | 261 | 2,436 | 1,042 | 308 | 231 | 263 | 536 | 18 | 110 |
| 1948 | 4,887 | | 37 | 247 | 230 | 2,216 | 825 | 288 | 229 | 259 | 442 | 13 | 101 |
| 1949 | 4,382 | 285 | 22 | 184 | 195 | 1,897 | 686 | 224 | 185 | 211 | 406 | 16 | 71 |
| 1950 | 3,679 | 247 | 29 | 176 | 159 | 1,571 | 585 | 179 | 153 | 171 | 313 | 15 | 81 |
| 1951 | 3,481 | 256 | 17 | 126 | 134 | 1,553 | 579 | 158 | 156 | 146 | 292 | 9 | 55 |
| 1952 | 2,538 | 175 | 24 | 94 | 100 | 1,108 | 398 | 115 | 104 | 125 | 214 | 5 | 76 |
| 1953 | 1,861 | 111 | 13 | 72 | 69 | 844 | 311 | 89 | 87 | 68 | 146 | 5 | 46 |
| 1954 | 1,593 | 105 | 10 | 76 | 51 | 714 | 307 | 71 | 42 | 63 | 123 | 2 | 29 |
| 1955 | 1,403 | 82 | 6 | 48 | 43 | 608 | 242 | 72 | 57 | 81 | 143 | 3 | 18 |

Source: Wherrett, *Miracle of the Empty Beds*, 253.

Table A14
Mortality Rates for All Forms of Tuberculosis, 1921–55 (per 100,000)

| | Canada | NF | PEI | NS | NB | QC | ON | MB | SK | AB | BC | YT | NT |
|---|---|---|---|---|---|---|---|---|---|---|---|---|---|
| 1921 | 87.7 | | 144.4 | 134.0 | 106.4 | 123.2 | 71.0 | 68.8 | 42.5 | 53.2 | 77.8 | | |
| 1922 | 86.0 | | 125.8 | 133.1 | 107.5 | 121.3 | 66.4 | 61.0 | 44.5 | 52.7 | 93.7 | | |
| 1923 | 87.2 | | 106.9 | 125.9 | 112.9 | 123.8 | 66.0 | 64.9 | 45.2 | 61.7 | 94.6 | | |
| 1924 | 84.1 | | 116.3 | 128.9 | 107.2 | 121.2 | 59.6 | 62.1 | 45.9 | 61.1 | 92.3 | | |
| 1925 | 80.5 | | 100.0 | 112.6 | 103.1 | 115.2 | 59.2 | 60.6 | 42.7 | 58.8 | 91.5 | | |
| 1926 | 84.0 | | 103.4 | 125.0 | 105.3 | 125.9 | 58.0 | 60.6 | 46.5 | 60.0 | 87.8 | | |
| 1927 | 81.1 | | 82.8 | 124.9 | 103.5 | 118.4 | 56.0 | 56.7 | 46.5 | 62.6 | 88.4 | 150.0 | 288.9 |
| 1928 | 80.5 | | 113.6 | 110.9 | 100.5 | 118.1 | 55.9 | 60.1 | 43.9 | 51.4 | 98.8 | 150.0 | 533.3 |
| 1929 | 77.9 | | 85.2 | 101.4 | 93.8 | 118.5 | 51.1 | 62.6 | 42.7 | 57.2 | 93.3 | 200.0 | 311.1 |
| 1930 | 79.8 | | 117.0 | 106.6 | 96.6 | 118.6 | 52.9 | 66.2 | 45.1 | 57.6 | 91.7 | 375.0 | 655.6 |
| 1931 | 73.7 | | 77.3 | 102.2 | 83.0 | 110.6 | 50.4 | 61.3 | 35.4 | 52.2 | 92.5 | 275.0 | 200.0 |
| 1932 | 68.5 | | 98.9 | 100.0 | 79.2 | 102.0 | 46.2 | 56.3 | 30.4 | 54.2 | 79.9 | 325.0 | 190.0 |
| 1933 | 65.7 | | 80.0 | 91.0 | 84.0 | 98.5 | 41.7 | 58.5 | 32.1 | 52.0 | 75.9 | 375.0 | 290.0 |
| 1934 | 60.3 | | 102.2 | 87.9 | 67.4 | 88.9 | 37.7 | 54.9 | 31.6 | 42.0 | 78.3 | 275.0 | 320.0 |
| 1935 | 61.4 | | 65.2 | 91.0 | 78.3 | 92.0 | 36.4 | 60.8 | 29.2 | 43.0 | 76.8 | 440.0 | 409.1 |
| 1936 | 62.5 | | 65.6 | 89.3 | 82.4 | 93.3 | 36.8 | 59.1 | 30.0 | 49.4 | 75.4 | 660.0 | 454.5 |
| 1937 | 60.9 | | 69.9 | 84.0 | 88.8 | 88.2 | 36.2 | 59.6 | 32.9 | 43.8 | 79.3 | 240.0 | 427.3 |
| 1938 | 55.3 | | 86.2 | 74.8 | 77.4 | 82.2 | 33.7 | 48.5 | 29.6 | 35.9 | 69.0 | 340.0 | 263.6 |
| 1939 | 53.6 | | 67.0 | 76.3 | 64.0 | 83.0 | 29.3 | 50.6 | 25.7 | 36.0 | 69.7 | 360.0 | 408.3 |
| 1940 | 51.4 | | 58.9 | 72.9 | 65.3 | 76.4 | 27.0 | 50.7 | 26.8 | 40.6 | 71.8 | 80.0 | 433.3 |
| 1941 | 53.5 | | 73.6 | 74.2 | 68.6 | 80.6 | 29.0 | 44.9 | 31.7 | 41.3 | 65.2 | 220.0 | 616.7 |
| 1942 | 52.0 | | 47.8 | 64.1 | 71.1 | 80.2 | 28.1 | 46.4 | 29.6 | 34.9 | 64.1 | 360.0 | 525.0 |
| 1943 | 53.1 | | 46.2 | 68.8 | 48.6 | 82.2 | 28.1 | 53.1 | 29.8 | 37.5 | 68.1 | 280.0 | 675.0 |
| 1944 | 49.0 | | 63.7 | 58.4 | 51.6 | 75.0 | 26.9 | 47.9 | 26.7 | 36.0 | 55.5 | 540.0 | 850.0 |
| 1945 | 47.2 | | 45.7 | 54.6 | 57.0 | 71.8 | 25.4 | 43.3 | 27.3 | 32.5 | 55.3 | 420.0 | 1,058.3 |
| 1946 | 48.3 | | 58.5 | 62.8 | 57.9 | 72.4 | 25.8 | 44.6 | 26.8 | 37.6 | 57.4 | 237.5 | 631.3 |
| 1947 | 44.4 | | 67.0 | 50.2 | 53.5 | 65.7 | 25.0 | 41.7 | 27.6 | 31.9 | 51.3 | 225.0 | 687.5 |
| 1948 | 38.1 | | 39.8 | 39.5 | 46.2 | 58.5 | 19.3 | 38.6 | 27.3 | 30.3 | 40.9 | 162.5 | 631.1 |
| 1949 | 32.6 | 82.6 | 23.4 | 29.3 | 38.4 | 48.9 | 15.7 | 29.6 | 22.2 | 23.8 | 36.5 | 200.0 | 443.8 |
| 1950 | 26.8 | 70.4 | 30.2 | 27.6 | 31.1 | 39.6 | 13.1 | 23.3 | 18.4 | 18.7 | 27.5 | 187.5 | 506.3 |
| 1951 | 24.8 | 70.9 | 17.3 | 19.6 | 26.0 | 38.3 | 12.6 | 20.4 | 18.8 | 15.5 | 25.1 | 100.0 | 343.8 |
| 1952 | 17.6 | 46.8 | 24.0 | 14.4 | 19.0 | 26.5 | 8.3 | 14.4 | 12.3 | 12.8 | 17.8 | 55.6 | 475.0 |
| 1953 | 12.5 | 29.0 | 12.9 | 10.9 | 12.9 | 19.8 | 6.3 | 11.0 | 10.1 | 6.7 | 11.7 | 55.6 | 287.5 |
| 1954 | 10.4 | 26.6 | 9.9 | 11.3 | 9.4 | 16.3 | 6.0 | 8.6 | 4.8 | 6.0 | 9.5 | 20.0 | 170.6 |
| 1955 | 8.9 | 20.2 | 6.0 | 7.0 | 7.9 | 13.5 | 4.6 | 8.6 | 6.5 | 7.4 | 10.7 | 27.3 | 100.0 |

*Source:* Wherrett, *Miracle of the Empty Beds,* 255.

Table A15
Ten Leading Causes of Death in Canada, 1933–42

| Year | Diseases of the Heart — No. of Deaths | Rating | Rate per 100,000 Population | % of Total Deaths | Cancer (All Forms) — No. of Deaths | Rating | Rate per 100,000 Population | % of Total Deaths | Accidental or Violent Deaths — No. of Deaths | Rating | Rate per 100,000 Population | % of Total Deaths | Nephritis — No. of Deaths | Rating | Rate per 100,000 Population | % of Total Deaths | Diseases of the Arteries — No. of Deaths | Rating | Rate per 100,000 Population | % of Total Deaths | Diseases Peculiar to the First Year of Life — No. of Deaths | Rating | Rate per 100,000 Population | % of Total Deaths | Tuberculosis (All Forms) — No. of Deaths | Rating | Rate per 100,000 Population | % of Total Deaths | Pneumonia (All Forms) — No. of Deaths | Rating | Rate per 100,000 Population | % of Total Deaths | Intracranial Lesions of Vascular Origin — No. of Deaths | Rating | Rate per 100,000 Population | % of Total Deaths | Influenza (All Forms) — No. of Deaths | Rating | Rate per 100,000 Population | % of Total Deaths |
|---|---|---|---|---|---|---|---|---|---|---|---|---|---|---|---|---|---|---|---|---|---|---|---|---|---|---|---|---|---|---|---|---|---|---|---|---|---|---|---|---|
| 1933 | 15,485 | 1 | 145.2 | 15.2 | 10,653 | 2 | 99.9 | 10.4 | 6,216 | 7 | 58.3 | 6.1 | 5,516 | 8 | 51.7 | 5.4 | 6,950 | 4 | 65.2 | 6.8 | 7,337 | 3 | 68.8 | 7.2 | 6,999 | 5 | 65.1 | 6.8 | 6,487 | 6 | 60.8 | 6.4 | 3,198 | 10 | 30.0 | 3.1 | 4,019 | 9 | 37.7 | 3.9 |
| 1934 | 16,352 | 1 | 151.3 | 16.1 | 10,581 | 2 | 97.9 | 10.4 | 6,469 | 6 | 59.8 | 6.4 | 5,643 | 8 | 52.2 | 5.6 | 7,379 | 3 | 68.3 | 7.3 | 6,936 | 4 | 64.2 | 6.8 | 6,431 | 7 | 59.5 | 6.3 | 6,530 | 5 | 60.4 | 6.4 | 3,124 | 9 | 28.9 | 3.1 | 2,004 | 10 | 18.5 | 2.0 |
| 1935 | 16,069 | 1 | 147.1 | 15.2 | 11,156 | 2 | 102.2 | 10.6 | 6,898 | 5 | 63.2 | 6.5 | 6,176 | 8 | 56.6 | 5.9 | 8,302 | 3 | 76.0 | 7.9 | 6,880 | 6 | 63.0 | 6.5 | 6,597 | 7 | 60.4 | 6.2 | 7,411 | 4 | 67.9 | 7.0 | 2,520 | 10 | 23.1 | 2.4 | 3,392 | 9 | 31.1 | 3.2 |
| 1936 | 16,424 | 1 | 149.1 | 15.3 | 11,694 | 2 | 106.2 | 10.9 | 7,463 | 4 | 67.8 | 7.0 | 6,402 | 8 | 58.1 | 6.0 | 9,112 | 3 | 82.7 | 8.5 | 6,605 | 7 | 60.0 | 6.2 | 6,763 | 6 | 61.4 | 6.3 | 7,313 | 5 | 66.4 | 6.8 | 2,248 | 10 | 20.4 | 2.1 | 3,113 | 9 | 28.3 | 2.9 |
| 1937 | 16,840 | 1 | 151.6 | 14.8 | 11,963 | 2 | 107.7 | 10.5 | 7,358 | 5 | 66.3 | 6.5 | 6,530 | 8 | 58.8 | 5.7 | 9,609 | 3 | 86.5 | 8.4 | 6,644 | 7 | 59.8 | 5.8 | 6,669 | 6 | 60.0 | 5.9 | 7,731 | 4 | 69.6 | 6.8 | 2,005 | 10 | 18.1 | 1.8 | 5,260 | 9 | 47.4 | 4.6 |
| 1938 | 17,373 | 1 | 156.2 | 16.3 | 12,038 | 2 | 107.5 | 11.3 | 7,205 | 5 | 64.4 | 6.7 | 6,492 | 7 | 58.0 | 6.1 | 9,970 | 3 | 89.1 | 9.3 | 6,598 | 6 | 58.9 | 6.2 | 6,126 | 8 | 54.7 | 5.7 | 7,432 | 4 | 66.4 | 7.0 | 2,016 | 10 | 18.0 | 1.9 | 2,362 | 9 | 21.1 | 2.2 |
| 1939 | 18,562 | 1 | 164.3 | 17.0 | 12,399 | 2 | 109.7 | 11.4 | 7,173 | 4 | 63.5 | 6.6 | 6,588 | 6 | 57.9 | 6.0 | 10,884 | 3 | 96.3 | 10.0 | 6,174 | 7 | 54.6 | 5.7 | 5,977 | 8 | 52.9 | 5.5 | 6,596 | 5 | 58.4 | 6.1 | 2,060 | 10 | 18.2 | 1.9 | 3,955 | 9 | 35.0 | 3.6 |
| 1940 | 20,278 | 1 | 178.3 | 18.3 | 13,322 | 2 | 117.2 | 12.0 | 7,418 | 4 | 65.2 | 6.7 | 6,835 | 5 | 60.1 | 6.2 | 11,742 | 3 | 103.3 | 10.6 | 6,318 | 6 | 56.6 | 5.7 | 5,789 | 8 | 50.9 | 5.2 | 6,132 | 7 | 53.9 | 5.5 | 2,290 | 10 | 20.2 | 2.1 | 2,789 | 9 | 24.5 | 2.5 |
| 1941 | 26,602 | 1 | 231.5 | 23.2 | 13,417 | 2 | 116.8 | 11.7 | 8,442 | 3 | 73.5 | 7.4 | 7,399 | 4 | 64.4 | 6.5 | 6,733 | 5 | 58.6 | 5.9 | 6,252 | 6 | 54.4 | 5.5 | 6,072 | 7 | 52.8 | 5.3 | 5,955 | 8 | 51.8 | 5.2 | 4,567 | 9 | 39.7 | 4.0 | 2,411 | 10 | 21.0 | 2.1 |
| 1942[1] | 27,506 | 1 | 236.4 | 24.4 | 13,643 | 2 | 117.2 | 12.1 | 8,127 | 3 | 69.8 | 7.2 | 7,222 | 4 | 62.1 | 6.4 | 6,511 | 5 | 56.0 | 5.8 | 6,020 | 6 | 51.7 | 5.3 | 5,991 | 7 | 51.5 | 5.3 | 5,771 | 8 | 49.6 | 5.1 | 4,467 | 9 | 38.4 | 4.0 | 1,219 | 10 | 18.3 | 1.1 |

Source: Heagerty, "Health of the People of Canada," 534.

Note: The figures are exclusive of the Yukon and Northwest Territories.

1 Preliminary figures. The effects of certain changes in the classification and rearrangement of titles provided in the fifth revision of the international list of causes of death are apparent in the following: tuberculosis, diseases of the heart, diseases peculiar to the first year of life.

# Notes

ABBREVIATIONS

CAPCAR   Canadian Association for the Prevention of Consumption
         and Other Forms of Tuberculosis, *Transactions*
CAPTAR   Canadian Association for the Prevention of Tuberculosis,
         *Annual Report*
  CJPH   *Canadian Journal of Public Health*
 CLIOA   Canadian Life Insurance Officers' Association
  CMAJ   Canadian Medical Association, *Journal*
  CPHJ   *Canadian Public Health Journal*
   CTA   Canadian Tuberculosis Association
 CTAAR   Canadian Tuberculosis Association, *Annual Report*
  CTAB   Canadian Tuberculosis Association, *Bulletin*
  CTSE   *Canadian Therapeutics and Sanitary Engineer*
  JAMA   *Journal of the American Medical Association*
NAC CTA  National Archives of Canada, Canadian Tuberculosis
         Association, Records
 NCWCY   National Council of Women of Canada, *Yearbook.*
   NOT   Quebec Provincial Committee for the Prevention of
         Tuberculosis, *Notes on Tuberculosis*
   PHJ   *Public Health Journal*

INTRODUCTION

1 Carr, *What is History*, 52.

CHAPTER ONE

1 Adami, "Presidential Address," *CAPTAR,* 1910: 158–9.
2 Long, *Therapy of Tuberculosis*, 47–8; Brancker, Enarson, et al, "Statistical
  Chronicle," 107.

3 Bryder, *Below the Magic Mountain*, 183; Brancker, Enarson, et al., "Statistical Chronicle," 105, 110.

4 Trudeau, *Autobiography*, 40. Koch himself noted the implications of his discovery: "Tuberculosis has so far been habitually considered to be a manifestation of social misery, and it has been hoped that an improvement in the latter would reduce the disease. Measures specifically directed against tuberculosis are not known to preventive medicine. But, in the future, the fight against this terrible plague of mankind will deal no longer with an undetermined something, but with a tangible parasite, whose living conditions are for the most part known and can be investigated further. See also Wain, *A History of Preventive Medicine*, 330; Bates, *Bargaining for Life*, 38–9; Cartwright, *A Social History of Medicine*, 120; Myers, *Captain of All These Men of Death*, 7, 10, 12; Vrooman, "Our Knowledge Concerning Tuberculosis," 597; R. Dubos and J. Dubos, *The White Plague*, 66; Teller, *The Tuberculosis Movement*, 5–18.

5 Boyars, "Treatment of Tuberculosis," 1–7.

6 Daniel, "Tuberculosis," 637–45; Comstock, "Epidemiology of Tuberculosis," 8–15; Bates, "Tuberculosis," 20–4; Fishman, *Pulmonary Diseases*, 1821–82.

7 Copp, *Anatomy of Poverty*, 88–9; MacDougall, *Activists and Advocates*, 11; Defries, *Public Health in Canada*, 15, 35, 49, 56, 69, 90, 101, 115, 131.

8 Brown and Cook, *Canada 1896–1921*, 50; Artibise, "The Urban West," 150, 152, 158.

9 Brown and Cook, *Canada 1896–1921*, 84–5.

10 Cook, *The Regenerators*, 3–6, 228–31.

11 Quoted in Rutherford, "Tomorrow's Metropolis," 378.

12 Playter, *Consumption*, 63.

13 Bryce, "The Struggle against Tuberculosis," NCWCY, 1908; 34.

14 Quoted in CTAAR, 1955, 102. See, for example, Mrs Adam Shortt, "Some Social Aspects of Tuberculosis," CAPTAR, 1912: 108, 110; Quebec, *Report*, 80; Crichton, "Greatest of All Triumvirates," 511.

15 Holbrook, "Forty Years of Advance," 31; "Hamilton Health Association," CAPCAR, 1908: 82; 1909: 88.

16 W.J. Dobbie, "The First Forty Years – And Then What?," CTAAR, 1940: 16.

17 Holbrook, "Forty Years," 40–1.

18 NCWCY, 1908: 28; Hopkins, *Canadian Annual Review of Public Affairs*, 1908: 145.

19 "Minutes," CAPCAR, 1907: 9; "Executive Council Report," capcar, 1907: 49; "Minutes," CAPCAR, 1908: 16; "The Montreal League for the Prevention of Tuberculosis," CAPCAR, 1909: 54.

20 Mrs P.D. Crerar, "Women's Work against Tuberculosis," CAPTAR, 1911: 77; Mrs Albert E. Gooderham, "What the Daughters of the Empire Are Doing Towards the Prevention of Tuberculosis," CAPTAR, 1913: 60.

21 "Bruchesi Institute," *CAPTAR*, 1913: 101; David Townsend, "Advantages of Early Sanatorium Treatment," *CAPTAR*, 1916: 98.
22 Holbrook, "Forty Years," 30.
23 Seymour, *Consumption*, 5.
24 Quebec, *Report*, 72; Fagan, pt. 2, 4.
25 Dr Laberge, "Some Essential Measures of Prophylaxis against Tuberculosis," *CAPCAR*, 1908: 114; "Committee No. 3: On Availability of Hospitals, Sanatoria, Care of Public Conveyances," *CAPCAR*, 1902: 49; Knopf, *A Preventable and Curable Disease*, 236; *Public Health Journal* 1 (Dec. 1910): 608.
26 *PHJ* 1 (Oct. 1910): 506.
27 "Dip Tank Milk," *CTSE* 1 (Aug. 1910): 409; *CTSE* 1 (June 1910): 317.
28 Knopf, *Preventable and Curable Disease*, 131–2. "Executive Council Report," *CAPCAR*, 1907: 50; Dr C. Eby, *NCWCY*, 1901: 48–9.
29 Knopf, *Preventable and Curable Disease*, 10; Waugh, "Some Household Insects," 337; *PHJ* 1 (Sept. 1910): 457, 464.
30 Hunter, "Tuberculosis and Insurance," 313.
31 "The Ottawa Association," *CAPTAR*, 1910: 147; "The Montreal League for the Prevention of Tuberculosis," *CAPCAR*, 1905: 31.
32 To prove the association between tuberculosis and alcohol, the commission cited a French doctor who showed the mortality from tuberculosis was twice as high in tavern-keepers as shopkeepers Quebec, *Report*, 80, 63.
33 "Bruchesi Institute," *CAPTAR*, 1913: 108.
34 Laberge, *CAPCAR*, 1908: 120; Dr Dubé, "Alcoholism and Tuberculosis," *CAPTAR*, 1910: 51–3.
35 Knopf, *Preventable and Curable Disease*, 214.
36 Quebec, *Report*, 80.
37 MacGregor, "Alcohol and Immune Defense," 1474–9.
38 Adams and Jordan, "Infections in the Alcoholic," 188–9.
39 Singh, Mehta, et al., "Susceptibility to Pulmonary Tuberculosis," 676–81; Ellner, "Immune Dysregulation in Human Tuberculosis," 142–9; Hwang, Khan, et al., "HLA-A, -B, and DR Phenotypes and Tuberculosis," 382–5.
40 Middlebrook, "Tuberculosis and Medical Science," 5.
41 Cassel, *The Secret Plague*, 101–21.
42 Pierce, *Common Sense Medical Advisor*, 499; Crichton, "The Greatest of All Triumvirates," 511.
43 King, *The Battle with Tuberculosis*, 216.
44 McLaren, *Our Own Master Race*, 15.
45 Ibid., 25, 49, 67.
46 Shortt, "Social Aspects of Tuberculosis," 108; Sir James Grant, "Address," *CAPTAR*, 1916: 27; Bryce, "Tuberculosis in Relation to Feeble-Mindedness," 369; Shortt, "Social Aspects of Tuberculosis," 110.

47 Barr, "Medicine of the Future," 416.

48 Ibid, 417.

49 Knopf, "Birth Control," 118.

50 Shortt, "Social Aspects of Tuberculosis," 108.

51 Shirreff, "Municipal Milk Supply," 260.

52 Quoted in Playter, *Consumption*, 328.

53 "Montreal League," CAPCAR, 1906: 57.

54 "Immigrant Question," CAPCAR, 1907: 28–30.

55 Ibid, 30–1.

56 Ibid, 35–6.

57 F. Montizambert, "Speech to the 1901 Tuberculosis Conference," NAC CTA IIb. (1901); Quebec, *Report*, 69.

58 Bryce, "Tuberculosis in Immigrants," CAPCAR, 1908: 127; "Minutes," CAPCAR, 1908: 16; "Executive Council Report,"CAPCAR, 1907: 49.

59 *PHJ* 1 (Aug. 1910): 425; A. J. Richer, "The Economic Aspect of the Tuberculosis Problem in Canada," CAPCAR, 1903: 19.

60 J.G. Adami, "The Modes of Treating Tuberculosis and Their Cost," CAPTAR, 1909: 151.

61 McLaren, *Our Own Master Race*, 25, 49, 67.

62 Campbell, *Holbrook of the San*, 57.

63 MacDougall, *Activists and Advocates*, 77.

64 Knopf, *Preventable and Curable*, 84, 87, 96–8.

65 *CTSE* 1 (Aug. 1910): 418.

66 "Report of the Special Committee on Matters Concerning the Public Health," NCWCY, 1906: 32.

67 Carl Berger notes this rural idealization in the thought of imperialists such as Denison, G.M. Grant, and Stephen Leacock; Paul Rutherford notes that although urban reformers were conscious of urban problems and sometimes nostalgically yearned after a supposedly more stable, happier rural life, they also nevertheless recognized that the city was a fact of Canadian life, and attempted to improve it. Berger, *Sense of Power*, 177–97; Rutherford, *Saving the Canadian City*, xvi; 368, 373–4.

68 P.H. Bryce, "The Duty of the Community in Checking and Preventing the Ravages of Consumption," NCWCY, 1898: 134; Seymour, *Consumption*, 7.

69 Holbrook, "Forty Years," 31; Knopf, *Preventable and Curable*, 156.

70 Quebec, *Report*, 17, 30, 84; Dr Dubé, "Alcoholism and Tuberculosis," CAPTAR, 1910: 53.

71 "Fighting the White Plague," 77.

72 A klondike bed was made up by putting several layers of heavy wrapping paper under the mattress, then layering the blankets both horizontally and vertically to form a snug shell that the patient had to crawl into through the one opening at the head. Then the pillows were

arranged in a V shape with the apex at the head and the other ends tucked under the bed-clothing to prevent the wind from blowing down the patient's back. And the patient wore loose, warm clothing Knopf, *Preventable and Curable Disease,* 75–8.

73 Holbrook, "Forty Years," 31; "Montreal League for the Prevention of Tuberculosis," CAPCAR, 1906: 63; *Sanatorium for Consumptives in Manitoba,* 13; Campbell, *Holbrook,* 76.

74 Laviolette, *Trembling Mountain, Laurentides,* 31–2.

75 Bates, *Bargaining for Life,* 37; Affronti, "Mycobacterial Antigens," 2.

76 A.F. Miller, "The Sanatorium Treatment of Tuberculosis; Its Methods and Results," CAPTAR, 1918: 44–5.

77 Bruce, "The Treatment of Pulmonary Tuberculosis by Means of Graduated Rest and Exercise," CAPTAR, 1912: 134; D.A. Stewart, "Retrospect and Prospect: Tuberculosis Ten Year Ago, Today and Tomorrow," CAPTAR, 1920: 22.

78 Quoted in Artibise, *Winnipeg,* 241n40.

79 Fiat, "A Kick at Slum Workers," 374.

80 See Jordan, *Machine-Age Ideology;* Cook, *The Regenerators.*

81 J.H. Holbrook, "Reasons Why Open Cases Should Be Isolated," CAPTAR, 1916: 38.

82 "Committee No. 1: On Compulsory Notification," CAPCAR, 1907: 19.

83 Wherrett, *Empty Beds,* 39.

84 Connor, *A Heritage of Healing;* Houston, *R.G. Ferguson.*

85 Stewart, *Things New and Old,* 3–4.

86 Dr Sheard, "Efforts to Check the Spread of Consumption," NCWCY, 1901: 45.

87 Campbell, *Holbrook,* 65; "Montreal League for the Prevention of Tuberculosis," CAPCAR, 1908: 91.

88 "Committee No. 2: Prejudice against Consumptives," CAPCAR, 1906: 95–9.

89 "Report of Executive Council," CAPCAR, 1903: 15.

90 Knopf, *Preventable and Curable,* 22.

91 S.A. Knopf, "The Mission of Societies for the Prevention of Consumption in the Anti-Tuberculosis Crusade," CAPCAR, 1902: 27.

92 Elizabeth Shortt, NCWCY, 1908: 30.

93 Hopkins, *Canadian Annual Review,* 1909, 452.

94 A.J. Richer, "The Sanatorium and Its Mission," CAPCAR, 1906: 87; Knopf, "Mission," 33–4.

95 C.S. Eby, NCWCY, 1901, 48.

96 Campbell, *Holbrook,* 77–8; Holbrook, "Forty Years," 32.

97 "Fighting the White Plague," 75.

98 Elliott, "The Anti-Tuberculosis Movement," 78.

99 "Montreal League," CAPCAR, 1905: 27. (The Laurentian Sanatorium was opened in 1911).

100 E.S. Harding, "Dispensary Treatment," *CAPTAR*, 1910: 43.

101 "Ottawa Association," *CAPCAR*, 1909: 78; "Ottawa Association," *CAPTAR*, 1910: 141; "Minutes," *CAPTAR*, 1910: 32; "Montreal League," *CAPCAR*, 1906: 62; Holbrook, "Forty Years," 32; "Toronto League," *CAPTAR*, 1910: 119.

102 J.G. Adami, "The Modes of Treating Tuberculosis," *CAPTAR*, 1909: 145–6; Knopf, *Preventable and Curable*, 334, 340–1.

103 Adami, "Modes of Treating Tuberculosis," 146–8; Dr Campbell Howard, "The Class Treatment of Tuberculosis," *CAPTAR*, 1910: 35–7.

104 "Reports of Committees," *CAPCAR*, 1902: 46–8; 1904: 51, 53; 1907: 22.

105 "Committee on Legislation," *CAPCAR*, 1902: 47. "Committee on the Relation of Governments to the Crusade against Tuberculosis," *CAPCAR*, 1904: 51. "Executive Council Report," *CAPCAR*, 1907: 49.

106 "Reports of Committees," *CAPCAR*, 1902: 47–9; 1904: 51, 54; 1906: 93; "Minutes," *CAPCAR*, 1906: 19–20; A.J. Richer, "The Sanatorium," *CAPCAR*, 1906: 88.

107 In the debate that ensued over the resolution in the House of Commons, it was pointed out that the federal government could deal with the problem under section 91 of the British North America Act; and even Sidney Fisher, the minister of agriculture, who was opposed to the federal government establishing or maintaining sanatoria, admitted "I would not go so far as to say that we might not have the power to do that work." R.L. Borden caustically pointed out in reply to the argument that the problem was in the provinces' jurisdiction under subsection 7 of section 92 of the BNA Act (the establishment of hospitals) that "we have interfered by assisting local enterprises in the shape of provincial railways, which are as much subject to the jurisdiction of the provinces as the establishment of sanatoria," bolstering his position with Lord Herschell's argument in the questioning of Ontario's Liquor License Act before the Privy Council. Canada, House of Commons, *Debates*, 1905, 69, 1351–85.

108 "Minutes," *CAPCAR*, 1908: 26. Canada, House of Commons, *Debates*, 72: 8635–7, 9392–4, 9522–3.

109 Canada, House of Commons, *Debates*, 1905, 69: 1374.

110 Richer, *Tuberculosis Problem*, 4.

111 Quebec, *Report*, 9–10.

112 Ibid, 32; Copp, *Anatomy*, 102.

113 "Minutes," *CAPCAR*, 1904: 8–9.

114 "Report of the Executive Council," *CAPCAR*, 1908: 30; "The Montreal League, *CAPCAR*, 1905: 32; "Report of the Executive Council," *CAPCAR*, 1909: 30; "Report of the Executive Council," *CAPCAR*, 1905: 19–21.

115 "Minutes," *CAPCAR*, 1908: 14; Elliot, "Anti-Tuberculosis Movement," 84–5; MacDermot, 3.

116 Toronto Association, *Report of Inaugural Meeting*, 6; "Inter Alia," *PHJ* 1 (Nov. 1910): 565; "Montreal League," *CAPCAR*, 1905: 31; Richer, "Tuberculosis Problem," 17–8.

117 NAC CTA, IIa, file 58, A.J. Richer (Montreal League for the Prevention of Tuberculosis) to every doctor in Montreal, 25 Nov., 1903.

118 Campbell, *Holbrook*, 61.

CHAPTER TWO

1 "Report of the Executive Council," *CAPTAR*, 1919: 14.
2 Morton and Wright, *Winning the Second Battle*, 9–10, 25.
3 J.A. Machado, "President's Address," *CAPTAR*, 1919: 69.
4 Morton and Wright, *Winning the Second Battle*, 17.
5 Ibid., 90–2.
6 After 1 April 1918 all men received the pay of their rank plus sanatorium treatment. An Order-in-council then had them treated as civilians, and they received a pension while in the sanatorium. A total disability pension gave a private $600 per year. (J.H. Elliott, "Tuberculosis in the Canadian Forces," *CAPTAR*, 1917: 63; Elliott, "How Canada is Meeting the Tuberculosis War Problem," 406).
7 Lt Col Thompson, "What the Military-Hospitals Commission Is Doing for the Tuberculous Soldier," *CAPTAR*, 1917: 80–1.
8 Editorial, "The Tuberculous Soldier," *CMAJ* 6 (Oct. 1916): 922.
9 Campbell, *Holbrook*, 112
10 Byers, "Pulmonary Tuberculosis," 3–4; "Vocational Training," *CAPTAR*, 1917: 68; Elliott, "Tuberculosis War Problem," 404–5.
11 Ibid., 136, 176.
12 Elliott, "Tuberculosis War Problem," 401.
13 "Report of the Executive Council," *CAPTAR*, 1919:10.
14 Stewart, "Retrospect and Prospect," 24.
15 J. Roddick Byers, "Diseased Teeth a Factor in the Production of Lung Disease," *CAPTAR*, 1920: 17–19.
16 Hart, "The Tuberculosis Problem," 337.
17 "Mountain Sanatorium-Hamilton Health Association," "Saskatchewan," *CAPTAR*, 1918: 85, 156; Ferguson, "Control of Tuberculosis," 130.
18 The approximate amounts spent by the federal government providing accommodation for the treatment of tuberculosis in Canada were as follows:

| BC | Tranquille Sanatorium | $405,767 (of which $50,547 was for equipment) |
|----|----------------------|------|
| AB | Bowness | 424,289 |
| MB | Ninette | 198,798 ($12,441 equipment) |

| SK | Ft Qu'Appele | 277,511 | ($33,697 equipment) |
|----|--------------|---------|---------------------|
| ON | Freeport | 41,351 | |
| | Queen Alexandra | 237,373 | ($31,850 equipment) |
| | Mountain | 80,043 | ($12,745 equipment) |
| | Calydor | 30,000 | |
| QC | Laurentian | 246,230 | ($82,525 equipment) |
| | Lake Edward | 98,105 | ($9,150 equipment) |
| | Ste Foy Rd | 9,000 | |
| | Royal Edward Inst. | 6,090 | |
| NB | Jordan Memorial | 115,649 | |
| | St John County | 112,325 | |
| NS | Kentville | 638,016 | ($76,285 equipment) |
| PEI | Dalton | 288,718 | |

In addition, the federal government spent money on other institutions that were later closed or used for hospitals or institutions for other diseases:

| BC | Balfour | $ 40,999 |
|----|---------|----------|
| AB | Frank | 20,540 |
| SK | Earl Grey, Regina | 86,434 |
| ON | Mowat, Kingston | 337,663 |
| QC | Laurentide Inn | 42, 230 |

(NAC CTA, IIa, file 93, E.H. Scammel, Secretary of the Federal Department of Pensions and National Health, to R.E. Wodehouse, 1 Oct. 1929; Campbell, *Holbrook*, 109.)

19 Bernstein, "Home Treatment of Tuberculosis," 47.

20 "Hamilton Health Association," *CAPTAR*, 1920: 68.

21 *PHJ* 2 (Feb. 1911): 85; Stewart, "Tuberculosis Problems of Today," 12; Editorial, "Tuberculosis in Children," *CMAJ* 5 (July 1915): 615; Parfitt, "Tuberculosis Often of Secondary Importance," 10.

22 J.A. Machado, "President's Address," *CAPTAR*, 191:71.

23 W.J. Dobbie, "What Should Be Taught To-day about the Prevention of Tuberculosis," *CAPTAR*, 1919: 37.

24 C.D. Parfitt, "The Utility of Artificial Pneumothorax in the Treatment of Phthisis," *CAPTAR*, 1918: 54.

25 C.D. Parfitt and D.W. Crombie, "Artificial Pneumorax in the Treatment of Phthisis," *CMAJ* 5 (Apr. 1915): 281.

26 Ibid., 283. Editorial, "Artificial Pneumothorax in the Treatment of Pulmonary Tuberculosis," *CMAJ* 3 (Mar. 1913): 230–2; Kendall, "Artificial Pneumothorax," 207.

27 They also began to do nontuberculosis surgery more frequently toward the end of the decade, realizing that the patient had a better chance of recovering if other debilitating conditions, such as diseased tonsils, gallbladder, or appendix, were removed and carious teeth were repaired (Stewart, "Retrospect and Prospect," 25).

28 Editorial, "Heliotherapy," CMAJ 7 (May 1917): 444; Elliott, "Heliotherapy in Abdominal Tuberculosis," 420–4; J.H. Pryor, "Heliotherapy by the Rollier Method as Applied to Surgical Tuberculosis," CAPTAR, 1918: 28–34; Byrd, Kaplan, and Gracey, "Treatment of Pulmonary Tuberculosis," 560–7; Nardell, "Environmental Control of Tuberculosis," 1315–34; Stead, Yeung, and Hartnett, "Role of Ultraviolet Irradiation," 11–13.

29 "Minutes," CAPTAR, 1915: 9–10.

30 "Report of the Executive Council," CAPTAR, 1919: 14.

31 C.D. Parfitt, in discussion, following Elizabeth E. Harris, "The Visiting Nurse," CAPTAR, 1919: 32; Eunice Dyke, "Tuberculosis or Public Health Nurses," CAPTAR, 1914: 117

32 Ibid., 114.

33 Brittain, "Toronto Department of Public Health," 368.

34 Dyke, "Tuberculosis in Toronto," 404.

35 "Minutes," CAPTAR, 1917: 14–5.

36 MacDougall, Activists and Advocates, 26, 27, 30.

37 "Minutes," CAPTAR, 1917: 14.

38 Roberts, "Prevention of Tuberculosis," 70.

39 J.A. Machado, "President's Address," CAPTAR, 1919: 70.

40 "Hamilton Health Association," CAPTAR, 1915: 198; "Minutes," CAPTAR, 1913: 27.

41 Black, "Federal Bureau of Health," 335.

42 Hattie, "Some Medico-Sociological Problems," 254; Reid, "Heredity," 484.

43 Cassel, The Secret Plague, 238, 243.

44 "Bruchesi Institute," CAPTAR, 1919: 105.

45 Vrooman, "Responsibility for the Advanced Case," 581.

46 Miller, "The Canadian Practitioner's Diagnosis," 796–7.

47 Vrooman, "Responsibility for the Advanced Case," 576–8; Currey, "Some Problems for the New MOH," 513.

48 "Manitoba Sanatorium," CAPTAR, 1918: 194; "Bruchesi Institute," CAPTAR, 1916: 106.

49 Hastings, "Public Health Administration," 133.

50 "Minutes," CAPTAR, 15; Sutherland, "The Nationalization of Medicine," 6.

51 PHJ 4 (Jan. 1913): 47.

52 J.W. Daniel, "President's Address," *CAPTAR*, 1917: 87.

53 Morton and Wright, *Winning the Second Battle*, 19–21, 141, 177.

54 Parfitt, "Our Present Attitude," 484.

55 "Minutes," *CAPTAR*, 1912: 18.

56 "Minutes," *CAPTAR*, 1912: 21–2.

57 "May Court Club (Ottawa)," *CAPTAR*, 1918: 80.

58 "Minutes," *CAPTAR*, 1917: 17.

59 "Report of Committee of Resolutions," *CAPTAR*, 1917: 105; "Mountview Hospital, Calgary," *CAPTAR*, 1919: 156.

60 Elliott, "Diseases of the Respiratory System," 59; Stewart, "Tuberculosis Problems of To-Day," 8.

61 Morton and Wright, *Winning the Second Battle*, 224.

62 "Mt Sinai Sanatorium," *CAPTAR*, 1916: 143.

63 Hastings, "Democracy and Public Health Administration," 103.

CHAPTER THREE

1 Quoted in Connor, *A Heritage of Healing*, 96.

2 Miller, "The Forward Movement in Public Health," 120–1.

3 Holbrook, "Tuberculosis Campaign," 466.

4 Campbell, *Holbrook*, 149.

5 "Secretary's Report," *CAPTAR*, 1920: 8.

6 Porter, "Presidential Address," 272.

7 Thompson and Seager, *Decades of Discord*, 82, 83, 89, 342, 343, 347.

8 Ibid., 98, 101.

9 See Cook, *The Regenerators*.

10 Stewart, *Things New and Old*, 16.

11 Ferguson, "Tuberculosis Prevention," 204.

12 "Essex County Sanatorium" *CTAAR*, 1934: 86.

13 Stewart, *Things New and Old*, 5–6, 9–16.

14 Ibid., 6.

15 Fleming, *What You Should Know*, 4–5.

16 J.H. Elliot, "Tuberculosis in the Child: Preventive Role of the Open Air School, the Summer Camp, the Preventorium," *CTAAR*, *Papers on Tuberculosis*, 1925: 101.

17 R.G. Ferguson, "President's Address," *CTAAR*, 1936: 16.

18 Fleming, *What You Should Know*, 25–6.

19 Stewart, "The Challenge of Tuberculosis," 112.

20 D.A. Stewart, "The Red Man and the White Plague," *CTAAR*, 1936: 20.

21 Ferguson, "Control of Tuberculosis," 134.

22 Collins and MacMillan, "Tuberculosis and the Student Nurse," 649–54.

23 Wherrett, "Tuberculosis and the Student Nurse," 620.

24 Cruikshank, "Tuberculosis among Toronto Children," 71.

25 Wherrett, "The Need for Uniformity," 77–80.
26 Grant Fleming had asked George Wherrett if he had any information on the increasing prevalence of tuberculosis as one descended the economic scale. Wherrett replied that the only definite data available for Canada was information "on a number admitted to institutions in Canada by occupation," and "I find that it is difficult to work out an incidence from the Occupational Census, as the last census only includes those who are gainfully employed, and many who are admitted to tuberculosis institutions give an occupation but have not been 'gainfully employed' for years. The census also did not include those who were employed at home and were not given a definite salary." Nor, obviously enough, would this method of tabulation include those individuals who were not admitted to institutions; and this would *probably* be those least able to afford it. The Metropolitan Life Insurance Company reported that its industrial policyholders in Canada and the United States (those carrying less than $1,000 insurance and paying weekly premiums – mostly wage-earners) had a death rate of 81.3 per 100,000 in 1930. Ordinary policyholders (those with $1,000 policies or more) had a rate of 48.7 per 100,000, while those with policies of $5,000 or more had a rate of 17 per 100,000. From this, one could infer that tuberculosis was a disease of "lower economic groups" NAC CTA IIa, file 23, G.J. Wherrett to A. Grant Fleming, 30 Sept. 1938; Dublin, "Incidence of Tuberculosis," 293.
27 Wherrett, "The Need for Uniformity," 80–1.
28 Ibid., 76.
29 Morris, "Survey of Tuberculosis Patients," 170; Crombie, "The Present Anti-Tuberculosis Program," 487; Cassidy, *Public Health and Welfare Reorganization*, 324.
30 "Saskatchewan Royal Commission," *CTAAR*, 1922: 209–10.
31 "Report of the Royal Commission in Saskatchewan," *CTAAR*, 1922: 110–14; A.F. Miller, "The Place of the Clinic in the Tuberculosis Campaign," *CTAAR*, 1922: 65.
32 "Report of the Royal Commission in Saskatchewan," *CTAAR*, 1922: 114–16. *CTAAR*, 1923: 161; Odilon Leclerc, "Preliminary Report of the Tuberculosis Survey Committee of Quebec," *CTAAR*, *Papers on Tuberculosis*, 1924: 103; A.H. Baker, "The Tuberculosis Survey of School Children in Alberta – 1924," *CTAAR*, *Papers on Tuberculosis*, 1925: 33; "Industrial Study," *CTAAR*, 1930: 14.
33 MacKay, "Tuberculosis and the Community," 476.
34 Louis Dublin of the Metropolitan Life Insurance Company had announced in 1931 that the death rate for industrial employees and their families was 97.3 per 100,000 in Canada, compared to 59 in the United States. In 1925 the respective figures had been 104.1 and 78.4,

and he attributed the slow Canadian decline to the high death rates in the industrial populations of Nova Scotia, New Brunswick, and Quebec. Otherwise, the mortality was below that for white wage-earners in the United States. The editor of the *Bulletin* estimated that Montreal alone, with its hopelessly inadequate facilities, contained more than one-fifth of the country's industrial population. "Louis I. Dubilin," CTAB 10 (Dec. 1931): 3.

35  "Quebec Industrial Health Survey," CTAAR, 1934: 14.

36  "British Columbia," CTAAR, 1937: 41.

37  "British Columbia," CTAAR, 1936: 53; "Ontario," CTAAR, 1935: 75.

38  "Report of Executive Office," CTAAR, 1935: 12.

39  "British Columbia," CTAAR, 1939: 40; "Manitoba," CTAAR, 1939: 44; Boughton, "New Case Finding in Tuberculosis," 263.

40  CTA, *Community Campaign*, 5.

41  "Saskatchewan," CTAAR, 1936: 171; "Saskatchewan: Tuberculin," CTAB 14 (June 1936): 5.

42  Clarke, "Tuberculosis Control in New Brunswick," 106.

43  "Tranquille Sanatorium," CTAAR, 1929: 44.

44  Houston, *Ferguson*, 52.

45  "Manitoba," CTAAR, 1935: 56; "Nova Scotia," CTAAR, 1933: 57.

46  Stewart and Ross, "An Insidious Disease," 161.

47  Ross, "Diagnosis of Tuberculosis," 595.

48  Grant Fleming, "The Tuberculosis Problem," CTAB 19 (June 1941): 5.

49  "Queen Alexandra Sanatorium," CTAAR, 1934: 139.

50  Stewart and Ross, "Tuberculosis," 164.

51  Stewart, *Rest*, 4.

52  "Saskatchewan," CTAAR, 1925: 138; "Ontario: Calydor Sanatorium," CTAAR, 1922: 158; "National Sanitarium Association," CTAAR, 1924: 98; "Saskatchewan," CTAAR, 1926: 148; "Laurentian Sanatorium," CTAAR, 1928: 150.

53  Gaensler, "Surgery for Pulmonary Tuberculosis," 73–4.

54  Stewart, *Rest*, 3.

55  CTA, *What You Should Know*, 16.

56  Gale and Delarue, "Surgical History of Pulmonary Tuberculosis," 381–8.

57  Gaensler, "Surgery for Pulmonary Tuberculosis," 73–5, 77–9.

58  Ibid., 80; Brancker and Enarson, "Tuberculosis in Canada," 110.

59  Grace, "Surgical Procedures," 125; Kinsella, "Thoracic Surgery," 9, 10, 12.

60  James, "Pulmonary Tuberculosis," 389.

61  Fleming, *What You Should Know*, 30; Fleming, "The Tuberculosis Problem," 6.

62  "Nova Scotia," CTAAR, 1934: 67–8.

63  Bethune, "Early Compression," 40.

64 Sharpe, "Artificial Pneumothorax," 57; "Royal Ottawa Sanatorium," *CTAAR*, 1936: 133.
65 Crombie, "Anti-Tuberculosis Program in Ontario," 492; Brink, *Tuberculosis in Ontario*, 21; "New Brunswick," *CTAAR*, 1936: 70.
66 NAC CTA IIa, file 23, Montreal Medical Society, *Report of Tuberculosis Committee* 1936?): 2–3.
67 Gale and Delarue, "Surgical History of Pulmonary Tuberculosis," 381; Stewart, "What Is New in Tuberculosis?" 38; "Queen Alexandra Sanatorium," "Manitoba," *CTAAR*, 1936: 131, 60; "British Columbia," *CTAAR*, 1938: 34; "National Sanitarium Association," *CTAAR*, 1935: 110–11, 115.
68 "Saskatchewan Anti-Tuberculosis League," *CTAAR*, 1927: 129.
69 MacKenzie, "Renal Tuberculosis," 65; Editorial, "Intestinal Tuberculosis," *CMAJ* 17 (Sept. 1927): 1065–6.
70 Stewart, "Intestinal Tuberculosis," 599; "Saskatchewan," *CTAAR*, 1925: 138; 1926: 148; "Report of the Executive Council," "Department of National Health," *CTAAR*, 1930: 15, 24.
71 "Ontario: Provincial Board of Health," *CTAAR*, 1925: 72; Riddell, "Silicosis," 5–6.
72 Currie, "Montreal Anti-Tuberculosis and General Health League," 203.
73 McIntosh, "Cancer and Tuberculosis," 600–9, 360–1; Miller, "Comment on 'Cancer and Tuberculosis,'" 176.
74 Houston, *Ferguson*, 56–7.
75 "Saskatchewan," *CTAAR*, 1926: 149.
76 Holbrook, *CTAAR*, 1922: 95.
77 M. Hart, "Sheltered Employment for the Tuberculous in Canada," *CTAAR*, 1922: 92.
78 "Saskatchewan," *CTAAR*, 1937: 84–5.
79 Vancouver Survey Committee, *Survey of the Tuberculosis Situation*, 42.
80 Kirby, "Cases of Active Tuberculosis," 11.
81 Feldberg, *Disease and Class*, 160–1.
82 Ibid., 128–33.
83 Ibid., 156.
84 "National Research Council," *CTAAR*, 1935: 27–8; NAC CTA, III, file 6, W.J. Dobbie to R.E. Wodehouse, 31 Mar. 1930; Feldberg, *Disease and Class*, 138.
85 Ibid., 164.
86 Ibid., 200–7.
87 Use of BCG would also make it difficult to use future antibiotics for positive contacts, because all vaccinated persons would of course be positive (Houston, *Ferguson*, 98–101).
88 Stewart, "Anti-Tuberculosis Measures," 672.
89 Stewart, *Teaching about Tuberculosis*, 4.
90 Stewart, *Things New and Old*, 7.

91 "Mountain Sanatorium," *CTAAR*, 1927: 85.

92 "Nova Scotia Branch of the Red Cross Society," *CAPTAR*, 1920: 114; "Ontario," *CTAAR*, 1924: 78–9; "Ontario," *CTAAR*, 1923: 77; "British Columbia," *CTAAR*, 1923: 29; "Report of the Executive Council," *CTAAR*, 1925: 17.

93 Stewart, "Measures in Rural Districts," 670; G.C. Brink, "The Travelling Diagnostic Clinic for Diseases of the Lungs," *CTAAR, Papers on Tuberculosis*, 1925: 7.

94 "Royal Edward Institute," *CTAAR*, 1925: 125.

95 "Jessel and Powell: Summary (A) Canada," *CTAB* 9 (June 1931): 3.

96 "Ontario," *CTAAR*, 1935: 135; Meakins, "Tuberculosis and the Family," *NOT* 1 (Jan. 1939): 3; "Report of Executive Office," *CTAAR*, 1935: 11.

97 "Alberta," *CTAAR*, 1937: 35; Ferguson, "Diagnosis and Eradication of Tuberculosis," 528.

98 Dobbie, "Control of Tuberculosis," 494–5.

99 Stewart, "Challenge of Tuberculosis," 115.

100 "Quebec," *CTAAR*, 1938: 57; "Manitoba," *CTAAR*, 1931: 42.

101 Chown and Medovy, "Pulmonary Tuberculosis in Childhood," 364; Temple, "Routine Examination of Tuberculosis Contacts," 509.

102 CTA, *Community Campaign*, 3; CTA, *Protect the Contact*, 3–4.

103 "Ontario," *CTAAR*, 1933: 60; "British Columbia," *CTAAR*, 1935: 42; "Manitoba," *CTAAR*, 1937: 53–4; Brink, "Provincial Tuberculosis Program," 217.

104 Wodehouse, *Sanatorium Situation in Ontario.*

105 Stewart, "Measures in Rural Districts," 672; "Tranquille Sanatorium," *CTAAR*, 1928: 56.

106 Ibid.; "National Sanatarium Association," *CTAAR*, 1924: 98; Holbrook, "Tuberculosis Campaign in Canada," 467.

107 "Saskatchewan," *CTAAR*, 1925: 135; "Saskatchewan," *CTAAR*, 1928: 166.

108 This figure is for Manitoba. Jackson, "Public Medical Services," 616; R.G. Ferguson, "The Most Important Agencies in a Provincial Campaign against Tuberculosis," *CTAAR, Papers on Tuberculosis*, 1925: 36–7.

109 Stewart, *Teaching about Tuberculosis*, 5.

110 Ibid.

111 "British Columbia," *CTAAR*, 1930: 41.

112 Stewart, "Measures in Rural Districts," 672.

113 "Royal Ottawa Sanatorium," *CTAAR*, 1926: 114.

114 Fifty thousand dollars was a grant from the Ontario Government; the rest was voluntary donations. "Mountain Sanatorium," *CTAAR*, 1926: 88.

115 "Saskatchewan," *CTAAR*, 1929: 119; "Resident Tuberculosis Treatment Institutions of Canada, 1927," *CTAB* 7 (Sept. 1928): 3.

116 "British Columbia," *CTAAR*, 1929: 47.

117 "Resident Tuberculosis Treatment Institutions, 1927," 3.

118 This figure does not include Lake Edward (Quebec), a semiprivate institution with 90 percent paying patients, or Calydor, a private institution. Wodehouse, *Sanatorium Situation in Ontario*.

119 British Columbia was more complicated. Its rate in 1928 was 108.2, but 85.2 percent was due to native Canadians, over which the provincial government had no control. The balance of the population, including the Chinese, Japanese, and East Indians, who had a death rate twice that of the white population, had roughly a rate of 70, which compared favourably with the rest of the country. Nova Scotia, New Brunswick, and Quebec, however, could not make similar significant reductions. Wodehouse, *Sanatorium Situation in Ontario*.

120 CTA, *Tuberculosis Programs*, 2; NAC CTA, IIa, file 47, "Recommendations re Nova Scotia," 4.

121 Stewart, "What is New in Tuberculosis?" 37.

122 Eighty-six percent of the patients could contribute nothing to the cost of their treatment. "Brief Presented to Rowell Commission," *CTAB* 16 (Mar. 1938): 3; Fleming, "Tuberculosis Problem," 5.

123 "Ontario," *CTAAR*, 1934: 85.

124 Ferguson, "Tuberculosis Prevention," 205.

125 By this point, three beds per death was the standard required to isolate all cases. Both Ontario and Saskatchewan had achieved this level for their white populations and had no waiting lists at sanatoria. Wherrett, "Tuberculosis Control," 290–1.

126 "Manitoba," *CTAAR*, 1932: 37.

127 "Quebec," *CTAAR*, 1931: 109; 1932: 94; "Ontario," *CTAAR*, 1933: 66.

128 "Saskatchewan," *CTAAR*, 1932: 100; "Quebec," *CTAAR*, 1933: 125; "Quebec," *CTAAR*, 1932: 84.

129 "Alberta," *CTAAR*, 1931: 28.

130 Holbrook, "Tuberculosis Campaign," 461; Young, "Health Units in British Columbia," 136–7.

131 "Review of Year," *CTAAR*, 1928: 14; 1929: 11; "Secretary's Report," *CTAAR*, 1923: 12–3; "Minutes," *CTAAR*, 1919: 64.

132 Campbell, *Holbrook*, 135.

133 R.G. Ferguson, "The Most Important Agencies in a Provincial Campaign against Tuberculosis," *CTAAR*, *Papers on Tuberculosis*, 1925: 39.

134 Gibbon, *Three Centuries*, 340; Baudouin, "Activities of the French Health Centre," 222; Russell, "Nursing in Manitoba," 35.

135 "British Columbia," *CTAAR*, 1936: 56.

136 Fleming, *What You Should Know*, 43.

137 "Quebec," *CTAAR*, 1939: 59.

138 These confused answers reflect, as well, the wording of the question. "Gallup Survey of Tuberculosis," *CTAB* 17 (Sept. 1939): 3–4.

139 Rutherford, *Saving the Canadian City*, xxi.

140 Forbes, "Prohibition and the Social Gospel," 11; Allen, *The Social Passion*, 352.
141 See Cook, *The Regenerators.*
142 Thompson, "Defeat of Prohibition," 175–6, 179–86; Allen, *Social Passion*, 274–5.
143 Ibid., 352.
144 Miller, "Public Health," 121.
145 Stewart, *Social Ramifications*, 11.
146 "Report of Executive Office," *CTAAR*, 1939: 24.
147 NAC CTA, III, file 6; R.G. Ferguson, "Research in Vaccination against Tuberculosis" (enclosed with letter, R.G. Ferguson to G.J. Wherrett, 2 Feb. 1939).
148 McCann, "Public Health Activities," 258.
149 Fraser, "Man's Attitude towards His Physical Life," 590; R.G. Ferguson, "President's Address," *CTAAR*, 1936: 16.
150 Stewart, *Things New and Old*, 19.

CHAPTER FOUR

1 Miller, "Public Health," 121.
2 Melvin, "Our Voluntary Assistants," 457–61; Porter, "Presidential Address," 275; "Montreal Anti-Tuberculosis and General Health League," *CTAAR*, 1925: 121–2.
3 Hall, "Private Philanthropy," 42.
4 Melvin, "Voluntary Assistants," 461.
5 NAC CTA IIa, file 65, "Public Health Conference, May 27, 1924."
6 Governor-General of Canada, "What Can the Layman Do?" *CTAB* 2 (June 1924): 1.
7 George D. Porter, following Dr W.J. Dobbie, "On the Advisability of Reviving the Local Anti-Tuberculosis Societies of Canada," *CTAAR*, *Papers on Tuberculosis*, 1924, 88–9.
8 Weaver, U.S. *Philanthropic Foundations*, 39.
9 Fosdick, *Rockefeller Foundation*, 2.
10 Fosdick, *Rockefeller Foundation*, ix; Nielsen, *Big Foundations*, 48–9.
11 Fosdick, *Rockefeller Foundation*, 22–3; Howe, "Scientific Philanthropy," 38–9.
12 Nielsen, *Big Foundations*, 55.
13 Fosdick, *Rockefeller Foundation*, 34.
14 Ibid., 34.
15 Ibid., 36.
16 Ibid., 53.
17 Lessard and Nadeau, "County Health Units," 126–7.
18 Nadeau, "Organization of County Health Units," 91.

19 Lasalle Laberge, "The Work of the Anti-Tuberculosis Clinicians in 1941," *NOT* 4 (Apr. 1942): 1.

20 McCullough, "County Health Unit," 123; Lessard and Nadeau, "County Health Units," 131; Middleton, "Full-Time Health Districts," 145.

21 Lessard, "County Health Work," 454; Middleton, "Full-Time Health Districts," 144; Bow, "Public Health Services," 597.

22 Bernard Langdon Wyatt, "Some Suggestions Based on the Experience of the Commission for the Prevention of Tuberculosis in France," *CTAAR*, 1922: 53.

23 Miller, "Community Responsibility," 103.

24 "Three Rivers Demonstration," *CTAAR*, 1926: 23.

25 The Three Rivers Demonstration went from 1923 to 1927, the Maritime Tuberculosis Educational Committee from 1926 to 1930 (it included New Brunswick and Prince Edward Island), the Nova Scotia Tuberculosis Commission from 1926 to 1930, and the Montreal Anti-Tuberculosis and General Health League from 1924 to 1928.

26 The Three Rivers Demonstration received federal and provincial grants, however.

27 The Rockefeller Foundation was active in Canada throughout the twenties. It gave the New Brunswick Department of Health $27,000 a year for two years for medical inspection of schools in rural districts if the government voted an equal amount and took the program over after two years. It also, as previously mentioned, subsidized the development of county health units and erected the Dalhousie Public Health Clinic in 1924 in Nova Scotia. "New Brunswick," *CTAAR*, 1922: 140; Beckwith, "Tuberculosis Control Program," 483.

28 J.G. Fitzgerald, "The Functions of the Red Cross in Peace Time," *CAPTAR*, 1920: 43.

29 Ibid., 42; "Secretary's Report," *CTAAR*, 1924: 14–16; "Report of Executive Office," *CTAAR*, 1925: 16; "Nova Scotia Branch of the Red Cross Society," *CAPTAR*, 1920: 114–7; A.F. Miller, "The Place of the Clinic in the Anti-Tuberculosis Campaign," *CTAAR*, 1922: 62; "Nova Scotia," *CTAAR*, 1926:18.

30 Editorial, "Anti-Tuberculosis Work in Canada," *CMAJ* 15 (Aug. 1925), 844.

31 "Three Rivers Demonstration," *CTAAR*, 1926: 23.

32 "Three Rivers Demonstration," *CTAAR*, 1925: 30; "Three Rivers Demonstration," *CTAAR*, 1927: 19; 1928: 22.

33 "Review of Year," *CTAAR*, 1926: 8; Alphonse Lessard, "The Three Rivers Demonstration," *CTAAR*, *Papers on Tuberculosis*, 1925: 25.

34 Editorial, "Life Insurance," (Jan. 1924), 48.

35 His italics. NAC CTA, IIa, file 49, R.E. Wodehouse to V.R. Smith, 23 Jan. 1926.

36 "Review of Year," *CTAAR*, 1928, 14; "Review of Year," *CTAAR*, 1930, 15; "Review of Year," *CTAAR*, 1930, 14; 1926, 11; "Periodical Examinations," *CTAB* 8 (Mar. 1930): 7.

37 *CTAAR*, 1930, 7.

38 Other than the paradigm, the Rockefeller Foundation, or the temporarily modified Red Cross, the first agency formed in the new style was, ironically, the result of a disaster – the Halifax Explosion. With roughly $250,000 remaining from the Massachusetts donations which was mentioned briefly in chapter 2 (made in the aftermath of the Halifax Explosion), the Massachusetts-Halifax Health Commission was established with a tuberculosis specialist to run clinics (first just for explosion victims, then extended to any needy citizens) and nutrition classes, to clear patients for admission to sanatoria and hospitals, and to educate Dalhousie University medical students and nurses. In 1920 it took over running the clinics and supervising the visiting nurses from the Halifax County Anti-Tuberculosis League, which proceeded to devote itself to relief work. The main work of the commission was the establishment of a health centre in Halifax (associated with Dalhousie University and erected by the Rockefeller Foundation), although the number of clinics offered declined due to budget retrenchment in 1925. Nevertheless the tuberculosis death rate in Halifax fell from 211.5 per 100,000 in 1919–20 to 118.2 in 1924–25. The commission ceased operation in 1928. While it did not deal with the problem of tuberculosis in the province as a whole, more than anything else, it demonstrated a need.

39 "Maritimes," *CTAAR*, 1927: 14.

40 "Maritime Tuberculosis Educational Committee," *CTAAR*, 1927: 25; "Maritime Tuberculosis Educational Committee," *CTAAR*, 1930: 14; "Maritime Tuberculosis Educational Committee," *CTAAR*, 1928: 29; NAC CTA, IIa, file 47, Canadian Tuberculosis Association, *Report: Maritime Tuberculosis Educational Committee, 1926–31*, 1.

41 NAC CTA, IIa, file 52, R.E. Wodehouse, *Report*, (11 Jan. 1930): 2.

42 "Nova Scotia Tuberculosis Commission," *CTAAR*, 1930: 20.

43 Wodehouse, *Report*, (11 Jan., 1930): 2–3.

44 Walker, *Service for the Royal Edward Institute*, 4–5.

45 "Costs and Results," *CTAB*, 4 (Mar. 1926):5.

46 Currie, "Montreal Anti-Tuberculosis and General Health League," 106.

47 Ibid., 263–9.

48 "Montreal Anti-Tuberculosis and General Health League," *CTAAR*, 1928: 140; Editorial, "Montreal Sets an Example," (June 1928), 278.

49 Montreal Health Survey Committee, *Survey*, 69.

50 Editorial, "An Event of Importance," 302.

51 C.D. Parfitt, "The President's Address," *CTAAR, Papers on Tuberculosis*, 1924: 11.

52 Wodehouse, "Combat against Tuberculosis," 902; "Some Monies Spent This Year," *CTAAR*, 1929: 14; "Financial," *CTAAR*, 1927: 11.

53 NAC CTA, IIa, file 48, E.E. Reid, chairman of the CLIOA health committee, to Joseph Hayes, 27 June 1931.

54 The Rockefeller Foundation continued its activities in Canada throughout the thirties. It still contributed, although on a decreasing scale, to Quebec's county health units (it had begun contributing in 1925) and aided the New Brunswick Department of Health from 1932 onwards in training its eleven medical health officers in public health. In 1934 it paid for a survey of the Nova Scotia Department of Public Health made by an independent authority, who presented his report in 1935, advising that the province be divided into four health districts, each under a trained medical health officer. The foundation then aided the province in training its medical officers in public health and helped set up the districts. As well, Sun Life aided the campaign by donating $5,000 for research in 1932 and helping to organize the Quebec Industrial Survey. Lessard, "Rural Sanitation in Quebec," 106; Warwick, "Full-Time Health Districts in New Brunswick," 294; Hopkins, *Canadian Annual Review*, 1932: 521; "Report of Executive Office," *CTAAR*, 1931: 15; Campbell, "Full-Time Health Services in Nova Scotia," 385; NAC CTA, IIa file 50, R.E. Wodehouse to E.E. Reid, 26 May 1930.

55 NAC CTA, IIa file 48, R.E. Wodehouse to E.E. Reid, 9 Dec. 1931.

56 The distressing situation in Nova Scotia was, according to Wodehouse, compounded by the fact that the medical superintendent of the provincial sanatorium worked hand-in-glove with the government and ran the sanatorium as a private or semiprivate institution. NAC CTA, IIa, file 48, R.E. Wodehouse to E.E. Reid, 4 Apr. 1931; G.H. Murphy to R.E. Wodehouse, 1 Dec. 1931.

57 NAC CTA, IIa, file 48, R.E. Wodehouse to Mr Lea, Minister of Health, PEI, (n.d.).

58 NAC CTA, IIa, file 54, R.E. Wodehouse to Mayor of Charlottetown, n.d.

59 Ibid., R.E. Wodehouse to P.A. Creelman, 23 Jan. 1931.

60 NAC CTA, IIa, file 54, P.A. Creelman to R.E. Wodehouse, 25 Apr. 1931.

61 He advised her in a telegram (12 June 1931) to complete the school inspections and leave the problem of holidays in abeyance until he arrived at the island later. NAC CTA, IIa, file 54, Mona Wilson to R.E. Wodehouse, 10 June 1931; R.E. Wodehouse to Mona Wilson (telegram) 12 June 1931.

62 Ibid., Mona Wilson to R.E. Wodehouse, 9 Apr. 1931.

63 In reference to this ongoing problem, Wodehouse wrote to Creelman in May 1931 to have the cars ready for inspection by the insurance men so that they could make a decision. Ibid., R.E. Wodehouse to P.A. Creelman, 14 May 1931.

64 From 1 July 1931 to 1 July 1936, CLIOA gave PEI $15,000 a year for five years ($75,000) – half the cost of establishing full-time health services. To tide it over the transitional period, they arranged to give the new health department another $5,000 for the following year. "Report of Executive Office," *CTAAR*, 1931: 14. "Canadian Life Insurance Officers Association," *CTAAR*, 1935: 23.

65 NAC CTA, IIa, file 48, W.J. Macmillan to R.E. Wodehouse, 15 Jan. 1932. "Report of the Executive Office," *CTAAR*, 1937: 11.

66 The Provincial Committee for the Prevention of Tuberculosis, which was formed in 1937, was supported by $30,000 from CLIOA and a similar amount from the Department of Health. "Quebec," *CTAAR*, 1937: 67.

67 "Nova Scotia," *CTAAR*, 1933: 54; "New Brunswick," *CTAAR*, 1932: 44.

68 The Quebec Provincial Committee was a voluntary organization, funded by CLIOA with $30,000 for a three-year campaign and a similar amount from the provincial government. Quebec's ratio of beds per death was one-third that of the other provinces, as can be seen from the table that follows. It spent less than two-thirds of the amount the others did on treatment and prevention, and with 28 percent of the population, had 43 percent of the tuberculosis deaths. Many of the beds it did have were in establishments without access to pneumothorax and surgery. The payment system was faulty. Under the Quebec Public Charities Act a municipality was required to pay for the treatment of an indigent, but "indigent" excluded individuals with *any* assets and required them to pay the full rate. The per diem government grant was paid only for indigents.

Tuberculosis in Quebec and Other Provinces (1937)

| | Population | Percentage of Pop. | Deaths | Percentage of Deaths | Death Rate |
|---|---|---|---|---|---|
| Quebec | 3,096,000 | 28 | 2,890 | 43 | 93.3 |
| Other province | 7,918,000 | 72 | 3,873 | 57 | 48.8 |
| Canada | 11,014,000 | | 6,763 | | 61.4 |

| | Deaths | | Beds | Ratio of Beds/Death | |
|---|---|---|---|---|---|
| Canada | 6,763 | | 8,504 | 1.25 | |
| Quebec | 2,890 | | 1,735 | 0.6 | |
| Other provinces | 3,873 | | 6,769 | 1.8 | |

| | Total Spending on Prevention and Treatment | |
|---|---|---|
| | Average | Per Capita |
| Canada | $6,195,338.39 | 0.56 |
| Quebec | 1,041,752.91 | 0.41 |
| Other provinces | 5,153,586.02 | 0.65 |

In Montreal there was a division in the campaign along linguistic lines, evinced by the two subcommittees – one English, one French – appointed by the provincial committee to study the situation in that city (although both agreed that more beds were essential for the French-speaking population). The secretary of the CTA, G.J. Wherret, recognized this situation in replying to a letter from Grant Fleming asking if separate English and French sanatoria should be established – he advised that the "English group ... Confine their efforts ... to providing treatment for the English-speaking section of the province." And in another letter he asked Fleming to interview a man who might be of some use to the English-speaking group in Montreal, for although "he has stirred up a lot of interest among the French-speaking elements ... because of his nationality I am doubtful if the French-speaking group will find a place for him in the campaign."

A confidential CTA report observed in 1936 that the English newspapers in Montreal had carried only a few stories about the seal sale that winter, and although the French papers had given it more publicity, "experience with other campaigns in Montreal has shown that stories and ads, etc., must appear in the English papers if results are to be expected, in that the majority of the contributors come from the English-speaking section of the population." Lionel Brittle, the writer of the report, went on to suggest that this might be partly due to the Kiwanis running the seal sale, since it was generally regarded as an English club.

The Provincial Committee ran a campaign of popular education under a director, through pamphlets, films and radio, speakers, and newspapers. Attendance increased at clinics, and (with government aid) sanatorium accommodation, costing over $1 million increased almost 50 percent from 1937 to 1941. But Montreal still remained a problem. NAC CTA, IIa, file 14, Quebec Committee for the Prevention of Tuberculosis, *Report*, (1938): 4–5; Grant Fleming to G.J. Wherrett, 7 June 1938; G.J. Wherrett to Grant Fleming, 16 Apr. 1938, 13 June 1938. "Quebec," *CTAAR*, 1937: 67–79; 1938: 55–6; 1940: 66–71. "Quebec Committee," *CTAB*, 16 (June 1938): 5; Lionel Brittle, *Confidential Report for the Canadian Tuberculosis Association, Ottawa: On the Montreal Christmas Seal Sale Held in November and December*, 1936: 2, 4 (in NAC CTA, V, file 6).

69 Charles, *Service Clubs*, 9, 37.
70 Ibid., 126.
71 Ibid., 51.
72 Ibid., 45–6.
73 Ibid., 99.
74 Thompson and Seager, *Decades of Discord*, 175.

75 Ibid, 76.

76 The National Sanitarium Association, which had run its own seal sale for twenty years to raise money to treat the tuberculous poor at its sanatoria (selling upwards of $550,000 worth of seals throughout the twenties), was upset by the entry of the CTA into the Ontario field. It claimed that the public would be confused, especially if seals were sold for a less definite purpose than treatment. As a result, the CTA stayed out of the Toronto area, and the National Sanitarium Association continued to run its own campaign and print its own seals. NAC CTA, V, file 5, G.A. Reid, manager of the National Sanitarium Association and the Toronto Hospital for Consumptives, *Address* (Toronto, 29 May 1929): 4–6; "Review of the Fiscal Year," *CTAAR*, 1931: 13.

77 It was less universal in Montreal, for example, where it was associated with the English Kiwanis Club.

78 NAC CTA, V, file 6, R.E. Wodehouse to L.S. Colwell (not sent), 29 Jan. 1932; IIa, file 59, W.F. Stambach to G.J. Wherrett, 24 Feb. 1940.

79 This total does not include $33,021 raised by the National Sanitarium Association, which ran its own sale. "Christmas Seal Campaign," *CTAAR*, 1940: 42–3.

80 See Bothwell and English, "Pragmatic Physicians," 479–93.

CHAPTER FIVE

1 Grayson and Bliss, *Wretched of Canada*, 122, 176.

2 As quoted in "More Adequate Aid," *CTAB* 14 (Sept. 1935): 1. The 1938 *Report of Tuberculosis Institutions* found less than 9 percent of the patients paid in full or in part. Wherret, "Tuberculosis Control," 290.

3 Stewart, "Challenge of Tuberculosis," 114.

4 Editorial, "Progress in Tuberculosis Control," *CPHJ* 29 (Apr. 1938): 189.

5 Thompson and Seager, *Decades of Discord*, 131–3, 281, 331.

6 Montreal Health Survey Committee, *Public Health Activities*, 112.

7 Editorial, "Treatment and Prevention," 231.

8 Stewart, "Measures in Rural Districts," 674; Holbrook, "Hamilton Health Association," 221.

9 "Minutes of the Annual Meeting," *CTAAR*, 1924: 10; Stewart, "Measures in Rural Districts," 673.

10 "Mountain Sanatorium," *CTAAR*, 1926: 91.

11 "Relationship between Tuberculosis and Mothers' Allowances, 1922," *CTAB* 1 (June 1923): 2; McCullough, "Public Health," 172.

12 Black, "Federal Bureau of Health," 408.

13 Grenier, "Anti-tuberculosis Campaign," 731; A.F. Miller, "The Federal Control of Tuberculosis," *CAPTAR*, 1914: 68–73; Bryce, "Federal Department of Health," 1–10.

14 Sutherland, "Nationalization of Medicine," 6; *PHJ* 3 (Mar. 1912): 134; S. Adolphus Knopf, "The Modern Warfare against Tuberculosis As a Disease of the Masses," *CAPTAR*, 1914: 55.

15 R.W. Bruce Smith, "The Relation of the State to the Tuberculosis Problem," *CAPTAR*, 1914: 58.

16 McClung, "What Will They Do with It?" 38.

17 Pickard, "Organization in Public Health," 611; Reid "Sanatorial Treatment of Tuberculosis," 316.

18 Black, "Federal Bureau of Health," 334.

19 Wright, "Aspects of Tuberculosis," 793–4; Hastings, "Democracy and Public Health Administration," 104.

20 Brown, "The Relation of the Pediatrician to the Community," 50.

21 By 1913 Alberta had legislation promising local tuberculosis institutions one-quarter of the cost of the erection and maintenance allowance of $1.75 per week; Saskatchewan promised a $60,000 grant and payment of 50 percent of the costs per patient per day (with $1 per day coming from municipalities for pauper patients). These provinces opened provincial sanatoria in 1920 and 1917 respectively, partially funded by the federal government, since they accommodated soldiers. (The Alberta government and federal government each agreed to pay $200,000 to buy a site and erect a sanatorium in 1919). The BC government voted $75,000 for a building for advanced cases at Tranquille, Manitoba gave $60,000 to the Ninette Sanatorium, and Ontario gave up to $4,000, or one-fifth of the cost of erection of a sanatorium, and spent $32,000 from 1910 to 1919 alone just adding to or helping establish sanatoria. Quebec gave $10,000 for tuberculosis work, while New Brunswick and Prince Edward Island had sanatoria built by private philanthropy – the Jordan Sanatorium at River Glade and the Dalton Sanatorium, respectively. The average cost per patient per day in a Canadian sanatorium was roughly $1.55, or $10.85 per week, in 1914. British Columbia gave a maintenance grant of $7.00 per week for advanced cases and $4.55 per week for incipient cases, with those able to do so paying $15.00 per week. Saskatchewan granted $3.50 a week per patient, Manitoba $2.80, and Ontario $3.00 (this was raised to $3.50 in 1919), with the municipalities paying an additional $4.90 per week for indigents. At the Nova Scotia Sanatorium, the patient paid $5.00 per week, and the government made up the difference (about $7.00). In New Brunswick, the patients paid $7.00 per week, and the government paid the balance, while Quebec and Prince Edward Island had no maintenance grant. To care automatically for its indigents, the Union of Manitoba Municipalities placed a levy on organized municipalities outside the four cities. Tuberculosis workers in Quebec complained that there was no free accommodation for incipient tuberculosis

patients in the province, while annual maintenance grants in Ontario increased from $26, 073 in 1910 to $279,491.22 in 1919.

Other changes were occurring in related health legislation in this period. Provincial public health nurses were hired in Manitoba (1916), Saskatchewan (1919), Alberta (1918), British Columbia (1917), and Ontario (1919). Alberta passed a public health act in 1910; Manitoba and Ontario revised theirs in 1911 and 1912; and New Brunswick and Alberta created departments of health under a minister in 1918 and 1919. Ontario and Saskatchewan both had free distribution of public health biological products, such as antitoxin, by 1917. Provincial governments were accepting some responsibility for the health of their citizens – albeit reluctantly in some cases. "Royal Edward Institute," CAPTAR, 1912: 270; Campbell, Holbrook, 98–9; McCullough, "Public Health," 294; "Executive Council Report," CAPTAR, 1913: 41–3; 1914: 24; Editorial, "The Laurentian Society," 222–3; Sanatorium Board of Manitoba, Souvenir, 5; "Royal Edward Institute," CAPTAR, 1916: 85; Defries, Public Health in Canada, 50, 72–3, 77, 90, 94, 105, 117, 124, 138.

22 "Royal Edward Institute," CAPTAR, 1914: 243; Hastings, "Why a Municipality Can Best Control Tuberculosis," 68–9; Elliot, "Prevention of Tuberculosis," 28.

23 Hastings, "Democracy and Public Health Administration," 105.

24 Copp, Anatomy, 97.

25 "Bruchesi Institute," CAPTAR, 1914: 139.

26 "Royal Edward Institute," CAPTAR, 1914: 249–50.

27 "Bruchesi Institute," CAPTAR, 1919: 107.

28 Dyke, "Tuberculosis in Toronto," 403.

29 "Minutes," CAPTAR, 1912: 17; Hocken, "New Spirit in Municipal Government," 203–4.

30 The estimated population for Toronto in 1916 was 544,456 and 637,844 for Montreal. "Bruchesi Institute," CAPTAR, 1918: 101–2; Lovell's Montreal Directory for 1916–17 (Montreal: 1916): 23.

31 The takeover and maintenance of the Tranquille Sanatorium by the BC government in 1921 was a case in point – it was now continually in debt, running with a deficit of $1,500 per month ($20,000 in 1920). As J.D. McLean remarked in the legislature, "We are proposing to take over the institution therefore for two reasons: first, because it has become too large and important an undertaking to be managed and supported by voluntary effort and, secondly, because the care of contagious disease of this nature should be the duty of the province." The first reason was the deciding factor: the government was forced to take over the institution to save it from bankruptcy. "British Columbia," CAPTAR, 1921: 86.

32 A. Lessard, "Anti-tuberculosis and Child Welfare Dispensaries in the Province of Quebec," *CTAAR, Papers on Tuberculosis*, 1924: 82.

33 A.B. Cook, "President's Address," *CTAAR*, 1923: 10; R.O. Davison, "Tuberculosis in Saskatchewan," *CTAAR, Papers on Tuberculosis*, 1924: 32.

34 "Saskatchewan," *CTAAR*, 1925: 134.

35 Manitoba, *Report on Tuberculosis*, 46–7.

36 CTA, *Eastern Ontario Counties Sanatorium*; "Saskatchewan," *CTAAR*, 1929: 121; Middleton, "Tuberculosis Control," 509.

37 Middleton, "Tuberculosis Control," 509–10; "Saskatchewan," *CTAAR*, 1926: 145; 1927: 127.

38 The Act Respecting Sanatoria and Hospitals for the Treatment of Tuberculosis covered the following:

1 The Anti-Tuberculosis League continued to operate the sanatoria (although the government paid for most capital costs now).
2 The province paid $1.00 a day per patient, with the rural and urban municipalities contributing the balance. The league apportioned the cost borne by the municipalities on the basis of their total equalized assessment for the preceding year. (A further amendment in 1930 adjusted the amount each paid slightly, so that the urban municipalities paid 40 percent and the rural 60 percent).
3 Except for veterans, a person could not be admitted to a Saskatchewan sanatorium unless he or she had been a provincial resident for at least six months.
4 Otherwise, everyone with a doctor's certificate was entitled to receive care at the expense of the league.

The Act also provided that the league could arrange for vocational training or employment. It was in force from 1 January 1929. Middleton, "Health and Sickness Insurance," 604; "Evolution of Tuberculosis Control in Saskatchewan," 510; "Saskatchewan," *CTAAR*, 1928: 164.

39 "Saskatchewan," *CTAAR*, 1930: 104; Middleton, "Health and Sickness Insurance," 604; "Saskatchewan," *CTAAR*, 1929; 119; 1930: 102; "Saskatchewan," *CTAAR*, 1923: 152.

40 "Saskatchewan," *CTAAR*, 1930: 105.

41 Manitoba, *Report on Tuberculosis*, 58–99; "Manitoba," *CTAAR*, 1929: 52–3; 1930: 48–9.

42 Brink, "Control of Tuberculosis," 483; "New Brunswick," *CTAAR*, 1936: 63.

43 In Ontario a royal commission on public welfare presented a comprehensive and detailed report on health and welfare services in that province in 1930, but with the onset of the depression, no real action was taken on its recommendations in the case of tuberculosis until the

end of the decade. Brink, "Tuberculosis Control," 1–2; *CPHJ* 32 (Oct. 1941): 503–4; Brink, *Across the Years*, 21.

44 Jackson, "Public Health Nursing," 576–7; "Manitoba," *CTAAR*, 1934: 49.

45 Gibbon, *Three Centuries*, 340.

46 Dobbie, "A Provincial Program," 496.

47 *Vancouver Survey*, 42; "British Columbia," *CTAAR*, 1934: 34.

48 "British Columbia," *CTAAR*, 1935: 47; 1938: 32.

49 "British Columbia," *CTAAR*, 1936: 48; 1939: 40; G.M. Weir, "British Columbia Progress," *CTAB* 18 (Sept. 1939): 7.

50 "Report of Executive Office," *CTAAR*, 1937: 20.

51 Brink, "Recent Advances in Tuberculosis Control in Ontario," 503.

52 "Ontario," *CTAAR*, 1939: 51.

53 "Ontario's War on Tuberculosis," *CTAB* 18 (June 1939): 3; "Ontario," *CTAAR*, 1940: 61; Brink, "Recent Advances," 3–4.

54 "Ontario's War on Tuberculosis," *CTAAR*, 1937: 61.

55 "Report of Executive Office," *CTAAR*, 1936: 23–4.

56 "Report of Executive Office," *CTAAR*, 1935: 13–14; "Report of Executive Office," *CTAAR*, 1937: 19.

57 Wherrett, "Progress in Tuberculosis Control," 290.

58 "Report of Executive Office," *CTAAR*, 1938: 16.

59 "Saskatchewan," *CTAAR*, 1931: 120.

60 Native Canadians and cattle were the major sources of infection that, according to the league director, were slowing down the elimination of tuberculosis in Saskatchewan – the only fields where the federal government was, or should be, active. In 1936, two-thirds of the population were drinking untested raw milk, while as far as the aboriginal problem went, he acidly observed, "The Dominion government has not as yet seen fit to support the anti-tuberculosis work in Canada by providing leadership through an adequate programme for the prevention of this disease among its own wards." "Saskatchewan," *CTAAR*, 1937: 80, 81.

61 Cassidy, 301.

62 "Saskatchewan," *CTAAR*, 1938: 60; 1939: 63; 1940: 76.

63 Interest was shown in all provinces in health insurance during the thirties. In both Alberta (1935) and British Columbia (1936), health insurance acts were passed but never put into effect. The Alberta Act was repealed in 1942. In 1934 a committee of the Canadian Medical Association submitted a report on health insurance, setting up some guidelines. Doctors had a taste of it with relief schemes in Ontario and Winnipeg. Fleming, "Health Services," 15; Shillington, *Medicare in Canada*, 21–2, 35–8; Editorial, "Medical Relief," 187; Jackson, "Medical Care in Western Canada," 316–7. For more detailed information see, as well, Shillington, *Medicare in Canada*, chaps. 3–6; *Canadian Journal of Public Health*, 1934–39; Naylor, *Politics of Health Insurance*.

64 Estimates based on the number of beds per 100,000 population had definite and obvious limitations, for they did not take into account the extent of infection. A province such as Nova Scotia or Quebec, with a high mortality rate indicating widespread infection, required more accommodation to isolate all sufferers than one with a low rate. Thus, Nova Scotia could have 106 beds per 100,000 in 1932, and Alberta 31.4, while Nova Scotia had a tuberculosis death rate almost double Alberta's – 99.2 compared to 51.9. Estimates based on the number of beds per death was subject to criticism as well, especially in the Western provinces, where the aboriginal population was included in the death rate. This measurement masked, to a certain extent, the improvement occurring in the white population, especially when the Western provinces were compared to provinces with a much smaller native population. For example, Wodehouse calculated the 1931 tuberculosis death rate per 100,000 population, aboriginals and Metis excluded, to be the following:

| CAN | PEI | NS | NB | QC | ON | MB | SK | AB | BC |
|-----|-----|-----|-----|-----|-----|-----|-----|-----|-----|
| 68 | 76 | 100 | 81 | 110 | 47 | 47 | 27 | 31 | 70 |

In British Columbia the racial factor entered in again, since the Chinese, Japanese, and East Indian populations had higher rates. To what extent this was due to racial susceptibility and to what extent it was due to economic factors, however, was not determined. British Columbia was also supposed to attract more than its share of tuberculosis sufferers from other provinces, although this supposition was not determined either.

Wodehouse suggested as well that part of Quebec's poor showing as a province was the result of the situation in greater Montreal, which was bad enough to lower the provincial statistics. Wodehouse, "Tuberculosis Statistics," 434, 436–7; NAC CTA IIa, file 13, CTA Revised Table, Up to October 1, 1932.

65 "Report of Executive Office," CTAAR, 1935: 13; Wherrett, "Tuberculosis Control," 289.

66 "Report of Executive Office," CTAAR, 1935: 13; "Report of Executive Office," CTAAR, 1939: 24.

67 In 1938 Montreal had a rate of 74.8. Broken down by ethnic group the rate was as follows: French Canadians, 83.2; British, 53.9; and Jewish, 37.6. Dr Adelard Groulx, director of the Montreal Health Department, blamed inadequate facilities for the high French Canadian rate. Dr Gagnon also faulted the high birth rate, since it offered more opportunity for contacts, especially among the working class. "Public Support Sought," CTAB 17 (June 1939); 4; "Progress in the Cities,"

*CTAB* 17 (Mar. 1940): 3; "Tuberculosis in Montreal," *CTAB* 17 (Sept. 1938): 3.

68 "Public Support Sought," *CTAB* 17 (June 1939): 4.

69 Groulx, "Public Health in Montreal," 589–92.

70 See McGinnis, *From Health to Welfare.*

71 There was constant strife over the pensions until legislation in 1925 prevented a reduction greater than 20 percent, and only 20 percent, at intervals of at least six months. By 1929, the Board of Pension Commissioners, not the Department of Health, decided if a veteran deserved treatment, and the treatment branch of the department looked after him only if he received it. NAC CTA, IIa, file 93, H. Sloman (for Director of Administration) *Memorandum Regarding Tuberculous Ex-Soldiers,* (Ottawa: 4 May 1925). "Tuberculosis among Ex-Servicemen," *CTAAR,* 1926: 26; "Treatment of Tuberculous Ex-Soldiers," *CTAAR,* 1929: 28.

72 Canada, Acts of the Parliament of the Dominion of Canada, *An Act Respecting the Department of Health,* section 7, 1, Public General Acts (Ottawa: 1919): 89.

73 C.D. Parfitt, "The President's Address," *CTAAR, Papers on Tuberculosis,* 1924: 8.

74 Canada, House of Commons, *Debates,* 1919: CXXXV, 1374.

75 Ibid.

76 McCulough, "The Highway of Health," 145.

77 McGinnis, *From Health to Welfare,* 218–19.

78 Quoted in McGinnis, *From Health to Welfare,* 220.

79 Ibid., 231.

80 "Manitoba," *CTAAR,* 1932: 37.

81 Stewart, "Challenge of Tuberculosis," 109.

82 Stewart, "The Red Man and the White Plague," 19–20; Stewart, *Address to the Convention of the Union of Manitoba Municipalities,* 3.

83 "Report of the Executive Office," *CTAAR,* 1936: 29.

84 NAC CTA, IIa, file 34, D.A. Stewart to John Bracken, 14 Nov. 1934: 12.

85 "Brief Presented to Rowell Commission," *CTAB* 16 (Mar. 1938): 4.

86 R.G. Ferguson, "President's Address," *CTAB* 16 (Sept. 1937): 2; Watson, "Racial Incidence of Tuberculosis," 195.

87 Stewart, *Social Ramifications,* 8.

88 It carried this research out at the federal Department of Agriculture (Ottawa), the University of Alberta, Queen's, the University of Montreal, McGill, the University of Toronto, the Queen Alexandra Sanatorium (London, Ontario) and the Fort Qu'Appelle Sanatorium (Saskatchewan). The research in Saskatchewan was among the Plains Indians, the information being, it was explained candidly, "of first importance in the operation of tuberculosis campaigns among the

more immunized whites." "Review of Year," *CTAAR*, 1926: 8; "Saskatchewan Anti-Tuberculosis League," *CTAAR*, 1927: 130.

89 In 1937 the associate committee on medical research of the NRC was
formed, and the old associate committee on tuberculosis work was
transferred to it, under a new subcommittee on tuberculosis. "National
Research Council," *CTAAR*, 1934: 19–25; NAC CTA, III, file 6, C.B.
Stewart, Assistant Secretary, Associate Committee on Medical Research,
NRC to G.J. Wherrett, 15 Nov. 1938.

90 NAC CTA IIa, file 88: Statistical Cards, Dominion Bureau of Statistics.

91 Editorial, "Government Assistance in Public Health," 478.

92 R.J. Collins, "Reviewing the Case for National Aid," *CTAB* 17 (Mar.
1939): 2; McCullough, "Highway of Health," 145.

93 McKinnon, "Tuberculosis," 520.

94 Stewart, "Challenge of Tuberculosis," 113.

95 Editorial, "Public Health and the Economic Depression," 139.

96 R.G. Ferguson, "President's Address," *CTAAR*, 1936: 16.

## CHAPTER SIX

1 Richardson, *Century of the Child*, 15.

2 Lowe, Daniel, et al., "Pulmonary Tuberculosis in Children," 223–4.

3 Canada, Commission on Conservation. *Control of Bovine Tuberculosis*;
International Commission on Bovine Tuberculosis, *Tuberculosis*.

4 Mazyck P. Ravenel, "Animal Tuberculoses and Their Relation to Human
Health," *CAPCAR*, 1904: 50.

5 Sutherland, *Children in English-Canadian Society*, 39, 139–88.

6 Ibid., 56–8.

7 Ibid., 60.

8 Copp, *Anatomy of Poverty*, 96–7.

9 Hopkins, *Canadian Annual Review*, 1909: 407. In 1910 the *Public Health
Journal* revealingly listed several ways of spotting impure milk, unconsciously commenting on the state of much of the milk sold in the
country:

If milk contains sediment, it is unfit for use.
If milk sours quickly, it is probably full of bacteria.
If milk keeps sweet a long time, it probably contains formaldehyde.
Milk, to be pure, should be free from shreds. Shreds in the milk indi-
cate a diseased cow.
Milk containing bits of dirt and hairs should be refused.
Gelatine in milk can be detected by a peculiar "sickish" taste. "Impure
Milk," *PHJ* 1 (Dec. 1910): ix.

10 "Committee No. 4: Inspection of Schools and Examination of Children," CAPCAR, 1906: 102.
11 Sutherland, "To Create A Strong and Healthy Race," 317–8.
12 Minns, "Tuberculosis in the Public Schools," 902.
13 "Royal Edward Institute," CAPTAR, 1917: 175; "Hamilton Health Association," CAPTAR, 1915: 201.
14 Sutherland, Children in English-Canadian Society, 51.
15 J.H. Elliott, "Tuberculosis in Childhood," CAPTAR, 1913: 79–85.
16 F.S. Minns, "School Work against Tuberculosis," CAPTAR, 1917: 33–4; Burke, "Forest Schools," 9.
17 MacDougall, Activists and Advocates, 193.
18 "Heather Club," CAPTAR, 1909: 60; "Hamilton Health Association," CAPTAR, 1911: 140; "Royal Edward Institute," CAPTAR, 1916: 87; "National Sanitarium Association," CAPTAR, 1915: 164.
19 Copp, Anatomy of Poverty, 99; Tessier, "Milk Depots," 65; "Report of the Executive Council," CAPTAR, 1919: 9; Blackader, "Infantile Death Rate," 371–5.
20 Pratt, Osler and Tuberculosis.
21 "British Columbia Association," CAPTAR, 1906: 80.
22 "Dispensary Treatment," CAPTAR, 1910: 46–7.
23 Machado, "President's Address," CAPTAR, 1919: 71.
24 34 R.W. Bruce Smith, "The Relation of the State to the Tuberculosis Problem," CAPTAR, 1914: 61.
25 H.E. Young, "Health Units in British Columbia," 137.
26 T.M. Sieniewicz, "Prevention of Tuberculosis Applied in the School Age," CTAAR, 1922: 46.
27 CTAAR, Papers on Tuberculosis, 1925: 120; "IODE Preventorium" CTAAR, 1928: 112.
28 Sutherland, Children in English-Canadian Society, 69.
29 Seymour, "Milk Problems in Canada," 243.
30 Ferguson, "Pure Milk Supply," 154; McCullough, "How to Safeguard the Milk," 256.
31 Seymour, "Milk Problems," 395.
32 The percentage of milk sold that was pasteurized was as follows: Calgary, 95 percent; Hamilton, 98 percent; Saskatoon, 100 percent; Toronto, 100 percent; Vancouver 95 percent; Regina, 65 percent; Edmonton, 66 percent; Montreal, 60 percent. Only 33 percent of the milk sold in Quebec City was pasteurized, but 100 percent of the milk sold was from tuberculin tested herds. "Tabulated City Activities," CTAAR, 1922, frontispiece.
33 Stewart, Medicine in New Brunswick, 118–9; McCullough, "How to Safeguard the Milk," 257.
34 Ravenel, "Transmission of Animal Diseases," 182.

35 Editorial, "Compulsory Pasteurization of Milk Supplies," 91.
36 "Ontario" *CTAAR*, 1934: 86; Alan Brown, "The Value of Pasteurization," *NOT* 1 (July 1939): 4; Adrien Plouffe, "Milk and Tuberculosis," *NOT* 3 (Dec. 1940): 4.
37 Berry, "Pasteurization in Ontario," 209.
38 Saywell, *Mitchell F. Hepburn*, 374; quoted in McKenty, *Mitchell Hepburn*, 174–6.
39 Ibid., 176–7.
40 Ibid., 210–11.
41 52.Editorial, "Compulsory Pasteurization," 90–1.
42 McLeod, "Public Health Nurse," 457.
43 In a letter to Dr Alphone L'Esperance, over a decade later, G.J. Wherrett, executive secretary of the CTA, opined that the associate committee on tuberculosis of the National Research Council, formed ostensibly to do research on tuberculosis in general, "was really formed with the idea of investigating BCG to determine whether it had any practical application in the eradication of bovine tuberculosis." NAC CTA, III, file 6, G.F. Wherrett to Alphonse L'Esperance, Medical Superintendent of the Lake Edward Sanatorium, Quebec, 1 Nov. 1938.
44 Wherrett, *Empty Beds*, 62.
45 Nadeau, "The Grancher System," 382–4; "Quebec: Bureau of Health," *CTAAR*, 1929: 100–1; Defries, *Development of Public Health*, 22.
46 As quoted ibid.
47 Nadeau, "The Grancher System," 383.
48 Stewart, *The Tuberculous Man at Home*, 3.
49 "Montreal Anti-Tuberculosis and General Health League," *CTAAR* 1925: 121.
50 "Minutes," *CAPTAR*, 1920: 15.
51 Browne, "Health Education in Rural Schools," 533–4; Russell, "Public Health Nursing," 33.
52 Flora C. Liggett, "Junior Red Cross in Nova Scotia," *CTAAR, Papers on Tuberculosis*, 1925: 13; Perry, "A Logical Highroad to Health," 61.
53 "St John County Hospital, IODE Preventorium," *CTAAR*, 1926: 63, 107.
54 The rate of infection of white school children in Saskatchewan was reduced from a probable 80 percent in 1910 to 10 percent in 1934. R.G. Ferguson, "President's Address," *CTAAR*, 1936: 16; NAC CTA, III, file 6, R.G. Ferguson, "Research in Vaccination Against Tuberculosis" (enclosed in letter to G.J. Wherrett, 2 Feb. 1939): 1; Stewart, *Tuberculosis*, 2.
55 "Mountain Sanatorium," *CTAAR*, 1936: 182; "Ontario, New Brunswick," *CTAAR*, 1935: 81, 63; NAC CTA, III, file 33, F.E. Lathe, "Notes on Preventorium Survey," memorandum to file 4-M4–28 (30 Mar. 1944).
56 MacDougall, *Activists and Advocates*, 196.

57 *Vancouver Survey*, 36, 39. The Vancouver Committee suggested turning the preventorium into a hospital to treat children with active tuberculosis and assessed the costs of preventorium treatment as it was and foster home treatment:

| *Relative Costs* | | *Per Annum,*<br>*for 26 Children* |
|---|---|---|
| Preventorium | | |
| ($1.41 7/8 per diem) | $43.14 per month | $13,460.00 |
| City foster homes ($4.00/week) | $17.33 per month | $ 5,407.00 |
| Children's aid foster homes | $14.50 per month | $ 4,524.00 |

The savings from placing these 26 children in foster homes would be $8,936.00 per annum according to the Vancouver Survey.

58 By 1936 family placement had sent 1,046 children, aged two to twelve years, to the country for a period of one to five years, at a rough cost of $125.00 per child. They were supervised by the visiting nurse and examined and x-rayed twice a year by the tuberculosis clinician. Out of the 1,046 children cared for by 1936, only 8 developed tuberculosis. Of the 671 children who left their foster homes after a year or more,

- 118 were recalled by their parents and returned to tubercular homes. The recall was supposedly motivated in most cases by a desire to obtain more relief money.
- 64 returned to infected homes after reaching the age limit (thirteen).
- 35 were adopted by their foster parents.
- 126 were institutionalized (e.g., in orphanages, convents, model farms).
- 307 returned home after the tubercular parent died.
- 10 left the foster homes as a result of illnesses other than tuberculosis.

Since children were returned home at the age of thirteen, it was obvious that the Grancher System, like the preventoria, failed to come to grips with the problem of tuberculosis in youths. Nor was it practised to the degree necessary to make a real dent in the Quebec tuberculosis problem – for in 1936 it was estimated that there were approximately 25,000 cases of active tuberculosis, which meant that roughly 20,000 dwellings were infected, with 25,000 to 30,000 children in danger of contamination. "British Columbia," CTAAR, 1934: 47; "Family Placement in Quebec," CTAAR, 1936: 151–6.

59 "Surveys of Young Canadians," CTAB, 15 (Dec. 1936): 8.

60 Fraser, "Man's Attitude," 591; Davidson, "Tuberculosis Contact," 259.
61 In Quebec the provincial government paid some compensation for animals slaughtered under this plan, as an incentive to farmers. "Department of Agriculture, Health of Animals Branch," CTAAR, 1934: 19.
62 "Department of Agriculture," CTAAR, 1933: 23; CTAAR, 1940: 44–5.
63 CTA, Intensive Community Campaign, 207.
64 Orr, "Role of the General Practitioner," 574.
65 J.A. Vidal, "Mass Detection Campaign Soon To Extend over Entire Province of Quebec," NOT 9 (Apr./May 1947): 1–2.
66 In 1947 at the request of the division of tuberculosis prevention, it became a junior sanatorium admitting only children with active tuberculosis for institutional care. In 1954 the number of admissions began to decline, and in 1959 the hospital ceased to function as a children's sanatorium. NAC CTA, IIa, file 63, G.J. Wherrett to F.E. Lathe, 11 Apr. 1944; Brink, Across the Years, 44.

CHAPTER SEVEN

1 R.J. Collins, "Address of the President," CTAAR, 1939: 12.
2 Adamson, "Canada Eliminates Tuberculosis from the Army," 163.
3 John McEarchern, "President's Address," CTAAR, 1940: 11.
4 Creighton, The Forked Road, 18, 19.
5 Ibid., 22, 24.
6 Ibid., 37.
7 John McEachern, "President's Address," CTAAR, 1940: 11. It cost $2.00 per person.
8 Editorial, "Halt Tuberculosis," 1.
9 The x-ray on discharge would clear up difficulties over pension claims, which had been such a problem after World War 1. "Report of Executive Office," CTAAR, 1940: 34.
10 Wherrett, "Tuberculosis in Wartime," 440; Jones, "Routine Chest X-ray Examination," 213; Editorial, "A New Attack on Tuberculosis," 562.
11 Adamson et al., "Tuberculosis in the Canadian Army," 127; NAC CTA IIa, file 73, R.J.Collins to H.H. Hale, 16 Jan. 1943.
12 Creighton, Forked Road, 48.
13 "The Pre-Employment Check-Up," CTAB 26 (Dec. 1947): 4; Fleming, "Public Health in Wartime," 146.
14 Editorial, "Health Training in Schools," 178.
15 Campbell, Holbrook, 158; "Tuberculosis and Industry," CTAB 20 (Dec. 1941): 2; "British Columbia," CTAAR, 1942: 40; Thomas, "Increased Tuberculosis Mortality," 19.
16 Ladoceur, "Fight against Tuberculosis," 24.
17 "Hens Suffer War Privations," CTAB 21 (Mar. 1943): 6.

18 "The Fifth Freedom" *CTAB* 21 (Dec. 1942): 6.

19 "More Mass Surveys," *CTAB* 21 (Sept. 1942): 8.

20 "Memorial to Federal Government," *CTAAR*, 1939: 9, "Sanatorium Changes during the War," *CTAB* 22 (June 1944):1.

21 J.H. Holbrook, "President's Address: Tuberculosis and the All-Out War Effort," *CTAAR*, 1942: 10.

22 "New Brunswick," *CTAAR* 1942: 49; "Manitoba," *CTAAR*, 1943: 42; 1944: 50; "Nova Scotia," *CTAAR*, 1943: 49; 1944: 55; "Ontario," *CTAAR*, 1943: 56.

23 "British Columbia," *CTAAR*, 1941: 34; Hatfield, *Tuberculosis in British Columbia*, vol. 2, 49–50, 52; "Nova Scotia," *CTAAR*, 1942: 63; "British Columbia," *CTAAR*, 1942: 40; Wherrett, "Challenge of Tuberculosis," *CTAAR*, 1943: 17.

24 The war had a double-edged effect on the pasteurization issue. Although the war made it difficult to obtain equipment, the requirements of the armed forces for safe milk supplies for the troops focused attention in many communities on the unsafe conditions, and led to the introduction of pasteurization plants and a program of milk control. By 1952 over 80 percent of all milk marketed in Canada was pasteurized. "Quebec," *CTAAR*, 1949: 85; Editorial, "Compulsory Pasteurization," 389–90; Groulx, "Pasteurization in the Province of Quebec," 17–21; Canada, *Tuberculosis Services in Canada*, 23.

25 "Minutes of Annual Meeting," *CTAAR*, 1942: 9; "Report of Executive Office," *CTAAR*, 1944: 17–8; "Minutes of Annual Meeting," *CTAAR*, 1944: 12; "Report of Executive Office," *CTAAR*, 1945: 14; "Sanatorium Changes during the War," *CTAB*, 22 (June 1944): 1.

26 Cassidy, *Public Health and Welfare Reorganization*, 140.

27 "Report of Executive Office," *CTAAR*, 1944: 18; "Quebec," *CTAAR*, 1944: 62–3.

28 "Saskatchewan," *CTAAR*, 1943: 69; The cost rose from $718,086.91 to $774,908.58; "Saskatchewan," *CTAAR*, 1944: 661–7, 1945: 45.

29 Creighton, *Forked Road*, 53.

30 Ibid., 78, 80, 82.

31 Ibid., 108.

32 Ibid., 115.

33 Ibid., 159, 160, 175.

34 J.H. Holbrook, "President's Address: Tuberculosis and the All-Out War Effort," *CTAAR*, 1942: 16.

35 Claxton, "Mapping Our New Frontiers of Health," 464.

CHAPTER EIGHT

1 Creighton, *Forked Road*, 243–4, 119, 121.

2 Dobbie, "The First Forty Years," 19; "Manitoba," *CTAAR*, 1940: 54; Wherrett, "Tuberculosis Problem," 298; "British Columbia," *CTAAR*, 1939: 40.

3 Wherrett, "Tuberculosis Problem," 298; "Ontarion," *CTAAR*, 1942: 63.

4 "Ontario," *CTAAR*, 1948: 71; NAC CTA, IIa, file 60, Montreal Anti-Tuberculosis League, letter.

5 "Minutes of Annual Meeting," *CTAAR*, 1943: 7; Ferguson, "Tuberculosis Control," 111; Miller, "Knowledge of Tuberculosis," 245.

6 Brink, "Tuberculosis Control," 3.

7 Wherrett, "First Aid in Tuberculosis," 7.

8 J.D. Adamson, "Presidential Address," *CTAAR*, 1946: 16.

9 NAC CTA, Ib, file 8, *Report of the Conference of Provincial Secretaries,* 10.

10 Holling, "Tuberculosis Case-Finding Techniques," 2, 3; "British Columbia," *CTAAR*, 1949: 42.

11 "Report of Executive Office," *CTAAR*, 1949; 20–1; Lee, "Patients in Sanatoria," 376; "Group X-raying Proves Its Worth," *CTAB* 27 (June 1949): 4; "Report of Executive Office," *CTAAR*, 1945: 16.

12 "Saskatchewan," *CTAAR*, 1947: 68; 1950: 91; "Manitoba," *CTAAR*, 1948: 50; "Ontario," *CTAAR*, 1942: 64; "Saskatchewan," *CTAAR*, 1949: 86.

13 "Quebec," *CTAAR*, 1949: 81.

14 Herman Gauthier, "Mechanized Anti-Tuberculosis Detection in Gaspesia," *NOT* 13 (Aug. 1950): 2.

15 "Saskatchewan," *CTAAR*, 1950: 91; "British Columbia," *CTAAR*, 1949: 42; *Tuberculosis Services in Canada,* 50.

16 J.D. Adamson, "Presidential Address," *CTAAR*, 1946: 17.

17 Editorial, "A New Attack on Tuberculosis," *CPHJ* 31 (Nov. 1940): 563.

18 Adamson and Edmison, "Immigration Tuberculosis," 432–4.

19 Bennett, "Tuberculosis in Recent Immigrants," 529.

20 NAC CTA, IIa, file 79, T.A. Crerar to G.J. Wherrett, 18 Dec. 1943; Adamson and Edmison, "Immigration Tuberculosis," 434.

21 "Report of Executive Office," *CTAAR*, 1950: 21; "Report of Executive Office," *CTAAR*, 1949: 20.

22 In Ontario, hospital admission x-rays were covered as well by workmen's compensation and most health insurance schemes and hospital prepayment plans. By 1949, 65 percent of the general hospitals in Ontario had miniature film equipment installed with the help of federal grants. "Nova Scotia," *CTAAR*, 1947: 52; "Ontario," *CTAAR*, 1948: 71; 1949: 66; "Manitoba," *CTAAR*, 1949: 46; "New Brunswick," *CTAAR*, 1949: 52–3; 1950: 54; "British Columbia," *CTAAR*, 1950: 42; "Group X-raying Proves Its Worth," *CTAB* 27 (June 1949): 4.

23 This figure excluded Prince Edward Island and Quebec, for which no figures were available. Wherrett, "Canada's Tuberculosis Services," 97.

24 Miller, "New Knowledge of Tuberculosis," 245.

25 Mayer, "Recent Advances in Tuberculosis," 565.

26 NAC CTA, IIa, file 94, G.J. Wherrett to Lt-Col E.J. Young, "Memorandum," 24 Aug. 1948.

27 "Report of Executive Office," CTAAR, 1948: 23; "Quebec," CTAAR, 1950: 87; Tuberculosis Services in Canada, 40.

28 Hatfield, "Tuberculosis Control," 424.

29 NAC CTA, III, file 7, F.E. Lathe to R.G. Ferguson, 16 Jan. 1946.

30 NAC CTA, III, file 6, G.J. Wherrett to Mary Dempsey, 15 Mar. 1945.

31 "Saskatchewan," CTAAR, 1946: 67.

32 "Ontario," CTAAR, 1947: 57; "Ontario," CTAAR, 1948: 71.

33 Lasalle Laberge, "The Work of the Anti-Tuberculosis Clinicians in 1941," NOT 4 (Apr. 1942): 1.

34 "Saskatchewan and Manitoba," CJPH 36 (Apr. 1945): 171; Nix, "Public Health Services," 182–3.

35 "Report of Executive Office," CTAAR, 1939: 24; J.H. Holbrook, "President's Address," CTAAR, 1942: 16; "Resolutions Committee," CTAAR, 1943:9.

36 Brink, "Tuberculosis Control," 3.

37 "Alberta," CTAAR, 1944: 39; "British Columbia," CTAAR, 1945: 28; "Manitoba," CTAAR, 1950: 49; A.R. Foley, "Tuberculosis and the War," NOT 5 (July–Aug. 1943): 4; "Undiagnosed Tuberculosis in Elderly Persons," NOT 6 (Nov. 1943): 1.

38 Specialists were finding that the "reinfection" form of the disease (chronic pulmonary tuberculosis) was developing even in those, such as medical and nursing students, who were definitely tuberculin negative before a recent exposure. Opinion varied as to what this meant. One school of thought claimed that this was still primary tuberculosis, which often took the form of a chronic process in adults and was no different from the "reinfection" form; another school thought the process was due to endogenous or exogenous reinfection quickly following the primary infection, assuming that the period of latency was shortened; and a third felt that it was reinfection following an evanescent type of primary infection that had occurred years ago, making the lesion appear as a cross between primary and reinfection disease. How much bearing this theoretical discussion had on medical practice was best expressed by Dr A.M. Jeffry in 1943. "After puzzling for a long time as to exactly what was meant by primary disease," he confessed," and "after vainly trying to fit it into what we saw at the clinics, I finally derived much peace of mind by just forgetting all about it ... In conclusion it would seem more reasonable to avoid classification of pulmonary tuberculosis and simply remember that granted that infection has occurred, then dangerous pulmonary tuberculosis follows

puberty rather than former benign disease." Mayer, "Recent Advances in Tuberculosis," 565–6; NAC CTA, III, file 34, A.M. Jeffry, "Classifications of Disease," (typed manuscript): 6–7.

39 Hatfield, *Handbook on Tuberculosis*, 25–31; Dr Carmichael, "President's Address," *CTAAR*, 1943: 13.

40 Grant Fleming, "The Tuberculosis Problem," *NOT* 3 (Apr. 1941): 2.

41 "Alberta," *CTAAR*, 1941: 32; "British Columbia," *CTAAR*, 1945: 28.

42 "Minutes of Annual Meeting," *CTAAR*, 1946: 11; "Report of Executive Office," *CTAAR*, 1946: 21; "Alberta," *CTAAR*, 1946: 36; "British Columbia," *CTAAR*, 1946: 40; "British Columbia," *CTAAR*, 1949: 41.

43 Brink, *Across the Years*, 52.

44 Adamson, "Presidential Address," *CTAAR*, 1946: 14

45 Burke, "Tuberculosis,"156–7.

46 Wherrett, *Tuberculosis in Canada*, 29–30.

47 "Ontario," *CTAAR*, 1945: 39.

48 Hatfield, "Tuberculosis Control," 423.

49 Wherrett, "The Challenge of Tuberculosis," *CTAAR*, 1943: 17.

50 Wherrett, "Tuberculosis Problem," 299; Hatfield, "Tuberculosis Control," 425.

51 Wherrett, "Tuberculosis in Wartime," 444; Mayer, "Advances in Tuberculosis," 568.

52 The BC division reported a 400 percent increase in surgery from 1946 to 1950. "British Columbia," *CTAAR*, 1950: 44.

53 "Manitoba," *CTAAR*, 1953: 57; NAC CTA, Id., file 2, G.J. Wherrett, "The Effect of New Treatments on the Organization of the Fight against Tuberculosis in Canada," (typewritten manuscript 1957?): 1.

54 "British Columbia," *CTAAR*, 1953: 35.

55 "Report of Executive Office," *CTAAR*, 1952: 26.

56 Brink, "Tuberculosis Control," 4.

57 Ibid.

58 Ibid.

59 "British Columbia," *CTAAR*, 1944: 44; "Tuberculosis Allowances in British Columbia," *CTAB* 25 (Sept. 1946): 6; "British Columbia," *CTAAR*, 1950: 47.

60 Fenton, "Public Health Nurse," 187–8.

61 Wicks, "Post-Sanatorium Care," 269.

62 Hatfield, "Rehabilitation," 217.

63 "Alberta," *CTAAR*, 1946: 34; "British Columbia," *CTAAR*, 1946: 43; 1949: 38; "Nova Scotia," *CTAAR*, 1949: 63; "New Brunswick," *CTAAR*, 1950: 54; "Ontario," *CTAAR*, 1950: 77; "Prince Edward Island," *CTAAR*, 1950: 79; *Tuberculosis Services in Canada*, 22, 30, 34, 36, 48, 51, 57, 61.

64 "Modern Conception of Rehabilitation," *CTAB* 25 (Sept. 1946): 7.

65 Collins, "After-Care and Rehabilitation," 215.

66 Ryan, "Mystic Order of the Bug," 17.

67 This conference was held in February 1951 and attended by representatives from the ten provincial governments and the national agencies, including the CTA. They stressed the need for an overall, national program and recommended that the federal government appoint a coordinator and form a national council. "Report of Executive Office," *CTAAR*, 1950: 21; "National Rehabilitation Program Recommended By Conference," *CTAB* 29 (Mar. 1951): 4.

68 NAC CTA V, file 5, G.J. Wherrett, "Present Concepts of the Best Use of Christmas Seal Funds." (Typed manuscript, n.d.): 5.

69 The provinces were organizing and extending their authority in the whole field of public health. Both Manitoba and Saskatchewan enacted new health legislation, the latter extending free treatment to those suffering from poliomyelitis, cancer, venereal disease, and mental illness and providing free medical and hospital care for recipients of old age pensions, blind persons' pensions, and mother's allowances and for wards of the Children's Aid Society. As well, the province would now give financial aid toward the construction of hospitals and health centres under a scheme that combined local control and initiative with centralized (provincial) direction and assistance. As a result Saskatchewan, the first to initiate free treatment for one chronic illness, had assumed total responsibility for other costly and chronic illnesses, along with the costs of medical care for those least able to pay. Vidal, "Mass Detection," 1; "Free Health Service Plan in Saskatchewan," *CJPH* 36 (Jan. 1945): 44; Sheps, "Saskatchewan Plans Health Services," 178, 180.

70 "Free Treatment in Winnipeg," *CTAB* 21 (Mar. 1943): 3; "Report of Executive Office," *CTAAR*, 1949: 22; "Alberta," *CTAAR*, 1942: 36; "Report of Executive Office," *CTAAR*, 1947: 23; "Ontario," *CTAAR*, 1950: 73; *Tuberculosis Services in Canada*, 55.

71 "British Columbia," *CTAAR*, 1943: 39; "Ontario," *CTAAR*, 1950: 77; "Ontario Takes Forward Step," *CTAB* 28 (Mar. 1950): 6; E.L. Ruddy, "Address," *CTAAR*, 1944: 16; "Report of Executive Office," *CTAAR*, 1947: 25.

72 "Alberta," *CTAAR*, 1950: 31.

73 "PEI Sets Good Example," *CTAB* 23 (Dec. 1944): 7; "Alberta," *CTAAR*, 1949: 36; "British Columbia," *CTAAR*, 1949; 37–8, 42; *Tuberculosis Services in Canada*, 35.

74 Hatfield, "Tuberculosis Control," 423.

75 NAC CTA, IIa, file 69: Non-residents. "British Columbia," *CTAAR*, 1944: 43.

76 NAC CTA, IIa file 69, J.J. Holbrook to G.J. Wherrett, 12 Jan. 1944.

77 "Reciprocity in TB Treatment," *CTAB* 24 (Mar. 1946): 8; Hatfield, "Some Thoughts on Tuberculosis Control," 427.

78 The provincial committee continued, as well, with an annual subsidy under Bill 31. "Quebec," *CTAAR*, 1946: 61–2; "Annual Meeting," *CTAAR*, 1947: 11; "Bill No. 31 – An Act to Combat Tuberculosis," *NOT* 8 (Apr. 1946): 1–2; "Quebec," *CTAAR*, 1949: 74.

79 The actual number of available beds rose from 2,957 in 1941 to 5,494 in 1950. "Quebec," *CTAAR*, 1941: 56, 58; 1950: 83–4.

80 "Report of Executive Office," *CTAAR*, 1947: 22; "Close-ups of TB in Montreal and Toronto," *CTAB* 28 (Dec. 1949): 4.

81 "Report of Executive Office," *CTAAR*, 1947: 22.

82 Dr A. Groulx, director of Montreal's department of health, further broke down the death rate in that city by race and language. In 1947 the total city rate was 56.4; but the mortality rate for French Canadians was 61.4; 43.8 for British (including English-speaking) Canadians 24.2 for the Jewish population; and 69.3 for other races. Groulx attributed the low rate among the Jewish people to the fact that "through the ages biological modifications had been acquired which conferred to the Jewish group a degree of natural immunity to various disease not shared by other ethnical groups." In other words, they had acquired some resistance to tuberculosis as a result of constant exposure. This "racial susceptibility" theory had been used in varying degrees before in Canada, notably to explain high rates in native Canadians and the Japanese and Chinese in British Columbia. It was supported by the epidemic course the disease often took in previously unexposed groups. (This is discussed further in chapter 10.)

   Another explanation would be that the Jewish community, which had a stringent hygienic code and which provided better treatment facilities and accommodation for its own community members, controlled the disease more effectively. Evidence to support this theory is found in the fact that although the 1910 Royal Commission suggested, as Terry Copp points out, a high incidence among the Jewish immigrants, the Montreal survey of 1928 reported them having the lowest rate of the three ethnic groups, *as well as* the most extensive facilities. The same was true in 1938, when Montreal's death rate was 74.8 per 100,000; the French rate was 83.2, the British 53.9, and the Jewish 37.6. Since the immigrants were seldom well-off, this indicated to some the importance of both personal hygiene and community responsibility in demanding adequate facilities to deal with the disease. This explanation would probably be less popular, however, as it reflected badly on the provisions made by the French Canadian community in Montreal for its own members. "Increase in Montreal," *CTAB* 22 (Sept. 1943): 2; "Close-ups of TB in Montreal and Toronto," 4; "Manitoba," *CTAAR*, 1949: 47; "Quebec," *CTAAR*, 1949: 74.

83 NAC CTA, IIa, file 12, G.J. Wherrett to J.F. Macdonald, 27 Jan. 1948.

84 Editorial, "Federal Government Assistance," 478; Editorial, "County Health Units," 30; Editorial, "Public Health Charter," 347.

85 Bothwell, "Health of the Common People," 191–220.

86 Editorial, "Federal Government Assistance," 479; Campbell, "Full-Time Health Services," 389.

87 CLIOA, "National Health Insurance," 150.

88 CTA, "Memorandum of Tuberculosis in Canada," submitted to the Select Committee of the House of Commons on Social Security, April 1943, *CTAAR*, 1942: 79–87.

89 NAC CTA, IV, file 3 G.J. Wherrett to Ian Mackenzie, 23 Oct. 1943.

90 NAC CTA, IV, file 3, J.J. Heagerty to G.J. Wherrett, 29 Aug. 1945; G.J. Wherrett to J.J. Heagerty, 29 Aug. 1945.

91 NAC CTA, IV, file 3, "Tuberculosis (Revised Copy)" (Typed manuscript, n.d.).

92 NAC CTA, IV, file 4, CTA, "Director of Division of Tuberculosis," (delivered to Dr Chisholm on 19 July 1945).

93 These included the departments of National Health and Welfare, Indian Affairs, Defense (Medical Services), Canadian Pension Commission, Bureau of Statistics, National Research Council, Northwest Territories Council. NAC CTA, IV, file 4, "The Division of Tuberculosis Control of the Department of National Health and Welfare" (enclosed with letter, G.J. Wherrett to Dr G.D.W. Cameron, 9 Oct. 1946): 1–3.

94 The grant was disbursed as follows:

| Province | Amount ($) |
|----------|-----------|
| PEI | 46,774 |
| NS | 182,585 |
| NB | 142,598 |
| QC | 1,069,564 |
| ON | 740,751 |
| MB | 187,998 |
| SK | 173,787 |
| AB | 183,203 |
| BC | 272,740 |

NAC CTA, IV, file 3, PC 3406, certified to be a true copy of a minute of a meeting of the Privy Council, appointed by His Excellency the Governor General on 28 July 1948, 1.

95 The Tuberculosis Control Grant and Hospital Construction Grant were only part of the National Health Program, which also included the following annual grants. When two figures are given, the first figure is the initial maximum amount disbursed, rising over a five-year period to the second, maximum amount.

1 *Health Survey Grants*: $625,000 (total, not annual, amount), to determine what each province needed.

2 National Health Grants
General Public Health Grant: $4,404,000 to $6,500,000, to prevent epidemic disease, lower child and maternal mortality, and fight polio, arthritis, and rheumatism.

| | |
|---|---|
| Tuberculosis Control Grant | $3,000,000 to $4,000,000 |
| Mental Health Care Grant | $4,000,000 to $7,000,00 |
| Venereal Disease Control Grant | $ 500,000 |
| Crippled Children's Grant | $ 500,000 |
| Professional Training Grant | $ 500,000 |
| Public Health Research Grant | $ 100,000 to $500,000 |
| Cancer Control Grant | $3,500,000 |

3 *Hospital Construction Grant*: up to $13,000,000 per year. (Martin, "A National Health Program," 220–3. "Report of Executive Office," CTAAR, 1948: 21; 1950: 22.

96 The estimate does not include the Hospital Construction Grants, which amounted to $4,761,000 by 1953–4. *Tuberculosis Services in Canada*, 9, 62.

97 Ibid.; "Quebec," CTAAR, 1949: 75; "Report of Executive Office," CTAAR, 1948: 22.

98 Layton, "National Health Grants," 370.

99 NAC CTA, IIa, file 12, G.J. Wherrett to J.K. Macdonald, 26 Feb. 1949.

100 The actual amount was $1,555,954. This total was exclusive of Montreal. "Christmas Seal Sale," CTAAR, 1950: 29.

101 "Ontario," CTAAR, 1948: 71; Holling, "Tuberculosis Case-Finding," 4.

102 "Alberta," CTAAR, 1947: 35.

103 "Annual Meeting," CTAAR, 1946: 11.

104 "Behind the Scenes of a City-Wide Survey," CTAB 22 (June 1944): 4; NAC CTA, Ib, file 8, *Mass Surveys: Report of the Conference of Provincial Tuberculosis Secretaries* (Ottawa: 26 May 1948): 11.

105 "City-Wide Survey," 4.

106 Ibid.: "Alberta," CTAAR, 1948: 38; NAC CTA, III, file 45, Leslie M. Rimes, manuscript of radio broadcast, enclosed with letter, Elizabeth Hodgson to G.J. Wherrett, 5 Mar. 1945.

107 "Mass Surveys in the Porcupine Area," CTAB 23 (Dec. 1944): 3; Dr Herman Gauthier, "Mechanized Anti-Tuberculosis Detection in Gaspesia," NOT 13 (Aug. 1950): 3.

108 Dr Herman Gauthier, a traveling diagnostician and the medical superintendent of the St Georges Sanatorium at Mont Joli, outlined the steps to prepare for a mass survey in Quebec, including assembling equipment and staff; notifying the curé, health unit staff, and local doctors; arranging for movies, sending out posters to the health unit and patch-

testing children under twelve. In all the detail he lists, however, there is no mention of the lay volunteers so crucial to the mass surveys in the rest of Canada. Their unimportance in the campaign in rural Quebec is striking. Ibid.

109 "City-Wide Survey," 4; "Alberta," *CTAAR*, 1948: 38; Rimes, manuscript of radio broadcast. Gauthier, "Mechanized Anti-Tuberculosis Detection," 2; "New Brunswick," *CTAAR*, 1947: 50; "Nova Scotia," *CTAAR*, 1949: 63; NAC CTA, IIa, file 70, G.J. Wherrett to Mrs K.L. Dawson, 15 Apr. 1946.

110 NAC CTA IIa, file 70, G.J. Wherrett to Mrs K.L. Dawson, 15 Apr. 1946.

111 NAC CTA, Ib, file 1, C. Robert Dickey to G.J. Wherrett, 27 Oct. 1943.

112 NAC CTA, IIa, file 26, A.R. Grant to G.J. Wherrett, 20 May 1944.

113 Ibid., 3 Oct. 1944.

114 Occasionally the seal sale got caught up in small-town prejudices and disputes that Grant had to try to untangle. In Woodstock, New Brunswick, for example, there was a fight with the postmaster over the return postage, which seemed to hinge on the fact that the seal sale director was not a native of the town – he had lived there only twenty-five years. Ibid., 10 Oct. 1944; Sept. 1944.

115 Nova Scotia, New Brunswick, Prince Edward Island, Quebec, and British Columbia had already formed provincial associations. The Ontario Tuberculosis Association was organized in 1945. In Manitoba and Saskatchewan, the whole campaign was run by the sanatorium board and league respectively. In 1946 the New Brunswick Tuberculosis Association was reorganized and the Nova Scotia Tuberculosis Commission was recognized as the Nova Scotia Association. Adamson, "Presidential Address," *CTAAR*, 1946: 13.

116 King, "Historical Study," 203.

117 NAC CTA, IIa, file 70, G.J. Wherrett to Mrs K.L. Dawson, 15 Apr. 1946; "Alberta," *CTAAR*, 1949: 33; 1950: 32–3; "Quebec," *CTAAR*, 1947: 65; "Ontario," *CTAAR*, 1946: 58.

118 "Alberta," *CTAAR*, 1950: 36.

119 Wherrett, *Provincial Committee on Tuberculosis*, quoted in King, "Historical Study," 288.

120 "Ontario," *CTAAR*, 1953: 92.

121 In Toronto the campaign was run by the National Sanitarium Association. It used CTA seals and paid the printer's cost plus 10 percent. It also paid for the educational material it used. The campaign in Montreal was essentially a subscription campaign. The CTA received a percentage of the seal sale, but few seals were sold there. NAC CTA, IV, file 5, "Excerpt from Minutes of Meeting of Executive Council, Canadian Tuberculosis Association, Calgary, 9 Sept. 1946," 1.

122 "Ontario," *CTAAR*, 1947: 56.

123 NAC CTA, IIa, file 59, G.J. Wherrett to Lionel Brittle, 29 Aug. 1942; G.J. Wherrett to Henry Fyon, 23 Jan. 1940.

124 NAC CTA, IIa, file 60, G.J. Wherrett to J.A. Couillard, 5 June 1943.

125 Ibid., C.O. Monat, president of the Montreal Anti-Tuberculosis League, to G.J. Wherrett, 25 Apr. 1944.

126 The Montreal Anti-Tuberculosis League president, C.O. Monat, insisted that the CTA was reimbursed for this, since the Montreal League gave the CTA $10,253.23 at the end of the first campaign. Ibid.

127 Ibid., quoted in Geo. Gregoire to C.O. Monat, 23 May 1944, 2.

128 Ibid. Geo. Gregoire to C.O. Monat, 23 May 1944, 2.

129 Ten percent of the receipts went to the CTA, 5 percent to the provincial committee.

130 NAC CTA, IIa, file 60, Gregoire to Monat, 23 May 1944, 1.

131 Ibid., J.M. Turgeon to G.J. Wherrett, 12 June 1944.

132 Wherret, *Montreal Anti-Tuberculosis League*, cited in King, "Historical Study," 355.

133 See NAC CTA, IIa file 6: Associated Canadian Travellers, especially G.J. Wherrett to R.G. Ferguson, 21 Oct 1946; and G.J. Wherrett to E.L. Ross, 4 Oct. 1946.

134 "Annual Report of Executive Office," *CTAAR*, 1942: 21; 1943: 28; Wherrett, "Health Conditions and Medical and Hospital Services," 49–60. NAC CTA, IV, file 4, B.D.B. Layton to G.J. Wherrett, 22 Dec. 1954.

135 "Report of Executive Office," *CTAAR*, 1946: 27; 1948: 25; 1949: 25.

136 The same seal was used in the United States, Great Britain, and Canada from 1943 onwards. From 1944–45 to 1945–46, particularly as a result of the Ontario Tuberculosis Association organizing more local associations, the number of seals used in Canada increased from 174 million to 236 million. Costs went from $33,995.48 to $48,407.59. "Christmas Seal Sale," *CTAAR*, 1941: 21; NAC CTA, IV, file 5, "Fiscal Review: Canadian Tuberculosis Association," 3–4.

137 NAC CTA, V, file 5, G.J. Wherrett to T.A.J. Cunnings, 4 June 1945.

138 "Report of Executive Office," *CTAAR*, 1948: 25; NAC CTA, IV, file 4, "Canadian Tuberculosis Association: Grant: $20,250," 2; C.J.W. Beckwith, "President's Address," *CTAAR*, 1950: 14.

139 "Report of Executive Office," *CTAAR*, 1943: 26–7; "Minutes of Annual Meeting," *CTAAR*, 1944: 10; "Report of Executive Office," *CTAAR*, 1947: 26; NAC CTA, IIa, file 12, Canadian Life Insurance Officers Association, "Annual Report of the Standing Committee on Public Health."

140 The Rockefeller Foundation, however, continued to be active in Canada through its International Health Division. From 1924, when it supported the establishment of a School of Hygiene at the university of Toronto to train public health workers, it had aided the development of health units and training programs for public health nurses at the

Universities of Toronto and British Columbia, aided surveys in Western Canada, helped develop Dalhousie University as a medical centre, erected the Dalhousie Public Health Clinic, and assisted in establishing the Cape Breton Island Health Unit and in organizing a metropolitan health area for Vancouver. As well, it made large contributions towards capital expenditures of Canadian universities' medical schools. In 1943 it surveyed and reported on health services in the city of Halifax. By 1945 the foundation had granted 166 fellowships for postgraduate training in public health to Canadian nurses and physicians, and its undertakings in Canadian public health represented an investment of several million dollars. That year the foundation opened a Canadian office in Toronto and appointed one of its senior members to direct its program in Canada. NAC CTA, IIa, file 12, G.J. Wherrett to J.D. Macdonald, 26 Feb. 1949; Editorial, "Rockefeller Foundation in Canada," 74–5; Beckwith, "Tuberculosis Control," 484; Editorial, "Rockefeller Foundation in Canada," 338–9.

141 Grant, "Health Education," 254.

142 "Our Knowledge and Our Efforts Have to Act on the Mass like a Tiny Portion of Yeast," *NOT* 11 (June–Aug. 1949): 1.

143 "The Seal Sale Comes of Age," *CTAB* 36 (Dec. 1947): 3.

144 "Nova Scotia," *CTAAR*, 1947: 55; 1949: 62; "Ontario," *CTAAR*, 1949: 70; "British Columbia," *CTAAR*, 1950: 41; *Tuberculosis Services in Canada*, 49.

145 NAC CTA, IIa, file 65, J. Limerick to J.J. Arsenault, 6 Mar. 1949.

146 "Report of Executive Office," *CTAAR*, 1948: 27; "OTA Reorganizes," *CTAB* 28 (Dec. 1949): 7.

147 Editorial, "Action is Needed," 40–1.

148 "Report of Executive Office," *CTAB*, 1950: 24.

149 Ibid., 20–1, 23.

150 NAC CTA, Id, file 2, G.J. Wherrett, "The Effect of New Treatments on the Organization of the Fight against Tuberculosis in Canada," 9.

151 G.C. Brink, "President's Report," *CTAAR*, 1952: 13; "Saskatchewan," *CTAAR*, 1949: 86.

152 "Ontario," *CTAAR*, 1953: 94.

153 "Report of Executive Office," *CTAAR*, 1953: 20, 23.

154 G.J. Wherrett, "The Changing Picture in Tuberculosis," *CTAAR*, 1955: 24.

155 J.A. Vidal, "President's Report," *CTAAR*, 1954: 12.

CHAPTER NINE

1 Kalbach and McVey, *Demographic Bases of Canadian Society*, 74. Primary occupations include agriculture, fishing, hunting, trapping, logging, mining and quarrying. Ibid., 241.

2 "Relief of Nursing Services," *CTAB* 27 (June 1949): 3.

3 Dubos, *The Mirage of Health*, 20, 127.

4 Galdston, "Humanism and Public Health," 1033.

5 Wilson, "Historical Decline of Tuberculosis in Europe," 366–96.

6 Wilson, "Tuberculosis in Minnesota," 16–52.

7 Sidel and Drucker, "Resurgence of Tuberculosis," 306.

8 Ibid., 306.

9 Dubos, *Mirage of Health*, 160.

10 Ibid., 71.

11 McKinnon, "Mortality Reductions in Ontario," 429.

12 Bates and Stead, "History of Tuberculosis," 1210.

13 Ibid., 1214.

14 Editorial, "Declining Tuberculosis Death Rate," 149–50.

15 H.E. MacDermot, "Is Tuberculosis a Hereditary or Contagious Disease?" *NOT* 2 (Feb. 1940): 3.

16 Buschman and Skamene, "Genetic Background," 59–80; Bates and Stead, "History of Tuberculosis," 1213.

17 Long, "Resistance to Tuberculosis," 6.

18 Dubos, *Mirage of Health*, 20.

19 Stewart, "Epidemiology of Tuberculosis," 110.

20 Dubos, *Dreams of Reason*, 71.

21 Ibid., 69, 74. Dubos, *Man, Medicine and Environment*, 82.

22 Kalbach, 53–5. Canadian specialists had noted the rise of cancer in conjunction with the fall of tuberculosis and speculated as to the cause. See "Statistics Comparing Cancer with Tuberculosis in the City of Saskatoon," *PHJ* 16 (May 1925): 216–19; McIntosh, "Cancer and Tuberculosis," 600–9; "Tuberculosis and Cancer," *CTAB* 19 (Dec. 1940): 7.

23 Stewart, *Tuberculous Man at Home*, 3.

24 Dubos, *The Dreams of Reason*, 95.

25 Carr, *What is History?* 52.

26 Croce, *Science and Religion*, vol. 1, 85–6, 102–3, emphasis added.

27 Ibid., 85–6, 102–3, 165, 170.

28 Jordan, *Machine Age Ideology*, 36.

29 Ibid., 24–5.

30 Ibid., 24–5, 66.

31 Ibid., 99–100.

32 Starr, *Social Transformation of American Medicine*, 140–1.

33 Wiebe, *Self-Rule*; Lasch, *Revolt of the Elites*.

34 Wiebe, *Self-Rule*, 148.

35 Ibid., 164, 169.

36 Ibid., 209.

37 Lasch, *Revolt of the Elites*, 166–7.

38 Ibid., 170.

39 Ibid., 167.

40 Ludmerer, *Learning to Heal*, 207.

41 Ibid., 214–17.

42 Ibid., 217, 222.

43 Starr, *Social Transformation*, 183–8.

44 Bliss, *Sir Joseph Flavelle*, 169.

45 Ibid.

46 Ibid., 450.

47 Ibid.

48 MacDougall, *Activists and Advocates*, 27–30.

49 McGinnis, *From Health to Welfare*, 36.

50 Ibid., n105, 193.

51 Letter, Wodehouse to Dr John A Ferrell, 19 Dec. 1936, quoted in McGinnis, *From Health to Welfare*, 181, 165.

52 MacDougall, *Activists and Advocates*, 189.

53 Ibid., 35.

54 Ibid., 66–7, 121, 35.

55 Ibid., 116.

56 Ludmerer, *Learning to Heal*, 192.

57 Fox, "Foundations and Medical Education," 476.

58 Rosenberg, *No Other Gods*, 122.

59 Ludmerer, *Learning to Heal*, 203.

60 McGinnis, *From Health to Welfare*, 218.

61 Houston, *Ferguson*, 86.

62 Ibid., 126.

63 Ibid., 130.

64 Edgley and Brissett, "A Nation of Meddlers," 41, 43, 45.

CHAPTER TEN

1 Miller, "Forward Movement in Public Health," 121.

2 Roberts, "Tuberculosis in Hamilton," 601.

3 William Osler in 1907, quoted in Campbell, *Holbrook*, 57.

4 D.A. Stewart, "Some Postulates," *CTAB* 13 (Sept. 1934): 7.

5 NAC CTA, IIa file, 93, Sloman, *Memorandum: Tuberculosis Ex-Soldiers*.

6 Stewart, *Things New and Old*, 5–6.

7 Stewart, *Social Ramifications of Tuberculosis*, 11.

8 Ferguson, "Recent Advances in Tuberculosis Control," 112.

9 Heagerty, "Wartime Control of Tuberculosis," 17.

10 C.H. Crooks, "Alberta: Report delivered at the ATA annual meeting in Calgary, 14–15 April 1951," *CTAAR*, 1950: 31.

11 *Tuberculosis Services in Canada*, 62.

12 "Report of Executive Office," *CTAAR*, 1954: 22.

13 "Annual Meeting," *CTAAR*, 1948: 10.

14　*Tuberculosis Services in Canada*, 62.

15　G.J. Wherrett points this out in *The Miracle of the Empty Beds*, 39.

16　Hastings, "Public Health Administration," 125.

17　*Tuberculosis Services in Canada*, 62.

18　Bates, *Bargaining for Life*, 246–7.

19　See McKeown, *Role of Medicine, Origins of Human Disease*; Sidel, Drucker, and Martin, "Resurgence of Tuberculosis," 304–5.

20　Wilson "Historical Decline of Tuberculosis," 366–96.

21　Wilson, "Tuberculosis in Minnesota," 16–52.

22　Bates, *Bargaining for Life*, 318.

23　Ibid., 329–30.

24　Ibid., 331.

25　Rothman, *Living in the Shadow of Death*, 233–34.

26　Ibid., 241.

27　Connor, *Heritage of Healing*, 93.

28　Ibid., 98.

29　Penney, *Inventing the Cure*, 120–1.

30　Mooney, *Shadow of the White Plague*, 194–5.

31　Maugham, "Sanitorium," 506.

32　Houston, *R.G. Ferguson*, 84.

33　Berger, *Sense of Power*, 6.

34　NAC CTA, IIb, file: 1905, C.J. Fagan, *State Aid to Assist in the Cure and Prevention of Tuberculosis*, (1905?), 1.

35　Canada, House of Commons, *Debates*, 1919 135 (Ottawa): 1374.

36　Ibid., 1905, 69, (Ottawa): 1380–3; Ibid., 1919, 135 (Ottawa): 1374.

37　C.D. Parfitt, "The President's Address," CTAAR, *Papers on Tuberculosis, 1924*: 8.

38　Editorial, "National Health Program for Canada," 248.

39　McGinnis, *From Health to Welfare*, 167.

40　The Dominion Council of Health passed a resolution to this effect in December 1928. The National Council of Women endorsed it in 1930. "Forward," CPHJ 20 (Mar. 1929); NCWCY, 1930, 44.

41　Editorial, "Federal Responsibility," 79.

42　McCullough, "The Highway of Health," 145.

43　NAC CTA, III, file 39 R.J. Collins to G.J. Wherrett, 6 Dec. 1937.

44　Editorial, "National Health Program for Canada," 248.

45　NAC CTA, IIa, file 94, (by authority of) Hon. Ian Mackenzie, Minister of Pensions and National Health, *Deaths among War Pensioners 1918–1936* (Ottawa: 1939): 6.

46　NAC CTA, IIa, file 64, G.J. Wherrett to Dr Clarence M. Hincks, 27 Oct. 1949.

47　Copp, *Anatomy of Poverty*. See "preface," 9; chap. 6, "Public Health," especially 100–3.

48　1910 Quebec Royal Commission, *Report*, 68, 79.

49 Montreal Health Survey Committee, *Survey*, 62.

50 Of the other two sanatoria, the Lake Edward Sanatorium was listed as "provincial." "Selected Information on Tuberculosis Institutions," *CTAAR*, 1950: 96.

51 Agnes M. Ferencz, in a 1945 study of the impact of urbanization on French Canadian medical attitudes pointed this out more generally. Ferencz, "Impact of Urbanization," 158, 160–1.

52 "Family Placement in the Province of Quebec," *CTAAR*, 1936: 156.

53 Adrien Plouffe, "Clinical Examination Preceding X-ray Examination," *NOT* 6 (Apr.–May 1944): 2.

54 Ibid., 3.

55 Stewart, *Things New and Old*, 8.

56 Each board had a representative of the provincial government on it. *Tuberculosis Services in Canada*, 47.

57 "Report of the Executive Office," *CTAAR*, 1952: 29.

58 Murrell, "Health Units in British Columbia," 392.

59 NAC CTA, IIa, file 70, G.J. Wherrett to Mrs K.L. Dawson, 15 Apr. 1946.

60 Heagerty, "Public Health in Canada," 59.

61 Wodehouse, "Prevention and Control of Tuberculosis," 670.

62 In *The Miracle of the Empty Beds*, Wherrett notes that the coming of free hospitalization and medicare did much to increase institutional costs for the treatment of tuberculosis. In earlier years sanatoria employed a limited number of graduate nurses and trained nurses' assistants. The regular medical staff did much of the day-to-day work – reading chest films for example – which would later be done by a radiologist. G.J. Wherrett, *Tuberculosis in Canada*, 65; *Empty Beds*, 45.

63 Porter, *Crusading against Tuberculosis*, 9.

64 Holbrook, "Hamilton Health Association," 164.

65 The 1910 Quebec Royal Commission noted this absence of a lay voluntary base. "Women might play a very important part in the campaign against tuberculosis," it commented. "Unfortunately, in our province, there is no general movement toward anti-tuberculosis organization among women." 1910 Quebec Royal Commission, *Report*, 101–2.

66 Ibid., 68.

67 Hastings, "Democracy and Public Health Administration," 105.

68 J.G. Adami, "Presidential Address," *CTAAR*, 1910: 165.

69 Danylewycz, "Nuns and Feminists in Montreal," 413–34.

70 Linteau, Durocher, and Robert, *Quebec*, 437–8, 533.

71 NAC CTA, IIa, file 23, G.J. Wherrett to Grant Fleming, 24 Feb. 1938.

72 Herman Gauthier, "Mechanized Anti-Tuberculosis Detection in Gaspesia," *NOT* 13 (Aug. 1950): 3.

73 NAC CTA, IIa, file 12, G.J. Wherrett to J.K. Macdonald, 27 Jan. 1948.

74 Hugh E. Burke and Geo. Gregoire, "Report of the Provincial Committee for the Prevention of Tuberculosis, 1949," *NOT* 13 (May 1950): 1.

75 Burke, "Tuberculosis – A Community Problem," 157.
76 "The Christmas Seal Campaign in Canada," *CTAAR*, 1937: 29; 1910 Quebec Royal Commission, *Report*, 68, 79.
77 Gagnon, "Tuberculosis in the Jewish Race," 13–15.
78 Playter, *Consumption*, 290.
79 Gagnon, "Tuberculosis in the Jewish Race," 14.
80 Ibid.
81 Buschman and Skamene, "Natural Resistance and Acquired Immunity to *M. Tuberculosis*," 59–79; Bates and Stead, "Tuberculosis as a Global Epidemic," 1205–17.
82 Letter, *Annals of Internal Medicine* 117, no. 4 (1 Nov. 1992): 796; Bates and Stead, "History of Tuberculosis," 1214.
83 Ibid.
84 Heagerty, "Wartime Control of Tuberculosis," 16.
85 NAC CTA, IIa, file 50, R.E. Wodehouse to E.E. Reid, 14 Nov. 1930.
86 Wodehouse, "Prevention and Control of Tuberculosis," 669.
87 *CTAB* 7 (Sept. 1928): 8.
88 NAC CTA, IIa, file 52, R.E. Wodehouse, *Report* (11 Jan. 1930) 2–3; NAC CTA, IIa, file 48, R.E. Wodehouse to E.E. Reid, 4 Apr. 1931.
89 However, these figures might not be specific enough – for just as the extent of the disease varied within the different ethnic groups, so might the distribution of wealth. Wherrett, "Tuberculosis Problem in Canada," 295–6.
90 Stone, Vannier, et al, "Meningitis Due to Iatrogenic BCG Infection," 561–63.
91 Thomas, *Lives of a Cell*, 33–4.
92 Stewart, *Teaching about Tuberculosis*, 3.
93 *Souvenir of the Laying of the Corner Stone of the New Children's Hospital for Consumptives by His Royal Highness the Duke of Connaught*, 27 May 1912: 4.
94 Lalonde, "Untold Epidemic," 280.
95 Playter, *Consumption*, 207.
96 Quoted in R.J. Needham, "A Writer's Notebook," *Globe and Mail*, 13 Apr. 1983.
97 Carr, *What is History?* 44.

# Bibliography

The annual reports of the associations cited in the notes, particularly those of the Canadian Tuberculosis Association in its various manifestations, included papers presented at annual meetings, in addition to brief reports from provincial organizations, sanatoria, and so forth. So that it does not become too unwieldy, these items are not included in the bibliography, and full references are given in the notes.

Adami, J.G. "Child Welfare Exhibitions and Their Value." *PHJ* 3 (July 1912): 371–5.

Adams, George B. "John George Adami: An Appreciation." *Southern Medical Journal* 22 (Feb. 1929): 172–7.

Adams, Harry G., and Colin Jordan. "Infections in the Alcoholic." *The Medical Clinics of North America* 68, no. 1 (1984): 185–9.

Adamson, J.D. "Canada Eliminates Tuberculosis from the Army." *Bulletin of the National Tuberculosis Association* 26 (Nov. 1940): 163–4, 171.

– "Osler and Tuberculosis." *The University of Manitoba Medical Journal* 20 (Feb. 1949): 119–24.

Adamson, J.D., and J. N. Edmison. "Immigration Tuberculosis." *CMAJ* 57 (Nov. 1947): 432–4.

Adamson, J.D., et al. "Tuberculosis in the Canadian Army, 1939 to 1944." *CMAJ* 52 (Feb. 1945): 123–7.

Alderson, W.H. "Rotary Means Service." *PHJ* 10 (Feb. 1919): 62–9.

Alexander, John. *The Collapse Therapy of Pulmonary Tuberculosis.* Springfield, IL: Charles C. Thomas, 1937.

Allen, Richard. "The Social Gospel and the Reform Tradition in Canada, 1890–1928." *Canadian Historical Review* 49 (Dec. 1968): 381–99.

– *The Social Passion.* Toronto: University of Toronto Press, 1973.

A.M. "Sleeping Out of Doors." *PHJ* 2 (Mar. 1911): 145–6.

Anderson, "Letter to the Editor." *PHJ* 8 (Nov. 1917): 309.

Archibald, Edward. "The Surgical Treatment of Pulmonary Tuberculosis." *CMAJ* 18 (Jan. 1928): 3–9.

Arnove, Robert F., ed. *Philosophy and Cultural Imperialism: The Foundations at Home and Abroad.* Boston: G.K. Hall, 1980.

Artibise, Alan F.J. *Winnipeg: A Social History of Urban Growth, 1874–1914.* Montreal: McGill-Queen's University Press, 1975.

– "The Urban West: The Evolution of Prairie Towns and Cities to 1930." In Stelter and Artibise, *The Canadian City,* 138–64.

"Artificial Pneumothorax in the Treatment of Pulmonary Tuberculosis." *CMAJ* 3 (Mar. 1913): 229–32.

Atherton, William H. "Child Welfare and the City." *PHJ* 2 (Oct. 1911): 461–6.

Atwater, Reginald. "The Control of Tuberculosis in Rural Areas." *CPHJ* 29 (Feb. 1938): 53–7.

Badeaux, Georgine. "L'infirmière et la lutte anti-tuberculeuse." *Canadian Nurse* 44 (Dec. 1948): 991–2.

Baker, A.H. "Alberta's Tuberculosis Problem." *CMAJ* 60 (June 1949): 572–4.

Ballantyne, A.C. "Tuberculosis in Waterloo County." *Canadian Nurse* 44 (Dec. 1948): 987–8.

Barr, Sir James. "The Medicine of the Future." *PHJ* 2 (Sept. 1911): 414–26.

Barrick, E.J. "How to Deal with the Consumptive Poor." *Canadian Journal of Medicine and Surgery* 6 (Sept. 1899): 254–61.

Bates, Barbara. *Bargaining for Life: A Social History of Tuberculosis, 1876–1938.* Philadelphia: University of Pennsylvania Press, 1992.

Bates, Gordon A. "Past and Future." *PHJ* 17 (Oct. 1926): 499–502.

– "Social Hygiene – A Broad Conception." *PHJ* 19 (Mar. 1928): 124–32.

– "Editorial: County Health Units." *CPHJ* 22 (Mar. 1931): 151–2.

Bates, Joseph H. "Tuberculosis: Susceptibility and Resistance." *American Review of Respiratory Disease,* 125, no. 3 (1982).

Bates Joseph H., and William W. Stead. "The History of Tuberculosis as a Global Epidemic." *Medical Clinics of North America* 77 (Nov. 1993): 1205–17.

Baudouin, J.A. "Pasteurization of Milk Supply." *PHJ* 9 (Jan. 1918): 11–26.

– "Report for 1925 on the Activities of the French Health Centre Conducted in Cooperation with the School of Public Health Nursing of the University of Montreal." *PHJ* 17 (May 1926): 222–5.

– "Vaccination against Tuberculosis with the BCG Vaccine." *CPHJ* 27 (Jan. 1936): 20–6.

– "Vaccination against Tuberculosis with the BCG Vaccine." *CPHJ* 31 (Aug. 1940): 362–6.

Bayer, Pat. "Canada's Fifty Year Old Battle against the 'White Plague.'" *Saturday Night* 51 (17 Nov. 1945): 34–5.

Beckwith, C.J.W. "The Tuberculosis Control Program in Halifax." *CJPH* 37 (Dec. 1946): 481–7.

Bendinelli, Mauro, and Herman Friedman, eds. *Mycobacterium Tuberculosis: Interactions with the Immune System.* New York: Plenum Press, 1988.

Benenson, Abram S., ed. *Control of Communicable Diseases in Man.* 12th ed. Washington: 1975.

Bennett, Charles F. "Tuberculosis in Recent Immigrants." *CPHJ* 31 (Nov. 1940): 515–30.

Berger, Carl. *The Sense of Power.* Toronto: University of Toronto Press, 1970.

Bernstein, D.H. "Home Treatment of Tuberculosis." *CMAJ* 8 (Jan. 1918): 38–48.

Berry, A.E. "Safeguarding the Milk Supply." *PHJ* 19 (Nov. 1928): 505–9.

– "Third Annual Report of the Committee on Milk Control." *CPHJ* 28 (Sept. 1937): 459–63.

– "Progress in Pasteurization in Ontario." *CPHJ* 32 (Apr. 1941): 208–12.

Bethune, Norman. "A Plea for Early Compression in Pulmonary Tuberculosis." *CMAJ* 27 (July 1932): 36–42.

Black, J.B. "A Federal Bureau of Public Health." *PHJ* 7 (Sept. 1916): 408–10.

– "The Establishment of a Federal Bureau of Health." *CMAJ* 8 (Apr. 1918): 333–5.

Black, Conrad. *Duplessis.* Toronto: McClelland and Stewart, 1977.

Blackader, A.D. "The More Important Causes Underlying the Heavy Infantile Death Rate in Large Cities and the Benefits to Be Derived from the Establishment of Milk Depots." *PHJ* 3 (July 1912): 367–71.

Bliss, Michael. *A Canadian Millionaire: The Life and Business Times of Sir Joseph Flavelle, Bart. 1858–1939.* Toronto: University of Toronto Press, 1992.

Board of Tuberculosis Sanatorium Consultants. *The Care and Employment of the Tuberculous Ex-Serviceman after Discharge from the Sanatorium.* Confidential report no. 6. Ottawa: 1920.

Bothamley, G.H. "The Koch Phenomenon and Delayed Hypersensitivity: 1891–1991." *Tubercle* 72 (1991): 7–11.

Bothwell, Robert S. "The Health of the Common People." In *Mackenzie King: Widening the Debate.* Edited by John English and J.O. Stubbs. Toronto: Macmillan, 1977, 191–220.

Bothwell, Robert S., and John R. English. "Pragmatic Physicians: Canadian Medicine and Health Care Insurance, 1910–1945." In S.E.D. Short, ed., *Medicine in Canadian Society: Historical Perspectives* (Montreal: 1981): 479–93.

Boughton, Harvey C. "New Case-Finding in Tuberculosis." *CPHJ* 28 (June 1937): 259–64.

Bow, M.R. "Public Health Services in Alberta." *CPHJ* 21 (Dec. 1930): 590–600.

Boyars, Michael C. "The Microbiology, Chemotherapy and Surgical Treatment of Tuberculosis." *Journal of Thoracic Imaging* 5, no. 2 (1990): 1–7.

Brancker, A., D.A. Enarson, S. Gryzbowski, E.S. Hershfield, and C.W.L. Jeanes. "A Statistical Chronicle of Tuberculosis in Canada: Part I. From the Era of

Sanatorium Treatment to the Present." *Health Reports* 1992. Statistics Canada 4: 103–123.

Brink, George Clair. "Physical Examination in Pulmonary Tuberculosis." *PHJ* 16 (Oct. 1925): 468–73.

– "The Travelling Diagnostic Clinic." *CPHJ* 22 (Apr. 1931): 163–8.

– "Influencing Factors in the Control of Tuberculosis." *CPHJ* 27 (Oct. 1936): 482–8.

– "Symposium on Tuberculosis: The Provincial Tuberculosis Program in Ontario." *CPHJ* 28 (May 1937): 216–20.

– "Recent Advances in Tuberculosis Control in Ontario." *CPHJ* 32 (Oct. 1941): 502–8.

– "Tuberculosis Control." *CJPH* 38 (Jan. 1946): 1–6.

– *Across the Years: Tuberculosis in Ontario.* Willowdale, ON: Ontario Tuberculosis Association, 1965.

Brink, George Clair, M.H. Brown, and K.G. Gray. "Tuberculosis Infection in 2492 Persons." *CPHJ* 24 (Oct. 1933): 471–8.

Brittain, Horace L. "Administration of the Toronto Department of Public Health." *PHJ* 6 (July 1915): 309–25; (Aug. 1915): 365–77; (Sept. 1915): 421–32; (Oct. 1915): 477–87.

Brown, Alan. "The Relation of the Pediatrician to the Community." *PHJ* 10 (Feb. 1919): 49–55.

Brown, E. Richard. *Rockefeller Medicine Men: Medicine and Capitalism in America.* Berkeley, CA: University of California Press, 1979.

Brown, Robert Craig, and Ramsay Cook. *Canada 1896–1921: A Nation Transformed.* Toronto: McClelland and Stewart, 1974.

Browne, Jean E. "Health Education in Rural Schools." *PHJ* 11 (Dec. 1920): 533–41.

– "Contribution of the Junior Red Cross to Public Health." *CPHJ* 22 (Feb. 1931): 99–100.

– "The Junior Red Cross: 'An Idea Whose Time Has Come.'" *CPHJ* 30 (Jan. 1939): 20–3.

Bruce, Oliver. "Pulmonary Tuberculosis." *CMAJ* 2 (Mar. 1912): 181–99.

Bryce, Peter H. "Report on Tuberculosis in Ontario." Paper presented to the Ontario Provincial Board of Health. Toronto, 1894.

– *Immigration in Relation to Public Health.* N.p.: 1906.

– "Tuberculosis in Canada as Affected by Immigration." *British Journal of Tuberculosis* 2 (1908): 264–7.

– "Maintenance of Public Health." *PHJ* 1 (Nov. 1910): 533–5.

– "County Officers of Health: Methods of Organization and Work." *PHJ* 2 (Aug. 1911): 357–60.

– "Immigration and Its Effects on Public Health." *PHJ* 4 (Dec. 1913): 641–7.

– "Tuberculosis in Relation to Feeble-Mindedness." *PHJ* 7 (Aug. 1916): 365–70.

- "Principles Involved in Notification of Tuberculosis." *PHJ* 8 (Jan. 1917): 1–5.
- "The Scope of a Federal Department of Health." *CMAJ* 10 (Jan. 1920): 1–10.
- "The Story of Public Health in Canada." In *Half a Century of Public Health: Jubilee Historical Volume of the American Public Health Association.* Edited by Mazyck P. Ravenel. American Public Health Association, 1921.

Bryder, Linda. *Below the Magic Mountain A Social History of Tuberculosis in Twentieth-Century Britain.* Oxford: Oxford University Press, 1988.

Bulmer, L.C. "Municipal Milk Inspector." *PHJ* 5 (July 1914): 500–3.

Burke, Donald S. "Of Postulates and Peccadilloes: Robert Koch and Vaccine (Tuberculin) Therapy for Tuberculosis." *Vaccine* 11 (1993): 795–804.

Burke, F.S. "Forest Schools as an Adjunct to School Health." *PHJ* 19 (Jan. 1928): 9–19.

Burke, H.E. "Tuberculosis – A Community Problem." *Culture* 2 (June 1950): 152–8.

Burke, Richard M. *An Historical Chronology of Tuberculosis.* 2nd ed. Springfield, IL: 1955.

Burnette, N.L. "Printed Material in Health Education." *CPHJ* 33 (Aug. 1942): 399–402.

Burnitt, Bailey B. "Raising the Standards of Living as a Weapon in the Anti-tuberculosis Campaign." *PHJ* 11 (Feb. 1920): 89–95.

Byers, J.R. "Occupation in the Treatment of Pulmonary Tuberculosis." *CMAJ* 8 (Jan. 1918): 1–7.

Byrd, Richard B., Peter D. Kaplan, and Douglas R. Gracey. "Treatment of Pulmonary Tuberculosis." *Chest* 66, no. 5 (1974) 560–7.

Caldwell, Stanley. "How to Stay Well." *Maclean's Magazine.* 58 (15 Feb. 1943): 18, 31–2.

Cameron, A.E. "The Prevalence and Extent of Bovine Tuberculosis in Canada." *CPHJ* 20 (Jan. 1929): 1–5.
- "Bovine Tuberculosis in Canada." *CPHJ* 29 (June 1938): 262–5.

Campbell, Marjorie Freeman. *Holbrook of the San.* Toronto: 1953.

Campbell, P.S. "Nostrum and Quack Evil." *PHJ* 13 (Sep. 1922): 400–10.

"Full-Time Health Services in Nova Scotia." *CJPH* 36 (Oct. 1945): 385–9.

Canada. Commission on Conservation. Committee on Public Health. *Report of the International Commission on the Control of Tuberculosis.* Ottawa, 1910.
- Department of National Health and Welfare, Research Division. *Tuberculosis Services in Canada.* Memorandum no. 11, General Series. Ottawa, 1955.
- House of Commons. *Debates,* 1905: 1351–85, 8636–7, 9392–4, 9522–3.
- *Debates,* 1919: 1366–80.
- *Journals,* 1905: 105, 445, 477, 506–8, 512.
- Special Committee to Consider Questions Relating to Pensions, Insurance and Re-establishment of Returned Soldiers, and Any Amendments to the Existing Laws in Relation Thereto. *Proceedings: Third and Final Report.* Ottawa, 1921.

Canada. Senate. *Debates*, 1905: 131–43, 232–52, 261–9, 416–17, 555, 769–70.
– *Journals*, 1905: 134, 175, 190, 288, 313, 339–42.
Canadian Association for the Prevention of Consumption and Other Forms of Tuberculosis. *Transactions*. 1902–1909.
Canadian Association for the Prevention of Tuberculosis. *How to Prevent Consumption*. Ottawa: 1910.
– *Annual Report*. 1910–21.
Canadian Life Insurance Officers Association. "The Public Health Aspects of the Proposed National Health Insurance Scheme for Canada: Memorandum Submitted to the Advisory Committee on Health Insurance of the Department of Pensions and National Health." *CJPH* 34 (Apr. 1943): 147–51.
Canadian Tuberculosis Association. *Annual Report*. 1922–55.
– *Bulletin* 1–29 (Sept. 1922–Mar. 1951).
– *What You Should Know About Tuberculosis*. Ottawa: 1922.
– *Canada's Experience in Tuberculosis Programmes*. N. p. [1929?].
– *Eastern Ontario Counties Sanatorium*. N.p.: n.d.
– *Protect the Contact*. Ottawa: [1934?].
– *How the Sanatorium Protects You*. Ottawa: [1937?].
– *Programme of an Intensive Community Campaign against Tuberculosis*. Ottawa: 1938.
Carmichael, D.A. "Tuberculosis in Childhood." *CMAJ* 32 (June 1935): 670–3.
Carr, E.H. *What is History?* Markham, ON: Penguin Books, 1964.
Cassel, Jay. *The Secret Plague: Venereal Disease in Canada 1838–1939*. Toronto: University of Toronto Press, 1987.
Cassidy, Harry M. *Public Health and Welfare Reorganization: The Postwar Problem in the Canadian Provinces*. Toronto: The Ryerson Press, 1945.
Cartwright, Frederick F. *A Social History of Medicine*. New York: Longman's 1977.
Chapman, Ethel M. "New Field of the Red Cross." *Maclean's Magazine* 33 (15 Sept. 1920): 73–4.
– "First Offensive in the Milk Campaign." *Maclean's Magazine* 34 (15 May 1921): 60–1.
– "Soundest Kind of Prevention." *Maclean's Magazine* 34 (Aug. 1921): 64, 68–9.
Charles, Jeffrey A. *Service Clubs in American Society: Rotary, Kiwanis and Lions*. Chicago: University of Illinois Press, 1993.
"Child Welfare Exhibition." *PHJ* 2 (July 1911): 336–7.
Chown, Bruce, and Harry Medovy. "Pulmonary Tuberculosis in Childhood." *CMAJ* 29 (Oct. 1933): 364–8.
Church, E. "Our Babies and the BCG." *Canadian Magazine* 76 (Sept. 1931): 7, 45.

Clark, M. "Closing the Gap in the Tuberculosis Program." *Canadian Nurse* 46 (Sept. 1950): 721–4.

Clarke, A.M. "Tuberculosis Control in New Brunswick." *CPHJ* 29 (Mar. 1938): 103–8.

Claxton, Brooke. "Mapping Our New Frontiers of Health." *CJPH* 36 (Dec. 1945): 455–64.

Collins, R.J. "Anti-Tuberculosis Activities in New Brunswick." *CPHJ* 25 (July 1934): 326–8.

– "After-Care and the Rehabilitation of the Tuberculous." *CPHJ* 31 (May 1940): 209–15.

Collins, R.J., and C.W. MacMillan. "Tuberculosis and the Student Nurse." *CMAJ* 34 (June 1936): 649–54.

– "Tuberculosis and the Student Nurse." *CPHJ* 31 (Dec. 1940): 579–83.

Comstock, George W. "Epidemiology of Tuberculosis." *American Review of Respiratory Disease* 125, no. 3 (1982).

Connor, J.H.T. *A Heritage of Healing: The London Health Association and its Hospitals 1909–1987*. London: London Health Association, 1990.

Cook, Ramsay. *The Regenerators*. Toronto: University of Toronto Press, 1985.

Copp, Terry. *The Anatomy of Poverty*. Toronto: 1974.

"Correspondence: The Employment of the Tuberculous." *CMAJ* 17 (May 1927): 605–8.

"Cows and Housing." *PHJ* 3 (July 1912): 401.

Cox, George H. *Consumption: Its Cause, Prevention and Cure*. NS: The Anti-Tuberculosis Leagues of the Island of Cape Breton, 1912.

Craig, D.A. "Tuberculosis Problems from a Public Health Standpoint." *PHJ* 6 (July 1915): 330–2.

"Creation of a New Health Unit in Alberta." *CPHJ* 31 (Apr. 1940): 204.

Creighton, Donald. *The Forked Road: Canada 1939–1957*. Toronto: McClelland and Stewart, 1976.

Crichton, J.E. "The Greatest of All Triumvirates." *PHJ* 4 (Sept. 1913): 509–13.

Croce, Paul Jerome. *Science and Religion in the Era of William James: Eclipse of Certainty, 1820–1880*. Vol 1. Chapel Hill, NC: University of North Carolina Press, 1995.

Crombie, D.W. "The Present Anti-Tuberculosis Program in Ontario." *CPHJ* 26 (Oct. 1935): 486–93.

– "Symposium on Tuberculosis: The Early Diagnosis of Tuberculosis." *CPHJ* 28 (May 1937): 211–15.

Cruikshank, G.L. "President's Address." *PHJ* 10 (Sept. 1919): 400–1.

Cruikshank, H.C. "The Problem of Tuberculosis among Toronto Children." *PHJ* 16 (Feb. 1925): 71–5.

Cummins, S. Lyle. "Contact with Infection in Tuberculosis." *CPHJ* 26 (Jan. 1935): 1–8.

Cunnings, T.A.J. "Rehabilitation of the Tuberculosis Patient – The Manitoba Program." *CJPH* 35 (Apr. 1944): 137–43.

Currey, D. V. "Some Problems for the New MOH" *PHJ* 10 (Nov. 1919): 511–14.

– "Community Milk Supplies in Ontario." *PHJ* 18 (July 1927): 301–11.

– "Utilizing Service Clubs, Women's Organizations, and Other Local Organizations in Public Health Education." *CPHJ* 33 (Nov. 1942): 552–4.

Currie, Sir Arthur W. "Montreal Anti-Tuberculosis and General Health League." *PHJ* 17 (May 1926): 199–204; 18 (Mar. 1927): 101–6; 19 (June 1928): 261–2.

Daniel, Thomas M. "Tuberculosis." In *Harrison's Principles of Internal Medicine.* 12th ed., 637–45. Toronto: McGraw-Hill, 1991.

Danylewycz, Marta. "Changing Relationships: Nuns and Feminists in Montreal, 1890–1925." *Histoire Sociale-Social History* 14 (Nov. 1981): 413–34.

Davidson, Miss. "Control of the Tuberculosis Contact." *CPHJ* 22 (May 1931): 258–61.

Defries, R.D. "Recent Health Legislation in Canada." *CPHJ* 29 (Apr. 1938): 180–7.

– *The Federal and Provincial Health Services in Canada.* 2nd ed. Toronto: 1962.

– ed. *The Development of Public Health in Canada,* Toronto: Canadian Public Health Association, 1943.

DeWitt, George E. "A Few Hints to the Medical Profession in Relation to Public Health Work." *PHJ* 7 (Feb. 1916): 63–8.

Dickson, E. MacPherson. "The Tuberculosis Hospital and Its Facilities for Teaching Health." *PHJ* 18 (Sept. 1927): 420–4.

Dobbie, W.J. "The Etiology of Tuberculosis." *PHJ* 12 (Aug. 1921): 337–51.

– "A Provincial Program for the Control of Tuberculosis." *CPHJ* 26 (Oct. 1935): 494–505.

– "Symposium on Tuberculosis: Discussion." *CPHJ* 28 (May 1937): 220–2.

Dolman, C.E. "The Health of the Nation." *CPHJ* 32 (Aug. 1941): 387–403.

Douglas, A.J. "Ways and Means in Public Health." *CPHJ* 21 (June 1930): 263–6.

Dowling, Harry F. *Fighting Infection.* Cambridge, MA: 1977.

Dublin, Louis I. "Incidence of Tuberculosis in the Industrial Population." *CPHJ* 23 (June 1932): 293.

Dubos, René. *The Mirage of Health.* New York: Harper and Row, 1959.

– *The Dreams of Reason: Science and Utopias.* New York: Columbia University Press, 1961.

– *Man, Medicine and Environment.* New York: 1968.

Dubos, René, and Jean Dubos. *The White Plague.* Boston: Little, Brown, 1952.

Dubovsky, H. "Artificial Pneumothorax in the Treatment of Lung Tuberculosis." *South African Medical Journal* 81 (1992): 372–75.

Duffy, John. "The American Medical Profession and Public Health: From Support to Ambivalence." *Bulletin of the History of Medicine* 53 (spring 1979): 1–22.

Dyke, Eunice. "Tuberculosis in Toronto." *PHJ* 4 (July 1913): 402–4.
- "The Registration of Tuberculosis." *PHJ* 6 (Oct. 1915): 500–1.
Edgley, Charles, and Dennis Brissett. "A Nation of Meddlers." *Society* 32 (May–June 1995): 36–46.
Editorial. "Dip Tank Milk." CTSE 1 (Aug. 1910): 414–5.
- "Reporting Cases of Tuberculosis." *CMAJ* 1 (Feb. 1911): 158–9.
- "Hygiene and the Ontario Legislature." *PHJ* 2 (Apr. 1911): 170–1.
- "Mortality Rates and Life Insurance." *PHJ* 2 (July 1911): 323–4.
- "The Laurentian Sanitarium." *CMAJ* 1 (Aug. 1911): 768–9.
- "The Final Report of the British Royal Tuberculosis Commission." *CMAJ* 1 (Oct. 1911): 978–82.
- "The Muskoka Sanitorium." *PHJ* 3 (Aug. 1912): 462–3.
- "Dr. Friedmann and His Cure." *PHJ* 4 (May 1913): 320.
- "Incipient Tuberculosis." *CMAJ* 3 (Sept. 1913): 797–9.
- "The Tuberculosis Problem." *PHJ* 4 (Dec. 1913): 675–6.
- "The Laurentian Society." *CMAJ* 4 (Mar. 1914): 221–3.
- "Tuberculosis in Children." *CMAJ* 5 (July 1915): 615.
- "The Tuberculous Soldier." *CMAJ* 6 (Oct. 1916): 922–3.
- "The Treatment of Soldiers Suffering from Pulmonary Tuberculosis." *CMAJ* 6 (Nov. 1916): 1010–12.
- "Heliotherapy." *CMAJ* 7 (May 1917): 443–6.
- "A Federal Department of Health." *PHJ* 7 (Nov. 1917): 308.
- "A Federal Department." *PHJ* 9 (Feb. 1918): 92.
- "Business and Public Health." *PHJ* 9 (May 1918): 245.
- "On Incomes." *PHJ* 9 (Aug. 1918): 391–2.
- "A Social Hygiene Programme for Canada." *PHJ* 10 (Jan. 1919): 42.
- "Opposition to the Federal Department of Health." *PHJ* 10 (Apr. 1919): 183–5.
- "The Fraternal Societies and Tuberculosis." *CMAJ* 9 (Mar. 1919): 258.
- "Public Health in New Brunswick." *PHJ* 11 (Apr. 1920): 191–4.
- "Modern Views on Tuberculosis." *CMAJ* 10 (Dec. 1920): 1137–40.
- "Regulars and Volunteers." *PHJ* 12 (Jan. 1921): 45–6.
- "A Unique Experiment." *PHJ* 12 (Feb. 1921): 91–2.
- "On the Treatment of the Tuberculous Ex-Service Man." *CMAJ* 12 (Apr. 1922): 253–5.
- "On the Diagnosis of Tuberculosis in Childhood." *CMAJ* 12 (July 1922): 497–8.
- "Health Machinery." *PHJ* 14 (May 1923): 238–9.
- "The New Order." *PHJ* 14 (Oct. 1923): 481–2.
- "Life Insurance and Public Health." *PHJ* 15 (Jan. 1924): 47–8.
- "The Causes of a Declining Tuberculosis Death Rate." *CMAJ* 14 (Feb. 1924): 149–50.
- "What of Rest in Tuberculosis." *CMAJ* 14 (July 1924): 640–1.

– "A New Treatment for Tuberculosis under Trial." *CMAJ* 15 (Apr. 1925): 409–10.
– "The Gold Treatment of Tuberculosis Again." *CMAJ* 15 (July 1925): 741–2.
– "Anti-Tuberculosis Work in Canada." *CMAJ* 15 (Aug. 1925): 843–4.
– "A Health Programme for Canada." *PHJ* 16 (Sept. 1925): 448–9.
– "The Greatest Need." *PHJ* 17 (Jan. 1926): 49–50.
– "Social Hygiene." *PHJ* 12 (Sept. 1921): 427–8; 17 (Mar. 1926): 197.
– "Human and Bovine Tuberculosis." *CMAJ* 16 (Apr. 1926): 438–9.
– "On the Value of the Sanatorium Treatment in Tuberculosis." *CMAJ* 14 (Oct. 1926): 1253–4.
– "Typhoid in Montreal." *PHJ* 18 (Mar. 1927): 149–50.
– "The Provision of Beds for Tuberculous Patients." *CMAJ* 17 (May 1927): 578–9.
– "Free Clinics in the West." *PHJ* 18 (July 1927): 349–50.
– "Montreal's Typhoid Epidemic." *PHJ* 18 (Aug. 1927): 399–400.
– "Intestinal Tuberculosis." *CMAJ* 17 (Sept. 1927): 1065–6.
– "Municipal Liberty." *PHJ* 19 (Apr. 1928): 175.
– "Montreal Sets an Example." *PHJ* 19 (June 1928): 278.
– "Federal Responsibility and Health." *PHJ* 19 (Feb. 1928): 79–80.
– "Treatment and Prevention." *PHJ* 19 (May 1928): 231.
– "The Experimental Investigation of Tuberculosis in Canada." *CMAJ* 20 (Jan. 1929): 47–9.
– "The Montreal Health Survey." *CPHJ* 20 (Apr. 1929): 196–7.
– "An Event of Importance." *CPHJ* 20 (June 1929): 302.
– "Montreal's New Board of Health." *CPHJ* 21 (Jan. 1930): 32–3.
– "The Development of County Health Units in Quebec." *CPHJ* 23 (Jan. 1932): 29–30.
– "Public Health and the Economic Depression." *CPHJ* 23 (Mar. 1932): 139.
– "Medical Relief." *CPHJ* 25 (Apr. 1934): 186–7.
– "The Campaign against Tuberculosis in College Students." *CMAJ* 35 (Sept. 1936): 313–6.
– "Compulsory Pasteurization of Milk Supplies." *CPHJ* 29 (Feb. 1938): 87–91.
– "Progress in Tuberculosis Control." *CPHJ* 29 (Apr. 1938): 188–90.
– "Halt Tuberculosis in the Army." *MacLean's Magazine* 51 (1 Nov. 1939): 1.
– "A New Attack on Tuberculosis." *CPHJ* 31 (Nov. 1940): 562–4.
– "The Need for Federal Government Assistance in Public Health." *CPHJ* 32 (Sept. 1941): 478–9.
– "The Development of County Health Units, Quebec." *CPHJ* 33 (Jan. 1942): 30.
– "Health Training in Schools." *CPHJ* 33 (Apr. 1942): 178–9.
– "A Public Health Charter for Canada." *CPHJ* 33 (July 1942): 344–55.
– "Army Shows the Way: X-ray Examination of Every Recruit." *Maclean's Magazine* 55 (15 Dec. 1942): 49.

- "The Halifax Health Survey." *CJPH* 34 (Mar. 1943): 140–1.
- "Efforts for the Compulsory Pasteurization of Milk in the Province of Quebec." *CJPH* 34 (Aug. 1943): 389–90.
- "Magnitude of the Problem of Prevention." *CJPH* 35 (Mar. 1944): 134–5.
- "The Rockefeller Foundation in Canada." *CJPH* 36 (Feb. 1945): 74–5; 51 (Aug. 1950): 338–9.
- "Tuberculosis Control in Nova Scotia." *CJPH* 38 (Feb. 1947): 100.
- "A National Health Program for Canada." *CJPH* 38 (June 1948): 246–8.
- Action is Needed." *CJPH* 42 (Jan. 1951): 40–1.
- "A Striking Reduction in Tuberculosis Mortality in Canada." *CJPH* 45 (Jan. 1954): 24–5.

Editorial Comment. *PHJ* 5 (July 1914): 472–3.

Elliott, Jabez H. "The Present Status of Anti-Tuberculosis Work in Canada (1908)." In Sixth International Congress on Tuberculosis, *Transactions.* vol. 4, part 1 (1908): 135–53.
- "The Anti-tuberculosis Movement in Canada." *British Journal of Tuberculosis* 4 (Apr. 1910): 73–89.
- "Shall We Have Pure Milk in Canada?" *PHJ* 2 (Aug. 1911): 353–7.
- "The Prevention of Tuberculosis." *PHJ* 4 (Jan. 1913): 28–30.
- "Heliotherapy in Abdominal Tuberculosis." *CMAJ* 7 (May 1917): 420–5.
- "How Canada is Meeting the Tuberculosis War Problem." *American Review of Tuberculosis* 2 (Sept. 1918): 400–8.
- "The Evolution of Dispensary Control of Tuberculosis." *American Review of Tuberculosis* 26 (Nov. 1937): 577–91.

Ellner, Jerrold J. "Immune Dysregulation in Human Tuberculosis." *Journal of Laboratory and Clinical Medicine* 108 (1986): 142–9.

Ewart, R.J. "The Influence of Dosage on the Reaction to the Tubercle Bacillus." *PHJ* 3 (Aug. 1912): 449–51.

Fagan, Charles J. *State Aid to Assist in the Cure and Prevention of Tuberculosis.* N.p.: [1905?].
- *Tuberculosis, or the Bacillus "At Home."* Parts 1 and 2. Victoria, BC: 1908.

"Fake Consumption Cures Make Millions of Profit." *PHJ* 4 (Nov. 1913): 638.

Farris, H.A. "Tuberculosis Hospitals and Dispensaries." *CMAJ* 9 (Sept. 1919): 830–4.

"Federal Bureau of Health." *PHJ* 4 (Nov. 1913): 634–5.

Fee, Elizabeth., and D.M. Fox. eds. *AIDS: The Burdens of History.* Berkeley, CA: University of California Press, 1998.

Feldberg, Georgiana D. *Disease and Class.* New Brunswick, NJ: Rutgers University Press, 1995.

Fenton, A. Edith. "The Public Health Nurse in the Tuberculosis Hospital." *CJPH* 39 (May 1948): 187–91.

Ferencz, Agnes M. "The Impact of Urbanization on French Canadian Medical Attitudes." Master's thesis, McGill University, 1945.

Ferguson, R.G. "A Tuberculosis Survey of 1,346 School Children in Saskatchewan." *CMAJ* 12 (June 1922): 381–3.
- "A Pure Milk Supply for the Farm Home." *PHJ* 18 (Apr. 1927): 151–5.
- "Activities in a Province-Wide Programme for the Control of Tuberculosis." *CPHJ* 26 (Mar. 1935): 130–7.
- "Some Simple Observations and Procedures of Assistance to the Practitioner in the Diagnosis and Eradication of Tuberculosis." *CMAJ* 32 (May 1935): 524–8.
- "Some Fundamentals in Tuberculosis Prevention." *CPHJ* 29 (May 1938): 203–12.
- "Recent Advances in Tuberculosis Control." *CJPH* 35 (Mar. 1944): 109–12.
- "BCG Vaccination in Hospitals and Sanatoria of Saskatchewan." *CJPH* 37 (Nov. 1946): 435–51.
Fiat, Justitia. "A Kick at Slum Workers." *CTSE* 1 (July 1910): 373–4.
"Fighting the White Plague." *Canadian Magazine* 36 (Nov. 1910): 74–8.
"Final Report of the English Committee on Tuberculosis." *PHJ* 4 (May 1913): 329–30.
Fishman, Alfred P. *Pulmonary Diseases and Disorders* 2nd ed. Toronto: McGraw-Hill 1988.
Fitzgerald, J.G. *An Introduction to the Practice of Preventive Medicine.* 2nd ed. St Louis, MO: 1926.
- "Some Aspects of Preventive Medicine." *CPHJ* 20 (Feb. 1929): 57–77.
Fleming, A. Grant. "Montreal Anti-Tuberculosis and General Health League." *PHJ* 17 (May 1926): 205–21; 18 (Apr. 1927): 156–70; 19 (June 1928): 263–9.
- "Health Services." *Canadian Congress Journal* 19 (Apr. 1940): 13–16.
- "Public Health in Wartime." *CPHJ* 33 (Apr. 1942): 145–7.
- ed. *What You Should Know about Tuberculosis.* Toronto: 1935.
Forbes. E.R. "Prohibition and the Social Gospel in Nova Scotia." *Acadiensis* 1 (Autumn 1971): 11–36.
Forbes, F.G. "Public Health Act – Its Scope and Application." *PHJ* 9 (Oct. 1918): 461–5.
Fosdick, Raymond B. *The Story of the Rockefeller Foundation.* New York: Harper & Brothers, 1952.
Fox, Daniel M. "Abraham Flexner's Unpublished Report: Foundations and Medical Education, 1909–1928." *Bulletin of the History of Medicine* 54 (winter 1980): 475–96.
Frappier, Armand. *Le Vaccin antituberculeux BCG: Sa découverte – Son innocuité.* Montreal: 1935.
Fraser, Roy. "Man's Attitude towards His Physical Life." *CPHJ* 23 (Dec. 1932): 587–96.
"Free Health Service Plan in Saskatchewan." *CJPH* 36 (Jan. 1945): 44–5.

Gaensler, E.A. "The Surgery for Pulmonary Tuberculosis." *American Review of Respiratory Disease* 125, no. 3, pt 2 (1982) 73–84.

Gagnon, Eugene. "The Low Mortality Rate from Tuberculosis in the Jewish Race." *CPHJ* 31 (Jan. 1940): 13–15.

Galdston, Iago. "Humanism and Public Health." *Bulletin of the History of Medicine* 8 (July 1940): 1032–9.

Gale, Godfrey L., and Norman C. Delarue. "Surgical History of Pulmonary Tuberculosis: The Rise and Fall of Various Technical Procedures." *Canadian Journal of Surgery* 12 (Oct. 1969): 381–8.

Gibbon, John Murray, and Mary S. Matheson. *Three Centuries of Canadian Nursing.* Toronto: Macmillan, 1947.

Gibson, D.M. "Prognosis in Minimal Pulmonary Tuberculosis." *CMAJ* 55 (July 1946): 1–4.

– "Tuberculosis Prevention." *CMAJ* 53 (Oct. 1945): 349–51.

Gilchrist, C.W. "Pioneer of Public Health." *Maclean's Magazine* 50 (15 Oct. 1937): 26, 28.

Goldbloom, Alton. "Tuberculosis in Children." *CMAJ* 28 (Mar. 1933): 286–9.

Goodchild, J.F. Fleming. "The State Medicine Factor of the Toronto Academy of Medicine." *PHJ* 2 (Jan. 1911): 5–10.

Gordon, P.H. *Fifty Years in the Canadian Red Cross.* Canadian Red Cross [1968?].

Grace, A.J. "Surgical Procedures in Pulmonary Tuberculosis." *CMAJ* 41 (Aug. 1939): 124–30.

Grant, Anne. *Grist for the Teacher's Mill.* 2nd ed. Ottawa: Canadian Tuberculosis Association 1947.

– "Health Education at the Local Level." *CJPH* 42 (June 1951): 254–6.

Grant, Sir James. "Our Race and Consumption." *Montreal Medical Journal* 29 (Sept. 1900): 673–9.

– "Tuberculosis and the Bacteriology of Everyday Life." *PHJ* 6 (Oct. 1915): 497–9.

Gray, A.L. "The Early Diagnosis and Prognosis of Pulmonary Tuberculosis by Roentgen Methods." *CMAJ* 4 (Nov. 1914): 979–82.

Grayson, L.M., and Michael Bliss, eds. *The Wretched of Canada: Letters to R.B. Bennett, 1930–1935.* Toronto: University of Toronto Press, 1971.

Great Britain. Royal Commission Appointed to Inquire into the Relations of Human and Animal Tuberculosis. *Report* Pt 1 London: 1911.

Gregoire, G. "Comité provincial de défense contre la tuberculose: Son origine, son programme." *Canada Français* 26 (Jan. 1939): 458–63.

Grenier, Eugene. "The Anti-Tuberculosis Campaign – A Social Campaign – The Role of Government – The Role of Private Effort." *CMAJ* 10 (Aug. 1920): 729–32.

Groulx, Adelard. "Developments in Public Health in Montreal during the Past Three Years." *CPHJ* 31 (Dec. 1940): 589–94.

– "Pasteurization in the Province of Quebec." *CJPH* 37 (Jan. 1946): 17–21.
Hall, Orlan. "Progress of Tuberculosis Eradication in Canada." *Canadian Journal of Comparative Medicine* 3 (Feb. 1939): 47–50.
– "Present Status of Tuberculosis Eradication in Canada." *Canadian Journal of Comparative Medicine* 5 (Mar. 1941): 75–7.
– "Tuberculosis Eradication in Canada." *Canadian Journal of Comparative Medicine* 6 (Feb 1942): 55–7.
Hall, Peter Dobkin. "Private Philanthropy and Public Policy: A Historical Appraisal." In *Philanthropy: Four Views*, ed. Robert Payton, New Brunswick, NJ: Social Philosophy and Policy Center, Transaction Books, 1988, 39–72.
Halpenny, J., and Lillian Ireland. *How to Be Healthy.* Toronto: 1911.
Hamilton Health Association. *The Mountain Sanatorium: Some Interesting Facts.* Hamilton, ON: [1940?].
Harris, D. Fraser. *The Prevention of Tuberculosis.* Halifax: 1913.
Harris, H. William, and John H. McClement. "Tuberculosis." In *Infectious Diseases*, edited by Paul D. Hoeprich, 351–78. Hagerstown, MD.
Harris, Norman M. "Presidential Address: Some Thoughts on the Organization and Progress of Public Health in Canada." *CPHJ* 20 (Aug. 1929): 375–85.
Harris, R.I. "Heliotherapy in Surgical Tuberculosis." *CMAJ* 12 (Nov. 1922): 799–805.
– "The Pathology of Bone Tuberculosis." *PHJ* 19 (Oct. 1928): 451–5.
– "The Menace of Raw Milk: 1. Milk-Borne Tuberculosis." *CPHJ* 23 (Jan. 1932): 1–5.
Hart, William M. "The Rural Health Officer's Relation to Pulmonary Consumption." *PHJ* 3 (Nov. 1912): 618–21.
– "The Tuberculosis Problem under After-War Conditions with Reference to Canada." *Journal of State Medicine* 27 (Nov. 1919): 336–9.
Hastings, Charles. "Democracy and Public Health Administration." *PHJ* 10 (Mar. 1919): 97–112.
Hastings, Charles J. "The Modern Conception of Public Health Administration." In Rutherford, *Saving the Canadian City.*
Hatfield, W.H. "A Tuberculosis Exhibit in Vancouver, BC." *CPHJ* 27 (Apr. 1936): 195.
– "Rehabilitation." *CPHJ* 31 (May 1940): 206–22.
– *Handbook on Tuberculosis.* Victoria, BC: Provincial Board of Health of the Province of British Columbia, 1944.
– *A History of Tuberculosis in British Columbia.* Vancouver, BC: 1952.
– "Some Thoughts on Tuberculosis Control in Canada." *CJPH* 35 (Nov. 1944): 423–30.
Hattie,W.H. "Some Medico-Sociological Problems Arising out of the War." *PHJ* 8 (Oct. 1917): 254–9.

– "The Co-ordination of State and Private Enterprises in Public Health Work." *PHJ* 11 (Sept. 1920): 418–21.

Hayes, Joseph. *The Control of Tuberculosis and Where the Responsibility Lies*. Nova Scotia: 1933.

Haygood, Lt Tamara Miner. "World War I Military Led the Way in Screening Chest Radiography." *Military Medicine* 157 (1992): 113–16.

Heagerty, J.J. "The Development of Public Health in Canada." *CPHJ* 25 (Feb. 1934): 53–9.

– "Wartime Control of Tuberculosis." *National Health Review* 10 (Jan. 1942): 16–18.

– "State of Health of the People of Canada in 1942." *CJPH* 34 (Dec. 1943): 529–42.

Hellyar, B. "The Approach to the Patient." *Canadian Nurse* 44 (Dec. 1948): 974–6.

Hill, H.W. "Tuberculosis." *PHJ* 9 (Oct. 1918): 457–60.

Hincks, Clarence M. "Letter to the Editor." *PHJ* 7 (Nov. 1917): 309–10.

Hocken, Horatio C. "The New Spirit in Municipal Government." In *Saving the Canadian City*, ed. Paul Rutherford.

Hodgetts, Charles A. *Consumption: General Precautions*. Ontario Provincial Board of Health: n.d.

– *Consumption, Personal Precautions*, Ontario Provincial Board of Health: n.d.

– "Relationship of the Medical Practitioner to Public Health." *PHJ* 3 (May 1912): 249–55.

– "A Survey of Public Health." *PHJ* 3 (Oct. 1912): 541–7.

Holbrook, John Howard. "Present Need of the Tuberculosis Campaign in Canada." *PHJ* 11 (Oct. 1920): 461–73.

– "Prevention of Tuberculosis in School Age." *PHJ* 14 (Jan. 1923): 19–26.

– "The Story of the Hamilton Health Association." *PHJ* 15 (Apr. 1924): 158–64; (May 1924): 219–21.

– "Forty Years of Advance." *The Canadian Hospital* 23 (Nov. 1946): 29–33, 92, 94.

Holbrook, John Howard, and A.S. Kennedy. "The Organization of a Medical Service within a Sanatorium." *CPHJ* 25 (May 1934): 234–7.

Holling, S.A. "A Tuberculosis Survey among Ottawa Federal Civil Servants." *CJPH* 36 (July 1945): 261–7.

– "Tuberculosis Case-Finding Techniques in the Province of Ontario." *CJPH* 40 (Jan. 1949): 1–6.

Hôpital du Sacré-Cœur pour les Tuberculeux et les Incurables. *Bénédiction de l'Hôpital par S.G. Mgr.-Gauthier.* [Montreal?: 1926?].

Hopkins, J. Castell. *The Canadian Annual Review of Public Affairs*, 1905–32. Toronto: 1906–33.

Houston, C. Stuart. "Ferguson's BCG Research – Canada's First Randomized Clinical trial?" *Clinical and Investigative Medicine* 16 (1993): 89–91.
– *R.G. Ferguson: Crusader against Tuberculosis.* Toronto: Dundern Press, 1991.
Howe, Barbara. "The Emergence of Scientific Philanthropy, 1900–1920: Origins, Issues and Outcomes." In *Philanthropy and Cultural Imperialism*, edited by Robert F. Arnove, 25–54. Boston: G.K. Hall, 1980.
Hunter, Arthur. "Can Insurance Experience Be Applied to Lengthen Life?" *PHJ* 6 (May 1915): 213–18.
Hunter, J. "Tuberculosis and Insurance." *Canadian Journal of Medicine and Surgery* 6 (Nov. 1899): 309–14.
Hutchinson, John A. "Public Health Legislation in the Province of Quebec." *PHJ* 4 (Sept. 1913): 502–4.
Hutchison, Woods. "The Conquest of Great Diseases." *PHJ* 2 (Apr. 1911): 153–5.
Hwang, Chen-Hong, Shanki Khan, Norman Ende, et al. "The HLA-A,-B, and DR Phenotypes and Tuberculosis." *American Review of Respiratory Disease* 132 (1985): 382–5.
"Impure Milk." *PHJ* 1 (Dec. 1910): ix.
Institute of Microbiology and Hygiene. *Notes on BCG.* Montreal: 1951.
"Inter Alia." *PHJ* 1 (Nov. 1910): 561–5; 3 (Mar. 1912): 133–4.
International Commission on the Control of Bovine Tuberculosis. *Tuberculosis: A Plain Statement of Facts Regarding the Disease, Prepared Especially for Farmers and Others Interested in Livestock.* Ottawa: 1911.
Jackson, F.W. "Public Medical Services in Manitoba." *CPHJ* 21 (Dec. 1930): 608–17.
– "Reorganization of Public Health Nursing Service in Manitoba." *CPHJ* 22 (Nov. 1931): 576–7.
– "The Provision of Medical Care in Western Canada." *CPHJ* 26 (July 1935): 315–20.
– "The Program of Medical Care in Manitoba." *CPHJ* 30 (Oct. 1939): 479–87.
– "Manitoba's Health Proposals." *CJPH* 34 (Apr. 1945): 131–4.
– "The Progress and Promise of the National Health Program." *CJPH* 40 (Oct. 1949): 427–30.
Janes, Robert M. "Surgery in the Treatment of Pulmonary Tuberculosis." *CMAJ* 33 (Oct. 1935): 389–92.
Jeffrey, A.M. "Childhood Tuberculosis." *CMAJ* 38 (Apr. 1938): 373–4.
Jemmott, John B. III, and Steven E. Locke. "Psychosocial Factors, Immunologic Mediation, and Human Susceptibility to Infectious Diseases: How Much Do We Know?" *Psychological Bulletin* 95 (1984): 78–108.
Johannesson, Sig Jul. "Alcohol and Tuberculosis." *PHJ* 3 (Oct. 1912): 563–8.
Jones, H.A. "Bilateral Artificial Pneumothorax in the Treatment of Pulmonary Tuberculosis." *CPHJ* 28 (Sept. 1937): 442–96.

Jones, J.H. Mowbray. "The Voluntary Health Agency." *CPHJ* 30 (Aug. 1939): 400–5.

Jones, W.A. "Routine Chest X-ray Examination of Recruits: A Survey of Results." *CMAJ* 43 (Sept. 1940): 213–17.

Jordan, John M. *Machine-Age Ideology: Social Engineering and American Liberalism, 1911–1939*, Chapel Hill: University of North Carolina Press, 1994.

Kalbach, Warren E., and Wayne W. McVey. *The Demographic Bases of Canadian Society.* Montreal: 1971.

Keifer, Zada. "System of Follow-Up Work for Tuberculosis." *PHJ* 13 (June 1922): 251–8.

Kendall, W.B. "Observations Relating to Diet in Tuberculosis." *CMAJ* 2 (Aug. 1912): 670–9.

– "Artificial Pneumothorax in the Treatment of Tuberculosis." *CMAJ* 5 (Mar. 1915): 206–11.

King, D. MacDougall. "What the Federal Government Might Do to Assist in the Control of Tuberculosis." *PHJ* 3 (July 1912): 383–7.

– *The Battle with Tuberculosis and How to Win It: A Book for the Patient and His Friends.* Philadelphia: J.B. Lippincott, 1917.

King, Floris Ethia. "Historical Study of the Voluntary Tuberculosis Community Health Program in Canada with Projective Emphasis." Ph.D. diss., University of North Carolina, Chapel Hill, 1967.

– "The Past and Future of the Canadian Voluntary Tuberculosis Association." *CJPH* 59 (Mar. 1968): 123–5.

Kinsella, Thomas J. "The Development of Thoracic Surgery in the Upper Mid-West." *Minnesota Medicine* (1972): 7–53.

Kinsey, H.I. "Diagnosis of Early Thoracic Tuberculosis in Children." *CPHJ* 25 (Mar. 1934): 134–40.

Kirkby, R.W. "Discovery of Cases of Active Tuberculosis amongst Ex-Patients in a Rural Province." *CPHJ* 28 (Jan. 1937): 10–12.

Klebs, Arnold C. *Tuberculosis.* New York: D. Appleton, 1909.

Knopf, S. Adolphus. *Tuberculosis: A Preventable and Curable Disease.* Toronto: McClelland and Goodchild, 1909.

– *Report to the United States Government on Tuberculosis with Some Therapeutic and Prophylactic Suggestions.* New York: National Tuberculosis Association, 1933.

– "Birth Control in Its Medical, Social, Economic and Moral Aspects." *PHJ* 8 (May 1917): 117–26.

Kobrinsky, Solomon. "Pregnancy and Tuberculosis." *CMAJ* 59 (Nov. 1948): 462–4.

Kohn, Robert. "Some Economic Aspects of Our National Health." *Public Affairs* 10 (1947): 88–91.

Laberge, L. "Danger de contamination massive chez les élèves." *Canada Français* 28 (Jan. 1941): 541–3.

– "Detection of Tuberculosis in School Teachers in the Province of Quebec."
    *CJPH* 34 (Mar. 1943): 125–9.

Ladouceur, Leo. "The Fight against Tuberculosis in Montreal." *CJPH* 36 (Jan.
    1945): 22–6.

LaHaye, Bruno. "The Development of County Health Units in the Province
    of Quebec." *CPHJ* 33 (Jan. 1942): 7–12.

Lalonde, Marc. "The Untold Epidemic: Heart Attacks and Strokes." *CJPH* 68
    (July/Aug. 1977): 277–81.

Langston, Hiram T. "Thoracoplasty: The How and Why." *Annals of Thoracic
    Surgery* 52 (1991): 1351–3.

Lasch, Christopher. *The Revolt of the Elites and the Betrayal of Democracy.* New
    York: W.W. Norton, 1995.

Laviolette, Camille. *Trembling Mountain, Laurentides, (Can.) 3,000 ft. A High
    Level Sanitarium for the Treatment of Tuberculosis.* Montreal: 1895.

Layton, B.D.B. "The Progress of the National Health Grants." *CJPH* 41 (Sept.
    1950): 366–73.

Lebœuf, Auguste. "The Prevention of Tuberculosis through Travelling Clin-
    ics." *CPHJ* 25 (Nov. 1934): 544–7.

Lee, Joseph H. "The Decrease in the Length of Stay in Patients in Sanatoria."
    *CJPH* 39 (Sept. 1948): 375–80.

Leibowitz, David. "Scientific Failure in an Age of Optimism: Public Reaction
    to Robert Koch's Tuberculin Cure." *New York State Journal of Medicine* 93
    (1993): 41–8.

Lerner, Barron H. "New York City's Tuberculosis Control Efforts: The Histor-
    ical Limitations of the 'War on Consumption.'" *American Journal of Public
    Health* 83 (1993): 758–66.

Lessard, Dr Alphonse. "County Health Work in the Province of Quebec." *PHJ*
    18 (Oct. 1927): 451–7.

– "Rural Sanitation in Quebec from the Provincial Standpoint." *CPHJ* 23 (Mar.
    1932): 103–8.

– "Presidential Address: Public Health Progress in Quebec." *CPHJ* 25 (Sept.
    1934): 411–16.

Lessard, Dr Alphonse, and Emile Nadeau. "County Health Units in the Prov-
    ince of Quebec." *CPHJ* 20 (Mar. 1929): 124–31.

Leutwyler, Kristin. "The Price of Prevention." *Scientific American* 272 (Apr.
    1995): 124–9.

Liddell, K.E. "Health Hucksters." *Canadian Business* 12 (May 1949): 56–7, 120.

Linteau, P.A., R. Durocher, and J.C. Robert. *Quebec: A History, 1867–1929.*
    Toronto: James Lorimer, 1983.

Linteau, P.A., R. Durocher, J.C. Robert, and F. Ricard. *Quebec since 1930.*
    Toronto: James Lorimer, 1991.

Little, G.M. "The Rural Health District." *CPHJ* 28 (July 1937): 333–8.

Long, Esmond R. "Acquired and Constitutional Factors in Resistance to Tuberculosis." In National Tuberculosis Association, *Transactions of 31st Annual Meeting* (1935): 1–6.

– *A History of the Therapy of Tuberculosis and the Case of Frédéric Chopin.* Lawrence, KS: University of Kansas Press, 1956.

Long, G. Roy. ed. *Kiwanis Club of Vancouver, 1919–1969 Golden Anniversary.* Vancouver, BC: Kiwanis Club, 1969.

Lowe, James E., Thomas M. Daniel, Charlotte Richer, and Walter G. Wolfe. "Pulmonary Tuberculosis in Children." *Journal of Thoracic and Cardiovascular Surgery* 80 (1980): 221–4.

Lucas, Alex. *Peter McArthur.* Boston: 1975.

Luce, P.W. "Free X-rays in Anti-tuberculosis Campaign." *Saturday Night* 59 (23 Oct. 1943): 29.

Ludmerer, Kenneth M. *Learning to Heal: The Development of American Medical Education.* New York: Basic Books, 1985.

MacDermot, H.E. *History of the Canadian Medical Association, 1867–1921.* Toronto: Murray, 1935.

– *Sir Thomas Roddick.* Toronto: Macmillan, 1938.

– *A Short History of the Royal Edward Institute.* Montreal: 1965.

– *One Hundred Years of Medicine in Canada.* Toronto: McClelland and Stewart, 1967.

MacDougall, Heather. *Activists and Advocates.* Toronto: Dundern Press, 1990.

MacGregor, Rob Roy. "Alcohol and Immune Defense." *Journal of the American Medical Association* 256, no. 11 (1986): 1474–9.

MacKay, T.W.G. "Tuberculosis and the Community." *PHJ* 18 (Oct 1927): 476.

MacKenzie, David W. "Renal Tuberculosis." *CMAJ* 12 (Sept. 1922): 620–5.

Mackenzie, Margaret. "Sydney Kiwanis Health Camp." *CPHJ* 20 (July 1929): 344–8.

MacKinnon, Andrew Pritchard. "The Association of Pulmonary and Bone and Joint Tuberculosis." *CMAJ* 14 (Feb. 1924): 124–9.

MacLeod, Wendall, Libbie Park, and Stanley Ryerson. *Bethune: The Montreal Years.* Toronto: James Lorimer, 1978.

MacTavish, W.L. "Special Grant by British Columbia for TB Sufferers." *Saturday Night* 63 (1 Nov. 1947): 12.

Magill, W.S. "New Methods in Diagnosis and Treatment of Infectious Diseases." *PHJ* 2 (Oct 1911): 469–73.

Maheux, A. "Lutte à la tuberculose." *Canada Francais* 28 (Dec. 1940): 397–400.

Manitoba Sanatorium. *Medical Histories and History Writing with Special Reference to Tuberculosis: A Few Notes and an Outline.* Manitoba: n.d.

Marshall, Marion. "My Personal Experience of Tuberculosis." *PHJ* 4 (Sept. 1913): 491–8.

Martin, Paul. "A National Health Program for Canada." *CJPH* 39 (June 1948): 219–26.
– "Canada's National Health Program." *CJPH* 39 (Dec. 1948): 478–85.
Mason, F.E. "Protection from Tuberculosis is Given by New Vaccine." *Saturday Night* 52 (30 Aug. 1947): 9.
Massachusetts-Halifax Health Commission. *Final Report ... with Appendices: October 1919 to October 1929.* Halifax, NS: 1932.
Maugham, W. Somerset. "Sanatorium." In *The Complete Short Stories of W. Somerset Maugham.* Vol. 2, 505–27. Garden City, NY: Doubleday, 1952.
Mayer, Edgar. "Recent Advances in Tuberculosis." *CMAJ* 43 (Dec. 1940): 565–70.
McCann, James. "Some Public Health Activities and Needs in Ontario." *CPHJ* 25 (June 1934): 255–9.
– "Canada's War Effort for the Health of Her People." *CPHJ* 32 (Dec. 1941): 587–93.
– "Our Wartime Health." *CPHJ* 33 (July 1942): 315–19.
McCarthy, Mrs MacDonald. "The Royal Edward Institute." *PHJ* 3 (May 1912): 248–9.
McClelland, James C. "Present Conceptions of Renal Tuberculosis." *CMAJ* 29 (Nov. 1933): 514–20.
McClung, Nellie. "What Will They Do With It?" *Maclean's Magazine* 29 (July 1916): 36–8.
McCuaig, Katherine. "'From Social Reform to Social Service': The Changing Role of Volunteers: The Anti-tuberculosis Campaign, 1900–1930." *Canadian Historical Review* 61 (Dec. 1980): 480–501.
McCullough, J.W. "Municipal Sanatoria." *PHJ* 2 (June 1911): 253–9.
– "The Ontario Public Health Act." *PHJ* 3 (Oct. 1912): 253–4.
– "The Public Health Act of Ontario." *PHJ* 4 (July 1913): 405.
– "Industrial Hygiene." *PHJ* 11 (June 1920): 245–58.
– "A Decade of Public Health Progress." *PHJ* 11 (July 1920): 293–300.
– "The Greatest Public Health Need in Canada." *PHJ* 16 (Apr. 1925): 171–4.
– "How to Safeguard the Milk We Use." *PHJ* 18 (June 1927): 255–7.
– "The Promotion of Rural Health in Ontario." *PHJ* 19 (July 1928): 35–62.
– "The County Health Unit." *CPHJ* 20 (Mar. 1929): 114–23.
– "The Highway of Health." *Social Welfare* 13 (Apr. 1930): 145–7, 154.
McCurdy, David G. "The Recalcitrant Tuberculosis Patient." *CJPH* 45 (Aug. 1954): 350–2.
McEachern, J.P. "Tuberculosis Cervical Adenitis in Children." *CMAJ* 13 (Dec. 1923): 866–71.
McGinnis, Janice P. Dickin. "The Impact of Epidemic Influenza: Canada 1918–1919." Canadian Historical Association, *Historical Papers,* 1977: 120–40.

–  "From Health to Welfare. Federal Government Policies Regarding Standards of Public Health for Canadians, 1919–1945." Ph.D. diss., University of Alberta, 1980.

McIntosh, J.W. "Cancer and Tuberculosis." *CPHJ* 20 (Dec. 1929): 600–9; 21 (July 1930): 360–1.

McKay, T.W.G. "Tuberculosis and the Community." *PHJ* 18 (Oct. 1927): 475–81.

McKenty, Neil. *Mitch Hepburn.* Toronto: McClelland and Stewart, 1967.

McKeown, Thomas. *The Origins of Human Disease.* Oxford: Basil Blackwell, 1988.

–  *The Role of Medicine.* Princeton, NJ: Princeton University Press, 1979.

McKinnon, N.E. "Tuberculosis – Our Great Public Health Problem." *CPHJ* 22 (Oct. 1931): 520.

–  "Symposium on Tuberculosis: The Extent of the Rural Health Problem in Ontario." *CPHJ* 28 (May 1937): 209–11.

–  "Mortality Reductions in Ontario, 1900–1942: 4 Tuberculosis." *CJPH* 36 (Nov. 1945): 423–9.

McKone, Barclay. "Post-Sanatorium Rehabilitation." *Canadian Nurse* 44 (Dec. 1948): 971–3.

McLaren, Angus. *Our Own Master Race.* Toronto: McClelland and Stewart, 1990.

McLeod, K.J. "The Public Health Nurse in Tuberculosis Work." *PHJ* 13 (Oct. 1922): 455–7.

McPhedran, F. Maurice. "The Diagnosis and Classification of Pulmonary Tuberculosis in Childhood and Adolescence." *The American Review of Tuberculosis* 20 (Oct. 1929): 532–636.

–  "Tuberculosis in Childhood as a Problem in Preventive Medicine." *CPHJ* 21 (Oct. 1930): 475–90.

McRae, D.F. "Tuberculosis Concepts Then and Now." *CMAJ* 51 (Aug. 1944): 139–41.

Meakins, Jonathan C. "Tuberculin in the Diagnosis of Tuberculosis." *CMAJ* 1 (Mar. 1911): 223–31.

–  "Metabolic Factors in the Treatment of Tuberculosis." *CMAJ* 17 (Mar. 1927): 277–81.

Medawar, Sir Peter. *The Threat and the Glory: Reflections on Science and Scientists.* New York: Oxford University Press, 1991.

Melvin, Geo. G. "Our Voluntary Assistants." *PHJ* 19 (Oct. 1928): 456–62.

Meyer, John A. "Tuberculosis, the Adirondacks, and Coming of Age for Thoracic Surgery." *Annals of Thoracic Surgery* 52 (1991): 881–5.

Michell, W.R. "The Evolution of Health Service Work, Medical, Dental, and Nursing, in Schools in Toronto with a Detailed Account of its Growth and Present Status." *PHJ* 15 (Dec. 1924): 541–6.

Middlebrook, Gardner. "Tuberculosis and Medical Science." *American Review of Respiratory Disease* 125, no. 3 (1982).

Middleton, F.C. "The Nursing, Medical and Hospital Problems in the Rural West." *PHJ* 10 (July 1919): 297–308.
– "Full-Time Health Districts in Saskatchewan." *CPHJ* 20 (Mar. 1929): 140–8.
– "Health and Sickness Insurance in Saskatchewan." *CPHJ* 21 (Dec. 1930): 601–7.
– "Evolution of Tuberculosis Control in Saskatechewan." *CPHJ* 24 (Nov. 1933): 505–13.
Miller, A.F. "The Canadian Practitioner's Diagnosis of Pulmonary Tuberculosis." *CMAJ* 4 (Sept. 1914): 793–8.
– "Community Responsibility with Regard to Tuberculosis." *PHJ* 14 (Mar. 1923): 99–109.
– "The New Knowledge of Tuberculosis." *CMAJ* 50 (Mar. 1944): 243–7.
Miller, A.F., and Jane Mortimer. *The War on Tuberculosis*. Halifax: 1921.
Miller, Dr Clarence. "The Forward Movement in Public Health and Its Relationship to Social Advance." *PHJ* 12 (Mar. 1921): 120–6.
Miller, James. "A Comment on Cancer and Tuberculosis." *CPHJ* 21 (Apr. 1930): 174–6.
"Milk Substitutes." *PHJ* 5 (Feb. 1914): 135.
Minns, F.S. "The Method of Dealing with Tuberculosis in the Public Schools of Toronto, Canada." *CMAJ* 5 (Oct. 1915): 902–8.
– "The Method of Dealing with Tuberculosis in the Public Schools of Toronto." *PHJ* 7 (Mar. 1916): 145–8.
Mitchinson, W., and J.D. McGinnis. *Essays in the History of Canadian Medicine*. Toronto: McClelland and Stewart, 1988.
Montreal Health Survey Committee. *Survey of Public Health Activities: Montreal, Canada*, Montreal: Metropolitan Life, 1928.
Montreal League for the Prevention of Tuberculosis. *On the Responsibility of the Federal Government in Relationship to the Prevention of Tuberculosis and upon Certain Measures Which Could Be Taken by it to Aid in the Prevention of Tuberculosis*. Montreal: 1905.
"Montreal Public School Health Report." *PHJ* 3 (Apr. 1912): 222.
Mooney, Elizabeth. *In the Shadow of the White Plague*. New York: Thomas Y. Crowell, 1979.
Morris, William. "Survey of Tuberculosis Patients in the Home, Vancouver, BC, 1936." *CPHJ* 29 (Apr. 1938): 166–70.
Morton, Desmond, and Glenn Wright. *Winning the Second Battle*. Toronto: University of Toronto Press, 1987.
Mullen, J.H. "History of the Organization of the Babies' Dispensary Guild, Hamilton (Inc.)." *PHJ* 6 (Nov. 1915): 542–4.
Murray, R.H. "Milk Sanitation in Canada." *CPHJ* 22 (June 1932): 259–66.
– "The Extent of Pasteurization in Canada." *CPHJ* 25 (Jan. 1934): 30–1.
Murrell, John F. "The Development of Health Units in British Columbia." *CJPH* 41 (Sept. 1950): 389–98.

Myers, J. Arthur. *Captain of All These Men of Death.* St Louis, MO: 1977.

Nadeau, Gabriel. "A TB's Progress: The Story of Norman Bethune." *Bulletin of the History of Medicine* 8 (Oct. 1940): 1135–71.

Nadeau, Emile. "Koch Bacillus Is Ordered to Leave." *PHJ* 4 (Mar. 1913): 158–9.

– "The Grancher System, as Applied in the Province of Quebec for the Protection of Childhood against Tuberculosis." *CPHJ* 21 (Aug. 1930): 382–6.

– "The Progress of the Organization of County Health Units in Quebec." *CPHJ* 22 (Feb. 1931): 90–1.

Naef, Andreas P. "The 1900 Tuberculosis Epidemic – Starting Point of Modern Thoracic Surgery." *Annals of Thoracic Surgery* 55 (1993): 1375–8.

Nardell, Edward A. "Environmental Control of Tuberculosis." *Medical Clinics of North America.* 77, no. 6 (1993): 1315–34.

National Archives of Canada. Records of the Canadian Tuberculosis Association.

National Committee for Mental Hygiene. Division on Public Health and Medical Services. *Study of the Distribution of Medical Care and Public Health Services in Canada.* Toronto: 1959.

National Council of Women of Canada. *Yearbook.* 1898, 1901, 1906–09, 1911–14, 1917, 1930.

"The National Health Grows." *CJPH* 39 (Aug. 1948): 348–9.

Naylor, C. David. *Private Practice, Public Payment: Canadian Medicine and the Politics of Health Insurance 1911–1966.* Montreal: McGill-Queen's University Press, 1986.

– ed. *Canadian Health Care and the State.* Montreal: McGill-Queen's University Press, 1992.

Nevins, Allan. *John D. Rockefeller: The Heroic Age of American Enterprise.* New York: Charles Scribner's Sons, 1940.

– *Study in Power: John D. Rockefeller Industrialist and Philanthropist.* Vol. 2. New York: Charles Scribner's Sons, 1953.

"New Government Program for Sanatorium Care of Tuberculous Patients in Ontario." *CPHJ* 29 (Sept. 1938): 472.

Nielsen, Waldemar. *The Big Foundations.* New York: Columbia University Press, 1972.

Nix, Margaret E. "Education and the Extension of Public Health Services." *CJPH* 37 (May 1946): 182–6.

Ogden, W.E. "The Difficulties in Prognosis in Pulmonary Tuberculosis." *CMAJ* 2 (Mar. 1912): 200–6.

Ogden, W.E., et al. "The Abolition of Clinical Tuberculosis by Anticipation and Control." *CMAJ* 40 (Mar 1939): 253–7.

One Who May Have Erred. "The Tuberculosis Problem." *PHJ* 4 (Dec. 1913): 683.

"The Only Safe Milk." *PHJ* 4 (May 1913): 328–9.

"Ontario and the Tuberculosis Exhibit." *PHJ* 2 (Feb. 1911): 73.

"Open Mail." *PHJ* 2 (June 1911): 284–6.

Orr, John. "The Role of the General Practitioner in the Prevention of Tuberculosis." *CMAJ* 41 (Dec. 1949): 571–4.

Osler, Sir William. "The Home in its Relation to the Tuberculosis Problem." *Canada Lancet* 38 (Mar. 1905): 600–12.

Ottawa Anti-Tuberculosis Association. *A Catechism on Tuberculosis.* Ottawa: 1908.

"Our Boards of Health and the Fly." *PHJ* 3 (Aug. 1912): 464.

Parfitt, Charles D. "The Recognition of Pulmonary Tuberculosis." *CMAJ* 2 (May 1912): 431–9.

– "Our Present Attitude towards Tuberculosis." *CMAJ* 2 (June 1912): 477–86.

– "The Examination of Sputum in Ontario." *PHJ* 4 (July 1913): 395–401.

– "Tuberculosis Often of Secondary Importance to Other Pathological Conditions." *CMAJ* 7 (Jan. 1917): 10–17.

– "The Prompt Diagnosis of Pulmonary Tuberculosis." *CMAJ* 14 (Nov. 1924): 1046–51.

– "Surgical Measures in the Treatment of Pulmonary Tuberculosis." *CMAJ* 22 (Feb. 1930): 170–5.

– "Osler's Influence in the War against Tuberculosis." *CMAJ* 47 (Oct. 1942): 293–304.

Parfitt, Charles D., and D.W. Crombie. "Artificial Pneumothorax in the Treatment of Phthisis." *CMAJ* 5 (Apr. 1915): 277–88; (May 1915): 373–88; (June 1915): 489–502.

Parsons, H.C. "History in Tuberculosis." *CMAJ* 12 (Apr. 1922): 216–18.

Paul, Frederick. "The Sub-Committee on Quack Advertising." *PHJ* 9 (Feb. 1918): 63–7.

– "The Trail of the Medical Vampire." *PHJ* 9 (June 1918): 249–54.

Payton, Robert, Michael Novak, Brian O'Connell, and Peter Dobkin Hall. *Philanthropy: Four Views.* New Brunswick, NJ: The Social Philosophy and Policy Center and Transaction Books, 1988.

Peirce, Surgeon-Cmdr Carleton B., et al. "The Incidence of Pulmonary Tuberculosis in the Royal Canadian Naval Service." *CMAJ* 51 (July 1944): 46–51.

Pemberton, R.E.K. "Layman Looks at Pasteurization." *Canadian Forum* 21 (Nov. 1941): 247–9; (Feb. 1942): 341–3.

Penney, Sheila M. *Inventing the Cure: Tuberculosis in Twentieth Century Nova Scotia.* PHD diss., Dalhousie University, 1990.

Penney, Sheila M. *Tuberculosis in Nova Scotia 1882–1914.* MA thesis, 1985.

Perry, Anne Anderson. "A Logical Highroad to Health." *Social Welfare* 13 (Dec. 1929): 60–3.

Petersdorf, Robert G. "The Evolution of Departments of Medicine." *New England Journal of Medicine* 303 (1980): 489–96.

Pickard, H.G. "The Need for More Complete Organization in Public Health Work." *PHJ* 4 (Nov. 1913): 610–11.

Pierce, R.V. *The People's Common Sense Medical Advisor in Plain English.* 78th ed. Bridgeburg, ON: 1914.

Pine, A. Howard. "Some Points in the Value of X-rays for Prognosis in Pulmonary Tuberculosis." *CMAJ* 14 (Oct. 1924): 953–5.

Playter, Edward. *Consumption: Its Nature, Causes and Prevention.* Toronto: William Briggs, 1895.

Porter, George. "Tuberculosis Mortality in Ontario." *PHJ* 2 (Mar. 1911): 111.

– "Tuberculosis and the Public." *PHJ* 3 (Oct. 1912): 561–3.

– *Tuberculosis and the Public.* N.p., 1912.

– *The Attitude of the Federal Government Towards Tuberculosis.* N.p., 1915.

– "The Tuberculosis Problem in Canada." *PHJ* 12 (Jan. 1921): 1–5.

– "Canadian Public Health Association: Presidential Address." *PHJ* 17 (June 1926): 271–6.

– "Pioneers in Tuberculosis Work in Canada." *CPHJ* 31 (Aug. 1940): 367–9.

– "Pioneers in Public Health." *CJPH* 40 (Feb. 1949): 84–6.

– *Crusading against Tuberculosis.* Ottawa: Canadian Tuberculosis Association 1953.

Postill, L. "Bed's Eye View." *Maclean's Magazine.* 59 (1 Nov. 1946): 24, 40, 42.

Pottenger, F.M. "The Evolution of Clinical Pulmonary Tuberculosis and Its Early Diagnosis." *CMAJ* 17 (Dec. 1927): 1429–34.

Power, Mary. "The Public Health Exhibit, Canadian National Exhibition, 1928." *PHJ* 19 (Dec. 1928): 563–89.

Pratt, Joseph. *Osler and Tuberculosis.* Reprinted from *Sir William Osler Memorial Volume.* 2nd impression. Bulletin no. 9, International Association of Medical Museums: 1927.

"The Present Status of Surgery in Tuberculosis." *CMAJ* 3 (Dec. 1913): 1087–93.

Prevost, Jules. "The Treatment of Pulmonary Tuberculosis after Forty." *CMAJ* 38 (Feb. 1938): 166–9.

Price, R.M. "The Incidence of Bovine Tuberculosis in Children." *CPHJ* 20 (July 1929): 323–330.

– "Milk and its Relation to Tuberculosis." *CPHJ* 25 (Jan. 1934): 13–15.

– "Bovine Tuberculosis in Children." *CPHJ* 29 (June 1938): 251–4.

Private Practice. "Tuberculosis and the Workshop." *PHJ* 2 (Mar. 1911): 145.

"Progress in Tuberculosis Control in British Columbia." *CPHJ* 27 (July 1936): 360–2.

"Proposed Measures for Health Insurance in Canada." *CJPH* 34 (July 1943): 338–42.

Province of Manitoba. Department of Health and Public Welfare. Health and Hospital Survey Committee of the Welfare Supervision Board. *Report on Tuberculosis.* Report no. 2. Winnipeg: 1929.

Pumphrey, Avis. "Rehabilitation of the TB Patient." *BC Bulletin* 2 (Aug. 1945): 9–11.

Quebec. Royal Commission on Tuberculosis. *Report.* Quebec: 1910.

Quebec Provincial Committee for the Prevention of Tuberculosis. *Notes on Tuberculosis* 1–18 (Sept. 1938 – Oct./Nov./Dec. 1955).

Race, Joseph. "Milk Supply in Relation to Tuberculosis in Ontario." *PHJ* 6 (Aug. 1915): 378–83.

Raney, Fraser. "What is a Patent Medicine?" *PHJ* 9 (Dec. 1918): 569–72.

Rankin, Allan C. "BCG Vaccine." *CPHJ* 22 (Sept. 1931): 459–66.

Ranney, A.E. "Tuberculosis and the Medical Officer of Health." *CPHJ* 27 (Oct. 1936): 477–81.

Ravenel, Mazyck. "Transmission of Animal Diseases to Man through Milk." *CPHJ* (Apr. 1941): 174–82.

"Recommendations from the Canadian Public Health Association to the Various Authorities Controlling the Administration of Public Health Matters in the Dominion." *PHJ* 3 (May 1912): 267–8.

Reid, A.P. "Sanatorial Treatment of Tuberculosis." *PHJ* 2 (July 1911): 309–16.

– "Sanitation As It Was." *PHJ* 7 (Nov. 1916): 481–5.

Reid, G. Archibald. "The Value of Heredity." *PHJ* 11 (Oct. 1911): 484

Reid, Helen R.Y. "Some Opportunities for Health Service from a Volunteer's Point of View." *PHJ* 10 (Sept. 1919): 409–17.

"Report Adopted and Presented to the Conference by the Section of Tuberculosis." *PHJ* 11 (Apr. 1920): 168–9.

"The Report of Dr Severin Lachapelle." *PHJ* 3 (Mar. 1912): 156–9.

*Report of the Conference of Provincial Secretaries: Mass Surveys.* Ottawa: 26 May 1948.

"Report of the Director of Medical School Inspection on the Teaching of Hygiene in Public Schools of Toronto." *PHJ* 12 (July 1921): 332–3.

"Report of the Royal Commission on Public Welfare in Ontario." *CPHJ* 21 (Oct. 1930): 507–12.

"Residence Rule Abolished for Patients in Ontario and Quebec." *CJPH* 37 (Jan. 1946): 39.

"Resolutions Proposed and Carried by the Canadian Public Health Association at the Annual Congress, Ottawa, Sept. 25 and 26, 1917." *PHJ* 7 (Mar. 1917): 307.

Richardson, Theresa R. *The Century of the Child.* Albany, NY: The State University of New York Press, 1989.

Richer, Arthur, J. *The Civic Aspect of the Tuberculosis Problem.* N.p., [1905?].

Riches, J.V. "An Experiment in Tuberculosis Control." *CJPH* 34 (Oct. 1943): 470–3.

Riddell, A.R. "Silicosis: Its Relation to Tuberculosis." *PHJ* 17 (Jan. 1926): 1–8.

– "The Spread of Adult Tuberculosis." *CPHJ* 23 (Sept. 1932): 411–15.

– "Tuberculosis in Industry." *CPHJ* 30 (Mar. 1939): 156–60.

Riddington, John. "The Role of Voluntary Societies in the Care of Public Health." *PHJ* 11 (Oct. 1920): 437–43.

Ritchie, John W., and Joseph S. Caldwell. *Primer of Hygiene.* Canadian Health Series. Revised Canadian edition. Toronto: W.J. Gage 1926.

Roberts, H.G. "The Prevention of Tuberculosis in the Country." *PHJ* 4 (Feb. 1913): 70–1.

Roberts, James. "Twenty-three Years of Public Health." *PHJ* 19 (Dec. 1928): 551–8.

– "Tuberculosis in Hamilton." *CPHJ* 22 (Dec. 1931): 600–5.

Robertson, J.S. "A Tuberculosis Survey in Bridgetown, Nova Scotia." *CPHJ* 31 (Apr. 1940): 194–7.

Rosenberg, Charles. *No Other Gods: On Science and American Social Thought.* Baltimore, MD: Johns Hopkins University Press, 1976.

– *Explaining Epidemics and Other Studies in the History of Medicine.* New York: Cambridge University Press, 1992.

Ross, C.B. "The Old Main." *The Sanatorium Sun.* N.p.: n.d. [circa 1950s].

Ross, Edward Lachlan. "Diagnosis of Tuberculosis Fifty Years Ago and Now." *CMAJ* 26 (May 1932): 593–6.

– "The Control of Tuberculosis in Manitoba." *CMAJ* 49 (Aug. 1943): 82–5.

– "Routine Chest Film of Patients Admitted to General Hospitals." *Manitoba Medical Review* 28 (Dec. 1948): 647–9.

Ross, Mary A. "Tuberculosis Mortality in Ontario." *CPHJ* 20 (Feb. 1934): 73–86.

Rothman, Sheila M. "Seek and Hide: Public Health Departments and Persons with Tuberculosis, 1890–1940." *The Journal of Law, Medicine and Ethics* 21 (fall–winter 1993): 289–95.

– *Living in the Shadow of Death: Tuberculosis and the Social Experience of Illness in American History.* New York: Basic Books, 1994.

Rousseau, Arthur. "Mémoire sur les conditions actuelles de la lutte anti-tuberculeuse dans la Province de Quebec." *Le Bulletin Medical de Quebec* 27 (Nov. 1926): 329–34.

Rousseau, Edmond. *Petit catéchisme de tempérance et de tuberculose.* 3rd ed. Quebec: 1915.

Roy, Octave. "BCG Vaccination in a Health Unit." *CJPH* 39 (Mar. 1948): 108–9.

Royal Edward Institute. *Report of the Opening of the Royal Edward Institute.* Montreal: 1909.

– *Annual Report.* Montreal: 1912.

Royer, Franklin. "The Public Aspect of Tuberculosis." *PHJ* 12 (May 1921): 213–20.

Russell, Elizabeth. "Provincial Public Health Nursing in Manitoba." *PHJ* 12 (Aug. 1921): 360–7.

– "Public Health Nursing in Manitoba." *PHJ* 17 (Jan. 1926): 33–6.

Rutherford, J.G. "Municipal Food Inspection." *PHJ* 5 (Jan. 1914): 13–20.

Rutherford, Paul. "Tomorrow's Metropolis: The Urban Reform Movement in Canada, 1880–1920." In *The Canadian City: Essays in Urban History.* Edited by Gilbert A. Stelter and Alan F.J. Artibise, 368–92. Toronto: Carleton University Press, 1977.

– ed. *Saving the Canadian City: The First Phase 1880–1920.* Toronto: University of Toronto Press, 1974.

Ryan, Clarence A. "The Tuberculosis Clinic." *CMAJ* 29 (Nov. 1933): 530–3.

Ryan, L.K. "Mystic Order of the Bug." *Maclean's Magazine* 54 (15 Nov. 1941): 17, 30–3.

Sanatorium Board of Manitoba. *Souvenir of the Twenty-fifth Anniversary of the Opening of the Manitoba Sanatorium at Ninette, Manitoba.* N.p.: n.d.

*Sanatorium for Consumptives in Manitoba.* N.p.: 1906.

Saskatchewan Anti-Tuberculosis League. *The People versus the White Plague.* Saskatchewan: [1961?].

"Saskatchewan and Manitoba." *CJPH* 36 (Apr. 1945): 170–1.

Saywell, John T. *"Just Call Me Mitch": The Life of Mitchell F. Hepburn.* Toronto: University of Toronto Press, 1991.

Savard, E.M. "Anti-tuberculosis Leagues in the Districts of Sanitary Inspection." *CMAJ* 9 (Sept. 1919): 823–9.

Schoales, J.S. "Importance of Housing and Lodging-House Inspection." *PHJ* 7 (Oct. 1916): 470–80.

Sellers, A.H., and K.M. Shorey. "Tuberculosis Trends in Ontario." *CJPH* 41 (Dec. 1950): 517–19.

Sepkowitz, Kent A. "Tuberculosis and the Health Care Worker: A Historical Perspective." *Annals of Internal Medicine* 120 (1994): 71–9. (See also correspondence, *Annals of Internal Medicine* 120 (1994): 971–2).

Seymour, M.M. *Consumption.* Public Health Branch, Department of Agriculture, Saskatchewan, Circular no. 6. Regina, SK: 1908.

– "Public Health in Saskatchewan: 1906–1912." *PHJ* 5 (May 1914): 300–4.

– "Presidential Address." *PHJ* 6 (Dec. 1915): 593–6.

– "A Study of Milk Problems in Canada." *PHJ* 17 (May 1926): 241–4; (June 1926): 295–301; (July 1926): 353–8; (Aug. 1926): 394–404.

Sharpe, W.C. "Artificial Pneumothorax in Pulmonary Tuberculosis." *CMAJ* 25 (Jan. 1931): 54–7.

Shaver, C.G. "A Basis for the Control of Tuberculosis in a Defined Area." *CPHJ* 26 (July 1935): 329–34.

– "Tuberculosis Mortality and Morbidity in the Counties of Lincoln and Welland, Ont." *CPHJ* 29 (Sept. 1938): 434–8.

Sheps, Mindel C. "Saskatchewan Plans Health Services." *CJPH* 26 (May 1945): 175–80.

Shillington, C. Howard. *The Road to Medicare in Canada.* Toronto: Del Graphics, 1972.

Shirreff, W.T. "Municipal Milk Supply." *PHJ* 3 (May 1912): 260–6.

Shortt, S.E.D., ed. *Medicine in Canadian Society: Historical Perspectives.* Montreal: McGill-Queen's University Press, 1981.

Sidel, Victor W., Ernest Drucker, and Steven C. Martin. "The Resurgence of Tuberculosis in the United States: Societal Origins and Societal Responses." *Journal of Law, Medicine and Ethics* 21 (fall-winter 1993): 303–16.

Singh, S.P.N., N.K. Mehta, H.B. Dingley, et al. "Human Leuocyke Antigen (HLA)-Linked Control of Susceptibility to Pulmonary Tuberculosis and Association with HLA-DR Types." *The Journal of Infectious Disease* 148, no. 4 (1983): 676–81.

Singh, Satinder Pal, and Nath Hrudaya. "Early Radiology of Pulmonary Tuberculosis." *American Journal of Radiology* 162 (1994): 846.

Slaughter, Sheila, and Edward T. Silva. "Looking Backwards: How Foundations Formulated Ideology in the Progressive Period." In *Philanthropy and Cultural Imperialism*, 55–86. Boston: G.K. Hall, 1980.

Smillie, Mrs N.C. "Some Advances in Medical Inspection." *PHJ* 3 (Mar. 1912): 118–22.

Smith, Barry. "Gullible's Travails: Tuberculosis and Quackery, 1890–1930." *Journal of Contemporary History* 20 (1985): 733–56.

Smith, F.B. *The Retreat of Tuberculosis 1850–1950.* London: Croom Helm, 1988.

"Souvenir of Laying of Cornerstone of the New Children's Hospital for Consumptives by His Royal Highness the Duke of Connaught," May 27, 1912.

Starr, F.N.G. "Surgical Tuberculosis." *CMAJ* 10 (Dec. 1920): 1096–1104.

Starr, Paul. *The Transformation of American Medicine.* New York: Basic Books, 1982.

"Statistics Comparing Cancer with Tuberculosis in the City of Saskatoon, Sask." *PHJ* 16 (May 1925): 216–19.

Stead, William W. "Genetics and Resistance to Tuberculosis." *Annals of Internal Medicine* 116 (1992): 937–41. (See also "Correspondence," *Annals of Internal Medicine* 117 (1992): 796).

Stead, William W., and Joseph Bates. "Tuberculosis." *Harrison's Principles of Internal Medicine.* 8th ed. Edited by George W. Thorn, et al., 900–12. Toronto: McGraw-Hill, 1977.

Stead, William W., Carole Yeung, and Carolyn Hartnett. "Probable Role of Ultraviolet Irradiation in Preventing Transmission of Tuberculosis: A Case Study." *Infection Control and Hospital Epidemiology* 17, no. 1 (1996): 11–13.

Stelter, Gilbert A., and Alan F.J. Artibise. *The Canadian City: Essays in Urban and Social History.* Ottawa: Carleton University Press, 1991.

Stewart, C.B., and C.J.W. Beckwith. "The Hazards in the General Hospital." *CJPH* 40 (Dec. 1949): 483–90.

Stewart, David A. *Rest.* N.p.: n.d.

– "The War and Tuberculosis." *American Review of Tuberculosis* 2 (Aug. 1918): 357–71.

– *The Social Ramifications of Tuberculosis.* Winnipeg, MB: 1920.

– "Tuberculosis Problems of To-Day: Doctrines, Conditions and Needs." *American Review of Tuberculosis* 4 (Mar. 1920): 1–11.
– "Work for the Tuberculous." *American Review of Tuberculosis* 4 (June 1920): 292–9.
– *The Tuberculous Man at Home.* N.p.: 1922.
– "Some Considerations Regarding the Diagnosis of Pulmonary Tuberculosis." *American Review of Tuberculosis* 5 (Feb. 1922): 981–93.
– "Pregnancy and Tuberculosis." *CMAJ* 12 (Jan. 1922): 1–3; (Feb. 1922): 103–6.
– "Tuberculosis of the Intestine – The Ulcerative Form, as a Phase of Pulmonary Tuberculosis." *CMAJ* 13 (Jan. 1923): 20–3.
– "Theses on Intestinal Tuberculosis." *American Review of Tuberculosis* 15 (May 1927): 588–600.
– "An Address on the Early Diagnosis of Pulmonary Tuberculosis." *CMAJ* 18 (Apr. 1928): 375–8.
– "Anti-tuberculosis Measures in Rural Districts." *CMAJ* 19 (Dec. 1928): 669–74.
– "The Epidemiology of Tuberculosis." *University of Manitoba Medical Journal* 1 (Mar. 1930): 109–14.
– *Teaching about Tuberculosis.* N.p.: [1930?].
– *Things New and Old.* Reprinted from *CMAJ* 24 (1931).
– "What is New in Tuberculosis." *CMAJ* 26 (Jan. 1932): 34–40.
– "The Challenge of Tuberculosis." *CPHJ* 23 (Mar. 1932): 109–17
– *The Robert Koch Anniversary – The Man and His Work.* N.p.: 1932.
– "Tuberculosis among Nurses – Part II." *American Journal of Nursing* 32 (Nov. 1932): 1165–8.
– "When a Province Tackles Tuberculosis." *CPHJ* 24 (June 1933): 269–75.
– *What the Teacher Should Know about Tuberculosis.* N.p.: [1934?].
– *Tuberculosis – Yesterday, Today and Tomorrow.* Ottawa: [1934?].
– *Address to the Convention of the Union of Manitoba Municipalities.* N.p.: 1934.
Stewart, David A., and E.L. Ross. "Tuberculosis: An Insidious Disease." *CMAJ* 31 (Aug. 1934): 160–4.
Stewart, W. Brenton. *Medicine in New Brunswick.* St John, New Brunswick: New Brunswick Medical Society 1974.
Stone, Margaret M., Ann M. Vannier, et al. "Brief Report: Meningitis Due to Iatrogenic BCG Infection in Two Immunocompromised Children." *New England Journal of Medicine* 23 (31 Aug. 1995): 561–3.
Struthers, Lina Rogers. *The School Nurse.* New York: G. Putnam, 1917.
Struthers, W.E. "Medical Inspection of Schools in Toronto." *PHJ* 5 (Feb. 1914): 67–78.
– "The Point of View in Medical Inspection of Schools." *PHJ* 4 (Feb. 1913): 67–70.

Sutherland, Dr Charles G. "The Nationalization of Medicine." *Maclean's Magazine* 27 (June 1914): 5–8.

Sutherland, Neil. "To Create a Strong and Healthy Race: School Children in the Public Health Movement, 1880–1914." *History of Education Quarterly* 12 (fall 1972): 304–33.

– *Children in English-Canadian Society: Framing the Twentieth-Century Consensus.* Toronto: University of Toronto Press, 1976.

Teller, Michael E. *The Tuberculosis Movement: A Public Health Campaign in the Progressive Era.* Westport, CT: Greenwood Press, 1988.

Temple, Allen. "The Results of Routine Examination of Tuberculosis Contacts." *CMAJ* 33 (Nov. 1935): 507–9.

Tessier, Mme Jule. "The Value of Milk Depots." *PHJ* 8 (Mar 1917): 65.

Thomas, F.E. "Increased TB Mortality: A By-Product of War?" *Saturday Night* 57 (4 July 1942): 19.

Thomas, Lewis *The Lives of a Cell.* New York: Penguin Books, 1978.

Thompson, John H. "'The Beginning of Our Regeneration': The Great War and Western Canadian Reform Movements." Canadian Historical Association, *Historical Papers*, 1972: 227–45.

– "The Voice of Moderation: The Defeat of Prohibition in Manitoba." *The Twenties in Western Canada.* Edited by S.M. Trofimenkoff. Ottawa: 1972: 170–90.

Thompson, John H., and Allen Seager. *Canada 1922–1939: Decades of Discord.* Toronto: McClelland and Stewart, 1985.

Thompson, S.E.L. "The Public Health Officer and His Relation to Public Health in Ontario." *PHJ* 10 (Sept. 1919): 393–6.

Thompson, J.J. "The Early Diagnosis of Pulmonary Tuberculosis." *CMAJ* 1 (Jan. 1911): 47–52.

Thomson, William A.R. *Black's Medical Dictionary.* 31st ed. London: 1976.

Tisdall, F.F., and Alan Brown. "The Relative Value of Different Tuberculin Skin Tests." *CMAJ* 16 (Aug. 1926): 939–43.

Toronto Association for the Prevention and Treatment of Consumption. *Report of Inaugural Meeting.* Toronto: 1900.

Tovell, H.M. "The X-ray Examination." *CMAJ* 12 (June 1922): 408–11.

Townsend, David. "Early Diagnosis of Tuberculosis." *CMAJ* 5 (Feb. 1915): 113–17.

– "Early Diagnosis of Tuberculosis." *PHJ* 6 (July 1915): 333–5.

Tracy, A.W. "The Eradication of Tubercular Cattle from Milch Herds." *PHJ* 7 (Feb. 1916): 80–1.

Trudeau, Edward Livingston. *An Autobiography.* New York: 1916.

"Tuberculosis and Ontario Hospitals." *PHJ* 3 (May 1912): 292.

Turgeon, J.M. "Comité Provincial de Defense Contre la Tuberculose." *Canada Français* 26 (Feb. 1939): 583–90.

Tyre, Robert. *The Cross and the Square: The Kinsmen Story, 1920–1970*, Canada Association of Kinsmen Clubs, 1970.

Valverde, Mariana. *The Age of Light, Soap and Water.* Toronto: McClelland and Stewart, 1991.

Vancouver Survey Committee. *Survey of the Tuberculosis Situation in Vancouver.* Vancouver: 1934.

Veterinary Hygiene. "Regulations Relating to Tuberculosis." *PHJ* 5 (July 1914): 495–6.

Vogel, Morris J., and C. Rosenberg, eds. *The Therapeutic Revolution.* Philadelphia: University of Pennsylvania Press, 1979.

Vrooman, C.H. "The Responsibility for the Advanced Case of Tuberculosis." *CMAJ* 3 (July 1913): 575–82.

– "Immunity in Tuberculosis." *CMAJ* 13 (June 1923): 411–14.

– "The Development of Our Knowledge Concerning Tuberculosis." Pts. 1–2. *CMAJ* 18 (May 1928): 594–9; (June 1928): 725–31.

Wace, C. "Queen Alexandra Solarium for Crippled Children." *Social Welfare* 12 (Dec. 1929): 67–8.

Wain, Harry. *A History of Preventive Medicine.* Springfield, IL: 1970.

Wakefield, A.W. "Trade Quackery in Medicine." *PHJ* 3 (Dec. 1912): 698–708.

Waksman, Selman A. *The Conquest of Tuberculosis.* Berkeley, CA: 1966.

Walker, W.F. *A Program of Service for the Royal Edward Institute, Based on a Study of the Tuberculosis Problem in Montreal, Canada.* Montreal: 1930.

Walters, L. "I Conquered TB" *Maclean's Magazine.* 56 (1 Mar. 1943): 18, 26–7.

Waltz, G.H. "New Foe for TB." *Maclean's Magazine* 61 (1 July 1948): 12, 32.

Warner, Lt Col W.P. "Tuberculosis in the Canadian Army." *CMAJ* 47 (Sept. 1942): 193–6.

Warwick, William. "Full-Time Health Districts in New Brunswick." *CPHJ* 30 (June 1939): 284–7.

Watson, Charles H.A. "A Study of the Racial Incidence of Tuberculosis in the Province of Manitoba." *American Review of Tuberculosis* 32 (Aug. 1935): 183–95.

Waugh, F.W. "Some Household Insects." *CTSE* 1 (July 1910): 337.

Weaver, John C. "'Tomorrow's Metropolis Revisited: A Critical Assessment of Urban Reform in Canada, 1890–1920." In *The Canadian City: Essays in Urban History*, edited by Gilbert A. Stelter and Alan F.J. Artibise, 393–418. Toronto: University of Toronto Press, 1977.

Weaver, Warren. *U.S. Philanthropic Foundations: Their History, Structure, Management and Record.* New York: Harper & Row, 1967.

Wherrett, George Jasper. "The Need for Uniformity in Tuberculosis Records and Statistics." *CPHJ* 28 (Feb. 1937): 75–81.

– "Tuberculosis and the Student Nurse." *CPHJ* 31 (Dec. 1940): 619–20.

– "The Tuberculosis Problem in Canada." *CMAJ* 44 (Mar. 1941): 295–9.

- "Progress in Tuberculosis Control in Canada." *CPHJ* 32 (June 1941): 287–92.
- "The Control of Tuberculosis in Wartime." *CPHJ* 33 (Sept. 1942): 438–45.
- "Survey of Health Conditions and Medical and Hospital Services in the North West Territories. *Canadian Journal of Economics and Political Science* 11 (Feb 1945): 49–60.
- "Industrial Medicine and Respiratory Diseases." *CMAJ* 52 (Mar. 1945): 271–5.
- "First Aid in Tuberculosis." *Canadian First Aid* 1 (Apr. 1945): 6–7.
- "Chassez-le de L'Usine." *Trades Labor Journal* 26 (Dec. 1947): 47.
- "Whither Tuberculosis?" *CJPH* 44 (May 1953): 185–6.
- "Recent Developments in Canada's Tuberculosis Services." *CJPH* 46 (Mar. 1955): 93–9.
- "The Effect of New Treatments on the Organization of the Fight Against Tuberculosis in Canada." International Union against Tuberculosis, 13th Conference. *Libro de Actos* 1957: 1082–8.
- "Changing Views on Tuberculosis as a National and International Problem." *CJPH* 50 (May 1959): 201–5.
- "The Diamond Jubilee of the Canadian Tuberculosis Association." *CMAJ* 84 (Jan. 1961): 99–101.
- *Tuberculosis in Canada.* Royal Commission on Health Services. Restricted for commission use only. Ottawa: 1962.
- "Emerging Patterns and Trends in Tuberculosis." *CJPH* 56 (Mar. 1965): 97–9.
- *The Miracle of the Empty Beds.* Toronto: University of Toronto Press, 1977.
Whitelaw, T.H. "Municipal Control of Milk Supplies." *PHJ* 3 (Nov. 1912): 621–5.
Wicks, C.A. "The Post-Sanatorium Care of Tuberculosis Patients in Ontario." *CPHJ* 31 (June 1940): 259–70.
Wiebe, Robert H. *The Search for Order.* New York: Hill and Wang, 1967.
- *Self Rule: A Cultural History of American Democracy.* Chicago: University of Chicago Press, 1995.
Wilkey, John R. "A Tuberculosis Fact-Finding Study in the London Secondary Schools." *CJPH* (Jan. 1943): 22–5.
Wilkins, W.A. "The Diagnostic Value of the X-ray Examination in Pulmonary Tuberculosis." *CMAJ* 9 (Apr. 1919): 333–8.
- "The Diagnostic Value of the X-ray Examination in Pulmonary Tuberculosis." *CMAJ* 10 (Nov. 1920): 999–1006.
Wilson, Leonard G. "The Historical Decline of Tuberculosis in Europe and America: Its Causes and Significance." *Journal of the History of Medicine* 45 (1990): 366–96. See also "Correspondence," *Journal of the History of Medicine* 46 (1991): 358–68.

– "The Rise and Fall of Tuberculosis in Minnesota: The Role of Infection."
*Bulletin of the History of Medicine* 66 (1992): 16–52.

Wilton, Peter. "The Toronto Free Hospital for Consumptive Poor." *Canadian Medical Association Journal* 146 (1992): 1812–14.

Wishart, F.O., and L.A. Pequenat. "Tuberculin Testing." *CJPH* 37 (Jan. 1946): 7–11.

Wodehouse, R.E. "Conditions in Canada in the Combat against Tuberculosis." *CMAJ* 13 (Dec. 1923): 901–2.

– "What is New in Tuberculosis." *PHJ* 17 (July 1926): 321–33.

– *The Sanatorium Situation in Ontario.* Ottawa: 1929.

– "How Sanatoria Can Help in the Prevention and Control of Tuberculosis." *CMAJ* 24 (May 1931): 668–71.

– "The Public Health Nurse in the Control of Tuberculosis." *CPHJ* 22 (Jan. 1931): 28–31.

– "Observations on Tuberculosis Statistics in Canada, 1921 and 1931." *CPHJ* 24 (Sept. 1933): 433–9.

– "Presidential Address." *CPHJ* 30 (Aug. 1939): 369–76.

Wright, J.S. "The Sociologic and Economic Aspects of Tuberculosis." *CMAJ* 8 (Sept. 1918): 791–6.

Yorke, K.M. "Saving Lives on the Wholesale Plan." *Maclean's Magazine* 26 (July 1915): 20–2, 93–6.

Young, H.E. "Full-Time Health Units in British Columbia." *CPHJ* 20 (Mar. 1929): 132–9.

Young, W.A. "Consumption Now a Communicable Disease." *Canadian Journal of Medicine and Surgery* (Mar. 1897): 129–32.

# Index

Abbott, Maude: on volunteers, 266
Adami, John George, 3; on immigration, 14, 17–18; on lay sisterhoods, 268
alcohol,12–13
anesthesia, interwar improvements, 72
antibiotics: and federal grants, 221–2; use of, 197
artificial pneumothorax, 43–4; historical experience, 71–2; during interwar period, 71, 80; refills, 79; role in noninfection, 98
Associated Canadian Travellers (ACT): and seal sale, 217–8

bacillus Calmette Guerin (BCG), 83–5; British Medical Council on, 85; ethical issues, 274; and Ferguson trials, 85, 193; lack of controls in Quebec, 192–3; liabilities, 85; Lubeck tragedy, 84; role of National Research Council, 84; in native peoples, 85; Quebec, 171–2; in Toronto, 84; and tuberculin, 61
Barr, Sir James: on immigration, 15
Baudoin, J.A., 84
Beck, Sir Adam, 26
bed shortages, 148, 194–7; resulting from emphasis on prevention, 94; World War 2, 183
beds: and death rate, 95, 148, 194
Bethune, Norman: on surgery, 78
Black, J.B.: on immigration, 48
Borden, R.L.: on federal responsibility, 32
bovine tuberculosis, 176–7; British commission on, 158

Brissett, Dennis, 244
British Columbia: industrial surveys, 66; mass surveys, 190; survey of health workers, 143; tuberculosis allowance, 199
British North America Act, 31, 151, 259, 262
bronchoscopy, 68
Bruchesi Institute: education, 51
Bryce, Peter, 7; on immigration, 17; on rural life, 21
Burke, Hugh E., 270
Byng, Governor General, 108

camps, 30–1
Canadian Army Medical Corps (CAMC), 38
Canadian Association for the Prevention of Consumption and Other Forms of Tuberculosis, 8
Canadian Association for the Prevention of Tuberculosis: on role of government, 53
Canadian Life Insurance Officers Association, 116; and CTA, 219; and federal health grants, 207, 209; and Maritimes, 117–8; and Prince Edward Island, 117–8
Canadian Medical Association, 8
Canadian Medical Association *Journal*: on volunteers, 52
Canadian society: 1900–14, 6; during interwar period, 57; post–World War 2, 186
Canadian Tuberculosis Association: Christmas Seal campaign, 124–5; and